LANGUAGE

and the Developing Child

by
KATRINA DE HIRSCH

Foreword by
JEANNETTE JEFFERSON JANSKY

THE ORTON DYSLEXIA SOCIETY
724 York Road
Baltimore, Maryland

MONOGRAPH NO. 4   1984

Other Writings By Katrina de Hirsch

1954. La dysléxie specifique. *Enfance* (Mars-Avril): 163–169.

1955. Prediction of future reading disabilities in children with oral language disorder. *Folia Phoniatrica* 7(4):231–248.

1961. Constitutional aspects of reading in *Changing Concepts in Reading Instruction.* ed. J.A. Figurel. Conference Proceedings of the International Reading Association. New York: Scholastic.

1962. Psychological correlates of the reading process in *Challenge and Experiment in Reading,* ed. J.A. Figurel. Conference Proceedings of the International Reading Association. New York: Scholastic.

1963. Reading: Total language disability in *Reading as an Intellectual Activity* ed. J.A. Figurel. Conference Proceedings of the International Reading Association. New York: Scholastic.

1964. With Jansky, J. and Langford, W. Oral language performance of two groups of immature children. *Folia Phoniatrica* 16: 109–122.

1964. With Jansky, J. and Langford, W. Oral language performance of premature children and controls. *Journal of Speech and Hearing Disorders* 29:60–69.

1966. With Jansky, J. and Langford, W. *Predicting Reading Failure: A Preliminary Study.* New York: Harper and Row.

1967. Speech and language disorders in *Comprehensive Textbook of Psychiatry,* II. ed. A. Freedman and H. Kaplan. Baltimore: Williams and Wilkins.

1968. With Jansky, J. Kindergarten protocols of high achievers, slow starters, and failing readers in *Dyslexia: Diagnosis and Treatment of Reading Disorders.* eds. A.H. Keeney and V.T. Keeney. St. Louis: C.V. Mosby.

1968. With Jansky, J. Early prediction of reading disability in *Dyslexia: Diagnosis and Treatment of Reading Disorders.* eds. A.H. Keeney and V.T. Keeney St. Louis: C.V. Mosby.

1972. With Jansky, J. *Preventing Reading Failure.* New York: Harper and Row.

1974. Early language development in *American Handbook of Psychiatry.* ed. S. Arieti. New York: Basic Books.

1975. Speech and language disorders in *Comprehensive Textbook of Psychiatry II.* eds. A. Freedman and H. Kaplan. Baltimore: Williams and Wilkins.

In Press. With Jansky, J. Assessment of specific language disabilities in *The Assessment of the Child and the Adolescent.* ed. E. Mahon and J. Saurs. New York: Jason Aronson Inc.

LANGUAGE *and the Developing Child*

The Orton Dyslexia Society
724 York Road
Baltimore, Maryland 21204

Printed in the United States of America

Cover design: Joseph M. Dieter, Jr.
Compositor: Brushwood Graphics Studio
Printer: Collins Lithographers

ISBN 0-89214-001-1

Contents

Preface

The Orton Dyslexia Society is honored to publish this collection of Katrina de Hirsch's papers. A pioneer in the field of learning disabilities, she speaks with authority to the clinician while giving to parents and teachers keen insights about children with special learning needs.

The papers in this volume encompass the work of over thirty years. In the course of those years de Hirsch employed her wide-ranging knowledge, her clinical experience, and her meticulous scholarly skills to develop an impressive body of work. Readers who compare papers on similar topics written at different times in her career will be impressed by their ever-increasing conceptual richness.

With the exception of much alterations as are required to conform to current usage, to achieve stylistic consistency, or to limit repetition, the papers appear as they were originally published. Where repetition of examples occurs, the editor considers them important to each context in which they appear.

When the papers first appeared each included its own reference list. Here the references are consolidated into a single list at the end of the book. We are grateful to the library staff, especially to Stanley Meyer, at Welch Medical Library of The Johns Hopkins University, without whose assistance this reference list would contain many more omissions than it does. Rebecca Hartwig gave valuable assistance in researching the citations and references; Jeannette Jefferson Jansky placed her knowledge of the literature as well as her unique understanding of Katrina de Hirsch and her work at our disposal throughout the publication process.

This collection introduces a new generation of teachers, clinicians, and parents to the work of one of the key figures in the continuing search for the causes and treatment of dyslexia, autism, stuttering, and other serious language disorders. Katrina de Hirsch is one of those rare individuals who not only has made original contributions to her field, but who has written about them with style and clarity.

Rosemary F. Bowler, Editor

Foreword

The diverse studies in this Monograph are the fruit of an extraordinary professional career.

Katrina de Hirsch grew up in Frankfurt surrounded by German philosophical and psychological thinking. After training at the West End Hospital for Nervous Diseases in London, she earned a Licentiate from the College of Speech Therapy. Soon after she emigrated to New York, she became Director of the Pediatric Language Disorders Clinic at the Columbia-Presbyterian Medical Center, and not long thereafter, one of the Founders of The Orton Society. Her contributions have been recognized in many ways: She is a Fellow of the British College of Speech Therapy, the American Speech-Language-Hearing Association, and the American Orthopsychiatric Association, and has been awarded Honorary Doctorates by Hood and Smith Colleges. Yet, it is noteworthy that she has usually functioned outside of the American establishment.

One of her earliest introductions was to Dr. Orton. His theory—that language disorders encompass a range of developmental oral and written deficits, and that language disabilities are inborn, often familial, and related to differences in the organization of the central nervous system—was consistent with her own orientation and clinical experience. Her detailed, subtle observations of the functioning of these children has extended our understanding of how oral language difficulties contribute to reading disabilities. Her first discussions along these lines were published during a period when professional journals were flooded with studies describing the mechanics of speech production. Her familiarity with the oral language problems of four- and five-year-olds was the matrix from which she began to make clinical predictions about their chances of learning to read. This clinical work was followed by a statistical investigation to determine which language tests, administered to kindergarten children, would predict reading status at the end of second grade. These early predictive studies led to a burgeoning of prediction research that continues today. For Mrs. de Hirsch the importance of these investigations lay in the attention they drew to early intervention.

With Lauretta Bender, Mrs. de Hirsch viewed many language disordered children as immature. When offered the opportunity to follow prematurely-born children and maturely-born controls, Mrs. de Hirsch was in a position to study a group which was by definition immature. She was able to document the ongoing lags in these children at a time when many educators and parents were convinced that they would "catch up," suggesting that it was not only acceptable, but desirable not to treat them.

Mrs. de Hirsch drew on her familiarity with German philosophical psychology in formulating her view of the reading process. Printed letters, words, and sentences were seen as Gestalten, or constellations of stimuli to be responded to as wholes. Difficulty maintaining Gestalten, that is to say, experiencing printed matter as fluid, was, she judged, a manifestation of developmental immaturity.

Her awareness of the complexity of the reading process, of how it works, is illustrated by an observation in a 1963 paper:

> . . . [E]voking the auditory image of the word during reading is only part of the process. If one analyzes the reading process, one finds a number of partial performances; there is the perceptual grasping of letter and word configurations, there is their evocation in inner speech, there is the comprehension of syntactical relationships, the construction of anticipatory schemata as to what the sentence is going to say, there is finally the assimilation of content into an already existing framework. All of this constitutes an integrated performance, one part influencing the other . . .

This anticipated by a decade those linguists of the 1970's who found that reading occurs as a function of multiple interactions, that both "top-down" and "bottom-up" approaches are brought into play.

Mrs. de Hirsch was curious about questions raised by difficult and unusual disorders. She considered dysrhythmic speech in various papers, returning to the possibility that the first signs of stuttering occur in linguistically vulnerable children when development suddenly opens the door to a seemingly infinite variety of lexical and grammatical combinations. Unfortunately, this linguistic explosion may coincide with the birth of a younger sibling or some interruption in communication between mother and child. Mrs. de Hirsch's analysis of the language of children with a rare autonomic nervous system disorder (familial dysautonomia) was the first that appeared in the literature.

Her lively case descriptions of children with severe receptive and expressive deficits were presented against the backdrop of theoretical speculations as to the nature and origin of the symptoms. Her reports have represented a valuable marriage of the clinical and the theoretical.

Her continuing work with individual children and their parents has revealed her acute awareness of the importance of the child's milieu for the resolution of his problems. Her appreciation of the significance of the child's psychological make-up for his management of his language disability was reflected in the 1965 manuscript describing differential improvement in two categories of adolescents. The report concluded that the ability to compensate is determined not only by the severity and pattern of weaknesses and strengths in language, but also by the strength of the psychological resources. A later article suggested that an awareness of neurophysiological dimensions of immaturity might help to explain lags in ego development viewed from the psychoanalytic framework. Mrs. de Hirsch indicated that these lags in ego development and delay in patterning perceptuomotor and linguistic stimuli should be regarded not as separate phenomena, but as manifestations of pervasive organismic immaturity that invades all aspects of the personality and interferes with the orderly organization of experience. She pointed out, moreover, that language is an important determinant in the differentiation of the ego itself. Elegant and humanistic applications were considered in a paper that described interactions between therapist and child, and explored what it is in the relationship that facilitates progress.

It is not only Mrs. de Hirsch's independence from the establishment that has freed her to write about what interests her and about essentials, but an independence that comes with an original and vital intelligence.

Jeannette Jefferson Jansky

Part I

THE CHILD'S DEVELOPING LANGUAGE

A Review of Early Language Development

Language pathology can be understood only in the framework of normal language development. This paper discusses some of the milestones in the process of language acquisition, a process which is part of the child's organismic growth within a given social matrix. To quote from Lewis (1963): "The linguistic growth of the child moves forward as a result of the interaction of two factors, those that spring from within the child himself and those that impinge upon him from the community. Children are richly endowed with the potentialities for symbolisation, the most potent of which is language."

From his earliest days the baby vocalizes. These vocalizations utilize the expiratory phase of the respiratory cycle. The airflow is modified by the vocal cords and by the various parts of the peripheral speech mechanism. This permits the resulting sound waves to be detected auditorily. The same process holds for all vocal productions, the baby's cry, his cooing and, at a later time, his speech. Lieberman (1967) has shown that the wave forms of the baby's cry have the same characteristics as adult sentences. Alterations in breathing produce the intonations that are instrumental in carrying messages long before the child uses words.

Hunger, pain, and discomfort will make the neonate cry. These discomfort cries approximate to narrow-front vowels and are usually nasalized. A few weeks later the baby will produce relaxed, open-back vowels in the range of *a-ae* during states of well-being. For the baby's mother, each characteristic vocal pattern has a distinctive meaning. Very early, then, the child uses the physiological mechanisms of respiration and phonation effectively for expressive purposes.

During the first months of life, the baby learns to associate his mother's voice with pleasant situations such as feeding. Her voice is probably at first experienced as part of a total constellation: a smiling face, the presence of caresses, the satisfaction of bodily needs. At three months the baby reacts positively to friendly tones and negatively to

Reprinted with permission of Spastics International Medical Publications, from *Developmental Medicine and Child Neurology* 12:87–97. 1970.

angry tones (Bühler and Hetzer 1935). Two or three months later he responds differentially to tones, to music, and to male and female voices. And long before he responds to the phonetic pattern of words, he responds to the prosodic features of language, to variations in intonation and pitch which carry the emotional load to communication.

The vocalizations the mother uses in her communication with the baby are tailored to his affective needs. They differ from those she uses in other situations in a number of features: in dynamic accent, in melody and rate, and in a marked tendency to rhythmic iterations (Grewel 1959). Di Carlo (1964) has made the pertinent observation that the mother caresses the child with her voice. Wyatt (1957) calls the dialogue between the mother and her baby a process of mutual feedback. The learning of the "mother language", she says, is achieved through unconscious identification. Infants are continually talked to in situations that are essential to their well-being. The vocal communication between mother and child during bathing, feeding, and dressing must of necessity play an important part in the shaping of the child's communicative behavior, of which language is but one aspect. The mother's voice, specifically, is bound to be heavily invested with affect for the baby, and one might assume that such an investment would have a bearing on his subsequent listening attitudes.

We know that with children brought up in institutions, maturational processes are delayed or interfered with. This is shown beautifully by Provence and Lipton in a study of such infants (1962), who were late in smiling, the handling of toys, and the differential response to people, and whose vocal and verbal development was often severely delayed. Well-mothered babies have a repertoire of most of the vowels and half of the consonants by the end of the first year. Brodbeck and Irwin (1946) compared frequency and variety of such children's vocalizations with those of children cared for in orphanages and found significant differences between the two groups as early as the first two months of life. The discrepancies became more marked by the fourth and sixth months. Similar findings are reported by Fisichelli (1950).

Between the fifth and tenth month of life, usually around the time the baby attempts to sit up, he begins to babble. The transition from expressive sounds to babbling is not well marked; the various stages of language development overlap. Babbling differs from expressive sounds in that it is not tied to specific situations such as hunger. Now the baby lies in his crib, plays with his fingers and toes, and plays with sounds that he produces spontaneously, for the sheer pleasure of making them. There is no mistaking the intense gratification the baby derives from the mouthing of sounds, and it is thus not surprising that analysts are impressed by the role this oral activity plays in early psychosexual development.

Every mother knows that she can stimulate long babbling exchanges between herself and her baby. It has been shown that nonsocial stimuli such as the sound of chimes do not increase infants' vocalizations. Nor does the mere presence of the human being result in more copious babbling (Todd and Palmer 1968). The human voice stimulates babbling and its effect is reinforced by the presence of the adult.

During babbling the baby "discovers" how to mould the outgoing breath stream so as to produce a whole repertoire of sounds. At the same time an auditory feedback loop is being established. As sound-producing movements are being repeated over and over again, a strong link is being forged between tactual and kinesthetic impressions on the one hand and auditory sensations on the other. A pattern of alternate hearing and uttering is set up. Sounds heard evoke more vocalizations that are no longer entirely random, but tend to resemble the phonemic and intonational configurations of the original model. One of the main functions of babbling is thus an intensive kinesthetic-proprioceptive-auditory learning experience resulting in primitive sound-movement schemata which are being established during babbling. The baby not only produces a whole range of different sounds, but he derives pleasure from imitating those he himself produces. This achievement reflects his growing capacity to store, if only for a limited time, and to retrieve the auditory-motor configurations which serve him as models for repetition. Recent research seems to show (Yeni-Komshian et al. 1968) that the auditory feedback monitoring system is already operative at the age of twenty-eight months and that the capacity to monitor one's own speech grows until the age of nine.

Intactness of the central nervous system is a prerequisite for the auditory-motor feedback loop. This loop does not become functional in babies who are deaf or hard of hearing. Deaf babies babble, but they discontinue after a while because they lack the feedback resulting from hearing their own sounds as well as those of the environment. Recent investigations have demonstrated (Fry 1966) that with amplification at the babbling stage, that is to say with the very early establishment of the auditory feedback loop, the language development of severely hard of hearing children approximates that of normal ones.

In the more advanced babbling stage, certain sounds which were produced during early babbling activities tend to drop out. Menyuk (1968) has found that during the first few months the sound repertoire of Japanese and American babies is very similar, but that by the ninth month the sounds used during babbling are similar to those produced by the children's respective language environment.

Around the tenth month and with the developing control over volume, pitch, and intonation, the baby enters the echolalic stage, when he attempts not only to imitate his own sounds but also the more patterned utterances he hears spoken around him. He begins to repeat words heard but not necessarily understood. Echolalia is a normal phase in language development and echolalic responses comprise a significant portion of children's speech up to twenty-nine months. Some toddlers repeat new words or new combinations of words for purposes of clarification. Echolalia is pathognomonic for mental retardation, autism, or aphasia only if it is the only response available to the child or if it occurs in older children.

Comprehension and production of language facilitate each other. However, comprehension, which places a lesser load on the immature organism, usually precedes production; passive control precedes active control. Before the baby uses words, he begins to interpret first the intonational and later the phonemic patterns of those around him. What happens when we say a child understands? He must be ready to make a modicum of sense out of the world that surrounds him; he must use some objects appropriately; he must have a rudimentary sense of self, of being separate. Probably he will then respond at first simply to the intonational configuration as part of a specific situation. Slowly the phonemic pattern becomes intertwined with intonational and situational features until very gradually, as further differentiation takes place, the phonemic pattern takes dominance irrespective of the situation.

We do know that in order to produce meaningful speech, the child must comprehend verbalizations directed to him. We do not, however, know which factors determine the ability to process linguisitc information. Nor do we know exactly what happens when the child uses his first meaningful utterances. McCarthy (1954) says there is a tremendous psychological gap to be bridged between the mere production of the phonemic form of a word and the symbolic representational use of that word in an appropriate situation.

During the past ten to fifteen years a good deal of disagreement has arisen between psychologists and linguists as to the relationship between babbling, that is to say nonsymbolic vocalization, and the first meaningful words. Psychologists say that language is slowly shaped out of the multitude of babbling sounds by means of selective reinforcement on the part of the parents who show their delight when the child produces sound combinations which resemble actual words. As a result of such reinforcement, the child gradually assembles a sound repertoire approximating that of the language he is reared in and begins to associate these sound combinations with specific situations, people, or objects. Linguists such as Jakobson and Halle (1956), on the other hand, draw a sharp dividing line between babbling and representational speech, while Brown (1958), in an intermediate position, suggests a "babbling drift" in describing the transition from babbling to language. We know that at the age of twelve months the child is able to imitate the intonational contours of his mother's speech. Many preverbal babies utter long strings of sounds which resemble those of adults in terms of melody and pitch. Mothers respond to these vocalizations as if they were definite messages, statements, commands, or questions. (That intonation plays a vital role in communication is testified to by the fact that autistic children's speech, which is devoid of communicative intent, is so often monotonous and poorly inflected.) A degree of meaning, a message, is thus associated with the modulated strings of sounds the baby produces before the emergence of single words. Advanced babbling *is* a kind of language and we cannot, therefore, talk of the emergence of symbolic utterances as a sudden event, but we must look on this development as an ongoing process. This process, the behaviorists say, is solely the result of continuous and selective reinforcement, while linguists maintain that it is a process reminiscent of embryonic development in the sense that it constitutes the unfolding of an inherent potential.

The baby's first words appear between the age of twelve and twenty months and are usually strongly affectively colored. They are by no means stabilized in terms of meaning, however. In the beginning, words are often simply by-products of action. The child frees himself only slowly from the constraint of specific situations and, as time goes on, learns to use words as substitutes for action. The growth of the child's vocabulary reflects a continuing process of modification that involves both the acquisition of new words and the expanding and refining of word meanings previously learned. *Doggie* is at first only the child's small fluffy toy dog; a little later the word is used to describe the real dog he sees at a neighbour's; and in the end it stands for all members of the species *dog*. The meaning of the word has been expanded. The opposite process takes place when the child says, for instance, *Me write a picture* (Cazden 1966b). In this case the child will find out that the word *write* refers only to those graphic activities which involve letters and numbers—the meaning of the word *write* has been contracted and refined.

By the age of two years, the average child has 200-300 words in his usage vocabulary; his understanding vocabulary is much larger. After the age of two he makes giant strides in the comprehension and production of meaningful words. However, we do not know whether the child's growing ability to use words symbolically depends on general organismic capacities that reach a critical minimum level around the age of eighteen months or whether there are factors *specific* to language which mature around that time, which are more or less independent of general processes. Lenneberg (1966) maintains that the ability to acquire language is a biological phenomenon relatively independent of that elusive property called intelligence. He suggests the possibility that intelligence is the *result* of the ability to comprehend and use language, rather than the other way around.

The enlargement of vocabulary, the growth of meaning which belongs to the semantic aspect of language, continues throughout the individual's entire life. The growth depends on the child's cultural background (the best single predictor of his recognition vocabulary is his mother's vocabulary score on the WISC), and on his inherent linguistic endowment. Above all, it depends on the affect tie between mother and child, the give and take between the two, and the constant and responsive guidance by the significant people who share his life experiences.

Around the time the child makes large strides in the acquisition of new words, he forges ahead towards mastery of the phonological system of his language. Phonology describes the matrix of features which differentiate one speech sound from another by virtue of certain characteristics; for instance, presence or absence of voice in the sounds *b* and *p*. Jakobson (1962) maintains that language development is characterized by the learning of successive contrasts in a more or less fixed sequence, the vowel-consonant contrast probably being the first to be learned.

We assume that children perceive linguistically significant contrasts and distinctions before they can produce them (the production of sounds is usually discussed under the heading of articulation). A four-year-old might say *dwess*, but he may shake his head when the adult uses the wrong form. According to Menyuk (1967a) there is little research on the perceptual distinctions children are able to make between the ages of one and three. Sounds for the young child are probably at first indistinguishable from one another. They acquire distinctiveness only slowly. Menyuk found that Japanese and American children acquire phonemic distinctions in approximately the same order, indicating that this hierarchy of distinctions depends primarily on the inherent developing perceptual and productive capacity of the child.

Children have to learn to distinguish not only between single features of sounds, but often between bundles of them. The child who says *dar* instead of *car* misses out both on place of articulation and on the voiced-unvoiced contrast. Young children whose articulation develops normally tend to substitute only one feature at a time, but older children with articulatory problems usually fail to distinguish several simultaneously, which raises questions as to possible gaps in memory and storage (Menyuk 1968). Articulatory errors may be due to a variety of factors: they may result from perceptual confusion, such as failure to recognize the diacritic feature which distinguishes a *t* from a *k*, or from inability to execute complex motor patterns such as the consonant

cluster *str* in the word *string*. That there is a strong link between auditory-perceptual and motor aspects of speech is stressed by Winitz (1967), who suggests that the road from perception to output is not a one-way street. Winitz, who adheres to the motor theory of perception, maintains that discrimination errors are frequently the result rather than the cause of misarticulation. Some articulatory errors, finally, are on a linguistic basis. A child may perceive the difference between sounds such as *f* and *v*, he may be able to produce both, but he may use the plural *leafs* because he has failed to incorporate the linguistic rule which requires a change from *f* to *v* in the pluralisation of certain nouns.

Articulatory competence varies from child to child at least within certain limits. Obviously not all forty-odd sounds of the phonological system of the English language crystallize at the same time. Development proceeds from crude and primitive to more complex and more differentiated forms. The child's earliest utterances contain only two or three phonemes. At eighteen months he may have mastered from eight to twelve of them, including diphthongs. From then on his production of the sounds of his language increases by leaps and bounds as a result of further differentiation. Sudden spurts are followed by phases of consolidation, but according to Templin (1966) the five-year-old child should produce 88 percent of all sounds correctly.

The order in which phonemic units are being mastered depends on several factors. One is degree of difficulty. The phoneme *s*, for instance, which requires intricate adjustments of the peripheral speech mechanism, may not be adequately produced until the age of seven. Frequency is another factor. The child will use those phonemes first that occur most often in the vocabulary he hears and uses.

As a rule children produce only those sound sequences which are part of their native language. An English child will not, for instance, produce the cluster *pf* which is a common one in German (as in the word *pferd*), but he will use the cluster *pl* which is acceptable in English. The sequence *ng* which occurs frequently during babbling in all positions becomes restricted to the middle and the final position of words. Children do not usually need formal training to incorporate these rules which they acquire fairly early. It is obvious that the mastery of the phonological system of the language requires a degree of central nervous system maturation. Beyond it we know that the child needs, if not systematic teaching, at any rate, a model. Without such a model he may falter on the road to mastery. It is the mother who serves as the primary language model, who literally feeds back to the child those sound sequences that are acceptable in his particular language environment. It is only later that the child learns to monitor his own speech. We assume that there are certain critical stages in language development when the model is of decisive importance, and we believe that imitation of and identification with a mother figure play an important role not only in the growth of vocabulary but also in the mastery of the phonological system.

In the acquisition of syntax and grammar, on the other hand, imitation, according to linguistic theory, is by no means of primary importance. The transition from nonrelational one-word utterances to relational speech consisting of two or more words represents a tremendous step in development. If one considers the enormous complexity of syntax and grammar one can only marvel at the fact that this process develops so rapidly; by the age of five, children use virtually all the structures they will ever use. They operate at first with stored fragments of speech heard. These imitations preserve word order, which is an important linguistic signal in English. Because of limitation in auditory memory span and, because, according to Brown and Bellugi (1964), this is as far as the child can "program," the early imitations are usually limited to a range from two to four units. More important, such imitations are not progressive in the sense that they are not applied to different contexts; they are not generalized.

The first nonimitative two- and three-word combinations which appear between twelve and twenty-four months are by no means random. They consist of content words—nouns, labels, verbs—open class words which carry the information, coupled with functors, pivot words, such as *off, more. More car* is an example. Such telegraphic speech, which is characterized by omission of most unstressed words conforms, nevertheless, to a regular pattern. The subsequent form, the noun phrase (*my big car*) as described by Brown and Bellugi (1964) is a cohesive grammatical unit that can be expanded through the use of modifiers. These early grammatical constructions reflect the child's discovery of basic phrase structure which leads to the formulation of kernel sentences. On this level one finds designative sentences (*this is a big car*), predicative sentences (*the car is broken*), actor-action sentences (*Mummy give milk*). From such kernel sentences new forms evolve through the use of transformations by means of additions, deletions, and rearrangements. Pronouns are substituted for noun phrases, serialisation is affected through the use of the word *and*, questions are formulated by prefacing sentences with *Wh* words. Thus, beginning with the simplest two-word combinations, one can trace the gradual emergence of phrases to the formulation of kernel sentences from which transformations can be derived. Three-and-a-half-year-olds use complete sentences of at least four words, including relational ones.

By means of a series of ingenious experiments, Berko (1960) investigated children's ability to make transformations. These experiments illustrate what is meant by "generating new forms." The experimenter, for instance, point to a doll and says: "Here is a man who knows how to wug, today he is . . . " and the child fills in *wugging* although he has never heard the present participle of *wug*. Children's very mistakes indicate that they do not simply imitate longer and longer bits of speech they hear. The limited linguistic corpus they are exposed to serves them as a source for grammatical generalizations and permits them to generate forms they have never heard. The child who says: "I have seen two mouses," proves that he has incorporated the rule that asks for the ending *ez* in the pluralisation of words such as house. The two-and-a-half-year-old who says, "Mommy, I want a chee," assumes that a *chee* is the singular of *cheese*. Both children have overgeneralized, but their mistakes show, nevertheless, that they have derived a set of abstract rules from a relatively small sample of linguistic input. These rules are basic to the decoding and encoding of language (Chomsky 1965). Mastery of these rules is a gradual process; the three-year-old, for instance, understands the contrast between subject and object in the active but not in the passive voice. The understanding and use of the passive voice belongs to an older age.

The impressive fact about normal language development is its universality and consistency. While children vary in the rate with which they incorporate the linguistic code, at least within certain limits, early speech milestones appear at roughly the same time. The large majority of children babble, use stress and intonation, utter two- to three-word combinations and acquire the basic rules of their language at about the same age. Without formal training, children incorporate a set of assumptions and rules regarding their language which allows them to understand and generate new forms. According to McNeill (1966), this proves that children are born with a set of "linguistic universals" as part of their innate endowment. Children, he says, are neurologically so "preprogrammed" with a language acquisition device that a minimum of stimulation is required for the realization of this potential. A less radical view assumes that children are born not so much with linguistic universals, but with propensities, *Anlagen*, which enable them to extract from the linguistic input the relevant data needed to organize language into a consistent system.

Children whose language development deviates pass through the normal grammatical stages later than do others. Menyuk (1967b) gives as an example the phrase *he no big boy*. This is a normal construction at age three, but may be used at age six by children with difficulties in the language area. Furthermore, speech defective children often fail to make the generalizations that are expected in normal language development. In fact, they may even perform linguistic operations which do not form part of their own language system. Their hypotheses as to the rules of grammar and phonology differ from those of children whose linguistic development runs smoothly. It may be of interest to mention in this context that grammar is relatively resistant to remedial help. Some very intelligent children need long-term assistance to achieve acceptable grammar.

While it is true that normal language development goes forward without formal training, "expansion" is an effective device in language learning (Brown 1964). Most mothers respond to children's telegraphic speech by presenting them with the nearest correct sentence, that is to say, they modify children's utterances by means of functor words, inflectional affixes, etc. Thus, a child may say, *Mummy lunch* and the mother may counter by saying: "Yes, Mummy is having her lunch." Such a response is far from being a correction. Cazden (1968a) has rightly pointed out that correction extinguishes communication altogether. Expansion, on the other hand, "supplies a model of more explicit encoding of intended meaning . . . at a time when the child's attention is directed to the significant clues of the message." It is, however, by no means easy to determine what is effective: *amounts* or *kinds* of stimulation.

There is a teaching device which supplies richer stimulation than does expansion. Expatiation consists of enlargement of the child's utterances. Thus when a child says *dog bark* the adult does not limit himself to the closest correct sentence, but adds: "He barks at the kitty, but he won't bite it." This kind of response provides a richer linguistic corpus to draw from than does expansion.

Mothers instinctively present to the children different language models at different stages in the language learning task. However, we know relatively little about what happens when a child is exposed precociously to advanced language models, nor are we entirely sure what occurs when he is presented with such models at a late stage.

There is, of course, no doubt that there is far less expansion and expatiation in deprived environments than there is in middle class ones. Lenneberg (1967) maintains, nevertheless, that not only the sequence of language milestones, but also the timing is relatively independent of environmental conditions. The onset of speech occurs more or less at the same time regardless of milieu; even children suffering from gross neglect learn to talk with relatively little delay. Lenneberg's position is open to question since there are many neglected children whose speech is deficient in the absence of a demonstrable neurological deficit. It would be foolish, furthermore, to deny that language dimensions such as richness and complexity of verbal output, ability to express feelings and ideas and level of abstraction, are heavily dependent on environmental support.

Bernstein (1961) has found that the speech of lower class individuals is characterized by rigidity of syntax and restricted structural possibilities for sentence organization. He states that middle class speech, in contrast, facilitates verbal elaboration and provides a complex conceptual framework for the organization of experience. This position is shared by Hess and his collaborators (1966) who found that the flow of language between mother and child varies according to social grouping. They view the mother as a teacher, a programmer of experience during the preschool years, and they have shown in a series of ingenious experiments that mothers from different social levels use different styles of processing information. This information processing is mediated through language. Hess's findings clearly demonstrate that the teaching style of lower class mothers is far less explicit and less effective than that of middle class mothers, and that teaching style is related to the cognitive functioning of the child.

The problem of language acquisition in disadvantaged children is even more complex for groups whose dialect differs from standard English. Differences in phonology and above all in grammatical structure in black children's speech are often wrongly viewed as language deficits. Cazden (1966a) in an excellent paper discusses the difference-deficiency issue. Disadvantaged children, she says, tend to be deficient in many measures of verbal skills. One must be sure, however, that developmental language scales do not distort the assessment of children who speak a nonstandard dialect. Povich and Baratz's study (1967) has shown that the proportion of linguistic transformations is the same in black children as in white middle class ones of comparable age. However, those transformations differ in kind. The form *he brother* for *his brother* for instance and the use of the double negative are typical transformations of the language code for adult blacks. Thus, these forms cannot be regarded as grammatically defective in the case of black children.

It is of interest that in all social groups, girls are more advanced in language development than boys, probably as a result of the relatively slower neurophysiological maturation of boys as compared to girls. First-born do better than younger children. Twins and triplets who have to share the mother's lap are worse off than are single babies, as elaborated on by McCarthy (1958).

It is impossible to overrate the importance of language in children's development. Language is our main tool in the construction of an organized universe. The preverbal child probably has some schemata, some ways of structuring the world, but these schemata can be assumed to be amorphous. The ability to use symbols permits the child to impose order on his experience and to arrive at some clarification of his outer and inner cosmos.

Language, Edelheit (1968b) states, is an obligatory component of human biological organization and plays a crucial role in the formation of the ego, which is the special human organism of adaptation. He adds that it is by no means clear to what extent ego organization is reflected in the language system and to what extent the internalized language system constitutes the regulatory organ of the ego. There is, however, no doubt as to the fact that ego development depends largely on an optimum level of verbal expression and that, conversely, ego defects of whatever origin are reflected in disturbances of language. As far back as 1946 Anna Freud has this to say: " . . . the attempt to master drive processes . . . by linking them to verbal signs which can be dealt with in consciousness was one of the . . . earliest and most necessary accomplishments of the ego, not one of its activities."

Things acquire stability and permanence by being named. Verbal signs anchor the significant people in the child's environment, they reassure him that the mothering person will return even if she is gone for a while, and they thus contribute to what is called object constancy.

Language helps the child to a clearer concept of self and nonself. The child probably has an emerging sense of self even before he begins to verbalize. But, as Peller (1966) points out, the distinction between self and nonself becomes much more differentiated when categories such as *I*, *mine*, and *self* emerge.

Language permits the child to express feelings, to externalize magical fantasies and thus to render them less dangerous. It makes possible the distinction between fantasies on the one hand and reality on the other, thus assisting reality testing, which is one of the essential functions of the ego (Katan 1961).

Words are needed for the direction of behavior and for impulse control. Planning ahead and postponing gratification is infinitely more difficult without the use of words. The formation of conscience is immensely facilitated when the child learns to internalize rules, and internalization remains precarious without the use of verbal concepts.

It has often been pointed out that language is an indispensable tool for cognition. By freeing the child from the here and now, by making possible operations such as classifying, serializing, and formulizing, words allow him to discover the common properties of separate perceptions and events which in turn permits the grouping of these single entities into new wholes. Language helps in the shift from associative to cognitive levels of functioning; it mediates, as pointed out by Luria (1961), even during nonverbal tasks.

It should be emphasized, however, that the potentialities of language are fully realized only during the later phase of ontogenesis. Ombredane (1951) distinguishes the affective, the ludic (playful), the practical, the representational, and the dialectic functions of language. In the young child, speech is as yet mainly a means of expressing feelings and demands, a thing with which to play, a device which substitutes for action, or an attempt to control and regulate the behavior of others. Kaplan (1959) describes young children's speech as governed by affective, playful, and practical needs and as highly charged and infused with personal meanings.

Freud (1946) said that language brings into being a higher psychical organization; one way to trace this road is to study the acquisition of language in the small child.

Concepts Related to Normal Reading Processes and Their Application to Reading Pathology

The Reading Problem

The literature on the physiology and psychology of normal reading is vast and, if one combines European and American research, probably goes into thousands of publications.

Historically, studies concerned with reading pathology were, until the last generation, mainly confined to work done by neurologists like Wernicke (1901–3), Pick (1913), Goldstein (1929,1948), and Conrad (1948,1951), who discussed the often gross reading disturbances arising from cerebral trauma. Of these neurologists, Orton (1932,1937), Schilder (1944), and Bender (1958) were the ones who were primarily concerned with the developmental reading disabilities found in children. However, the growing number of individuals involved in the research of children's reading difficulties has only recently begun to relate findings to what is known about normal reading processes.

What is reading? Reading is the successful response to the visual forms of language. The understanding of graphically fixed language units is the goal of reading. A large number of structures and functions are involved in the process. To begin with, there is the peripheral mechanism. The decisive organ for visual perception is, of course, the eye. But reading is obviously more than and different from seeing. The visibility of letters is not the same as their readability. Our dyslexic children do see letters, but they do not grasp their symbolic significance. Reading is not only concerned with visual perception; it is in the last instance an intellectual act.

There are, of course, some reading difficulties which are related to gross visual problems (Robinson 1958). Cleland (1953) feels that farsightedness and lack of binocular vision contribute significantly to reading difficulties. However, visual disturbances are probably far less frequently a factor in reading disabilities than is often assumed. A

Reprinted with permission of Heldref Publications, a publication of the Helen Dwight Reid Educational Foundation, from *The Journal of Genetic Psychology* 102:227–285. 1961.

report of the ophthalmological section of the Los Angeles County Medical Association published in 1940 still seems pertinent:

> Only if visual acuity is reduced 50 percent or more will the child have trouble with interpretation of symbols he can not see well. Except in far-sightedness of a marked degree, the child's power of focusing is sufficient to give adequate though not perfect vision. A small amount of myopia might be an advantage rather than a disadvantage. Crossed eye with normal vision in one eye has little or no effect on reading ability.

In reading the eye has a double task, a visual and motor one. The latter is served by a complex system of muscles and nerves. The eye does not rest on the text but glides along the printed line, not in a continuum but in a succession of movements and fixations.

The discussion whether or not fusion difficulties and/or faulty eye movements are responsible for reading difficulties is still going on. Orton (1943) and Tinker (1936) deny the significance of faulty eye movements in the etiology of reading disorders. Research has shown that the differences in number of eye fixations in excellent and in poor readers is surprisingly small. The Los Angeles report also states: "So-called faulty eye movements as judged by regressions depend primarily on poor understanding of subject matter, not on un-coordinated eye muscles; not the eye but the brain learns to read." Kainze (1956) in Vienna also maintains that the number of eye movements is a function of the ability to grasp meaning and not the other way around.

This is not the place to discuss cortical functions involved in reading. Suffice it to say that during the last generation the concept of what happens in the reading process has undergone considerable modification. Neurologists no longer believe that precisely pinpointed brain areas are responsible for specific performance. True, we do know that in lesions of the angular gyrus the interpretation of graphic signs is impaired or lost. We also know that the areas adjacent to it do stimulate processes involved in reading, which is a learned activity and needs a degree of maturation for functioning. However, we no longer believe that in reading we deal with separate and summative cortical excitations; rather, we assume the existence of highly complex activities involving the whole brain.

The angular gyrus clearly is not the only area significant in reading. We know, for instance, that in sensory aphasia characterized by inability to understand the spoken word, reading is often impaired as well. It appears thus that for reading comprehension auditory language centers are extremely important.

This leads to a question which has concerned research workers for some time. Does the printed word or letter act as a trigger which releases meaning directly? Is there a straight road leading from the visual graphic representation of the word to the concept? Or does the printed word trigger its oral counterpart, the spoken word, which in turn releases meaning? Does the printed word *mat*, a series of letters seen, a sequence in space, evoke directly the concept of *mat*? Or is the printed word consciously or unconsciously translated either overtly or in inner speech into a series of sounds heard, a sequence in time which in turn evokes the concept of *mat*? Kainz (1956) feels that the highly skilled reader proceeds directly from the printed symbol to the underlying concept, that he needs a minimum of inner sound. He believes that the familiar printed word is in itself a carrier of meaning, an assumption which has probably influenced the teaching of reading everywhere.

The opposite position is taken by people like Orton (1937) who say that the various levels of language function are so closely interrelated that they cannot be considered separately, that speech and reading represent a continuum in language development, that the visual and the auditory structure of the word are intimately bound up with each other. Schilder (1944) conceived of alexia as a disturbance involving the sound structure of the written word. Head (1926) felt that in reading the conventional graphic sign has to be translated silently or aloud into auditory verbal form. Unskilled readers find it necessary to form with their lips the spoken equivalent of the printed word; they have to *say* the word in order to grasp its meaning. There are many other workers in the field who maintain that even fluent readers evoke the auditory and motor images symbolized by printed letters but that these images are so fleeting and of so short a duration, the process goes so fast, that the individual is not necessarily aware of it. Even the practised reader will resort to vocalization when he meets an unknown word or tries to understand a difficult passage. It is likely that inner speech phenomena evoked by reading are never completely eliminated. How many vocal cues are needed is probably a matter of reading proficiency.

However, evoking the auditory image of the word during reading is only part of the process. If one analyzes the reading process, one finds a number of partial performances; there is the perceptual grasping of letters and word configurations; there is their evocation in inner speech; there is the comprehension of syntactical relationships, the construction of anticipatory schemata as to what the sentence is going to say; there is finally the assimilation of content into the already existing framework. All of this constitutes an integrated performance, one part influencing the other. It is only in unsuccessful reading experiences (as when someone reads a text aloud but does not grasp its significance) that one can separate out the partial performances. (Kainz 1956).

Whole-Part Learning

One of the basic problems in reading research is the question whether the skilled reader integrates letters or sounds into wholes, or whether the printed word is experienced globally. An answer to this question is obviously pertinent in terms of the battle now raging between the groups which teach reading in a global fashion and those who believe that words should be broken up into their phonetic elements and then blended into units. The theoretical philosophical foundation for the global approach is based on gestalt psychology, and it is imperative to discuss how this theory influenced the different systems of teaching reading.

Gestalt psychology as originally conceived by Wertheimer (1922,1944) defines gestalt as that function of the organism which responds to a given constellation of stimuli as to a whole. There is an innate tendency in human beings to experience whole configurations. We respond to a series of musical tones as to a tune, a melody, even if it is transposed into another key. The single elements, the separate notes, may be different, but the physiognomy of the configuration, the relationship of the parts to the whole, remains constant, the figure stays the same. We respond to a series of pencil strokes as to a square even if the square is presented at a different angle. As defined by gestalt psychology, visual forms obey certain laws:

(*a*) Form is characterized by being separated and standing out from the ground.

(*b*) The whole and its parts mutually determine each other's characteristics.

(*c*) The various parts of a form have different values, some are indispensable if wholeness is to be retained, others are relatively unnecessary.

(*d*) There is a tendency of the organism to complete unfinished gestalten.

These are only a few of the laws.

While the original gestalt experiments have been done with simple visual forms like circles and squares and while letters are, of course, much more complex, much of what is true for simple forms is true also for letters and words. We do not see all the single elements in a word, we see their characteristic features; words have a physiognomy, a particular relationship between the whole and the parts that makes it possible to recognize them, no matter if they are printed large or small, black or red, whether the print is good or relatively poor. We know that if one tears a word apart and prints it in separate syllables it takes 66 percent longer to read it because as a result of the separation the gestalt quality gets lost. In one of his experiments Korte (1923) presented words from a long distance so that they were at first quite indistinct and diffuse. The first impression of the word was a global one, including gestalt qualities like roundness, length, square-ness, and so forth. The second phase of recognition began with the moment when a characteristic single detail was recognized as de-cisively influencing the total gestalt.

In order to prove their point, which is that good readers are global readers, some gestalt adherents point to the fact that proficient readers make poor proofreaders since they are apt to overlook misprinted letters. It is quite true that such readers receive at best a slight shock on meeting the misprinted word because its physiognomy has somehow changed, it looks slightly unfamiliar. The skilled reader has to force himself to go back and check on each single letter. Since good readers are global readers, many educators and psychologists have concluded as a result that global reading is the correct method to teach children. However, as Daniels and Diack (1959) point out, the process of learn-ing to read is precisely a matter of turning an undifferentiated whole into a differentiated one. It is only the skilled and not the beginning reader who sees words in a structured and organized way. The child often does not. His ability to differentiate is as yet undeveloped.

Moreover, it would be unwise to underrate the importance of the determining letters as constituting elements of the whole con-figuration. It is not true that word configurations are necessarily and always experienced as ready and finished wholes. Many gestalt adher-ents admit that letters, too, are gestalten, partial gestalten, it is true, but possessing nevertheless the same quality as do whole words. We do not see all the single elements in a letter; what we do see is a characteristic configuration, which makes it possible for us to recog-nize a letter as such and enables us to discriminate, for instance, a T from an F, regardless of whether this T is large or small, printed in black or red, written in one handwriting or in another. Like the word, the letter has a gestalt also in the sense that it is structured, separate, that it stands out.

What it amounts to is this: in normal reading, analysis of wholes and integration of parts goes forward simultaneously and the com-bination of both makes for good reading.

One can describe these processes in different terms: it has been stated that both apperceptive and assimilative activities take place during reading. Under apperceptive reading one understands the ordering of perceived letters and letter groups into word con-figurations. Assimilative reading, on the other hand, is geared to large meaning units. In assimilative reading visual perception only acts as a stimulus. Reading processes go forward not only during eye fixations but also during eye movements. When one has to read a large number of books professionally, one only grasps the important words. All depends on the material and the goal. A research paper is read differently from a light novel. But even assimilative reading depends on smooth perceptive and apperceptive functioning (Kainz 1956).

To pull it together, both word and letter configurations are probably grasped on the basis of their determining features. Certain readers may tend to the apperception of larger gestalten, but even if they grasp them more or less as a whole they still must be able to analyze them into their elements quickly and reliably. Reading in other words requires both integrative and differentiating functions.

Normal children need only a few exposures of a particular printed word to recall it consistently. Langman (1960) describes it when she says that these youngsters easily perceive visual spatial gestalten, patterns which have a complex and distinct internal design as well as a general outline and configuration.

Whole-Part Disabilities

Children with severe reading disability have trouble with the very same functions that were found to be essential in normal reading, namely with integration and differentiation of visual patterns, or, to put it differently, with organization and structuring of visual spatial gestalten.

Hughlings Jackson (1958) calls alexia, the loss of reading ability resulting from brain injury, a functional regression of a highly organized activity to earlier stages of development. Leischner (1951) and Conrad (1948,1951) conceive of it as a result of a process of dedifferentiation. If this be so, if we think of alexia as a disruption or a breakdown of formerly well established schemata, we could postulate that the dyslexic child would find it difficult to learn to structure these schematas in the first place. It appears that the ability of these children to respond and organize visual gestalten is either inherently weak or lagging. Studies on normal development show a steady progression in differentiation and integration from early childhood through adolescence. The normal child will not be able to cope with as complex a skill as reading before he has reached a degree of maturation. Most youngsters are ready around the age of six and a half, and the large majority of them learn to master the process regardless of the method of teaching. There is no doubt that the spelling method of learning to read used so successfully in teaching children for generations was a poor one. *Cee Ai Tee* never did make *cat*, but most youngsters learned to read in spite of it. Why? Because they learned to integrate short units into longer ones and to analyze wholes into their determining parts simply because they were exposed to them.

Dyslexic children find these processes extremely difficult. We believe that their neurophysiological immaturity makes it hard or impossible for them to perceive and respond to complex gestalten. As a result of many years of clinical investigation we feel, moreover, that these youngsters reveal dysfunctions and immaturities not only in reading but in other areas as well (de Hirsch 1952).

Orton (1932) has shown how many dyslexic children are dyspraxic. Movement, like perception, requires patterning. A skilled motor act is not a succession of single isolated movements. A summation of separate movement units will not result in a fluid rhythmic performance. A motor act is a total gestalt and since dyslexic children's gestalt competence is often weak, it is not surprising that many of them are very clumsy.

The same children mostly have difficulty with spatial organization, to wit, their confusion in motor leads, their trouble with spatial sequences, their tendency to reversals, their difficulty with left to right progression, which have been described frequently (Harris 1957).

Bender (1938) has clearly shown the striking immaturity of gestalt functioning in dyslexic children in terms of visuomotor organization.

A large number of researchers, among them Orton (1937), Weiss (1950), de Hirsch (1961) and Arnold (1960), have discussed the poor motor speech patterns of these youngsters which reveal their difficulty with the organization of configuration in a temporal sequence. Their tendency to reverse sounds in words and words in sentences, their telescoping of long words, their omissions and substitutions, all bear witness to their trouble with differentiation and integration of complex auditory-motor patterns. The very monotony and dysrhythmia of dyslexic children's speech is symptomatic for their trouble with structuring temporal gestalten.

Gestalt psychology says that any coherent form is characterized by standing out in relief. Dyslexic children often lack the ability to differentiate figure from ground. Nothing on the page stands out for them; the printed symbols to them look like an undifferentiated, meaningless design (de Hirsch 1954).

To summarize, dyslexic children have trouble with various types of gestalten. Their patterning of motor, visuomotor, and perceptual configurations is often primitive. What then happens to them if they are confronted with the very abstract, very complex patterns represented by printed words and phrases?

Some dyslexic children have the greatest difficulty remembering even the shape of single letters. Not words only, but letters also are highly unstable. They look dangerously alike. They have no separateness, they lack a clear-cut physiognomy. These children cannot abstract the unessential features in a letter and pick out the determining ones, those which make, for instance, a letter look like an *F*.

After much drill they may learn to identify the letter, but only when it is presented in isolation: not when it is embedded in a word or when it is printed in another color, or when the size is enlarged or reduced. These children are unable to maintain the identity of the gestalt; they cannot transfer the characteristic gestalt quality into another configuration. Most unstable for them are, of course, those letters which actually look alike, as do *b* and *d*, and *p* and *b* and whose only differentiating feature is one of spatial arrangement.

If for dyslexic children short configurations like single letters are unstable, how much more must be longer ones, words?

Phonetic teaching does not only reduce the length and the complexity of gestalten; it is helpful also because it relates the visual to the auditory structure of the word and thus facilitates inner speech phenomena (Schilder 1944). In the teaching of phonetics single letters and sounds, partial visual and auditory wholes, are learned separately and are slowly fused into larger entities. However, no matter how children learn to read, in larger or smaller units, reading is never (even if taught phonetically) a process of adding one sound or one letter to another.

One of the gestalt laws says that the whole is more than and different from the sum of its elements. It has been shown in brain lesions, for instance, that a patient was able to read the two halves of the word *figure* and *head* but not the word *figurehead*. Some of our dyslexic children have immense difficulties fusing single sounds into longer units. Not unlike aphasiacs, they find it difficult to integrate parts into wholes. However, the majority does catch on when taught shorter units, and there comes a moment during the remedial process when the gestalt function seems to "jell," when the child no longer has to laboriously add and blend unit for unit, a moment when the process changes qualitatively and the youngster begins to integrate and differentiate spontaneously.

Thus in the final analysis there is no dichotomy between part and whole learning, since both are inherent in the reading process; it is rather a matter of which size configuration the child is ready for. Whole words and whole sentences are obviously more meaningful than sounds are. However, the point about dyslexic children is that their gestalt competence is weak to begin with; thus they do need additional help with the structuring and organization of wholes and often do better with shorter configurations.

There is another problem which can best be elucidated with the help of gestalt psychology. Why, for instance, do many dyslexic children sometimes recognize long and complicated words and have such trouble with short and seemingly easier ones? Why can they read a word like *courageously* but are confused between *there, then, when* and *where*? For two reasons: the abstract nature of the small grammatical words which represent spatial, temporal, and causal relationships makes them difficult to remember. Moreover, they are of about equal length, they lack physiognomy, the characteristic features which make for recognition.

Summary

I have tried to highlight briefly some aspects of normal reading processes which seemed pertinent in terms of children suffering from severe reading disturbances. It appears that skilled reading requires a high degree of integration and differentiation, an ability which is defined by gestalt psychology as competence in perceiving and responding to complex and highly organized configurations.

The very features which make for skilled reading, namely, integration and differentiation, are either deficient or lagging in dyslexic children. In fact, our clinical investigation seems to prove that these youngsters have trouble with organization not only of complex linguistic forms but also with more basic motor, visuomotor, and perceptual schemata.

Any remedial approach has to take into account the fact that dyslexic children have basic configuration difficulties. While the aim in reading undoubtedly is the assimilation of large meaning units, any method that facilitates the organization of small or large gestalten and which links the visual to the auditory image of the word will be helpful.

Early Language Development and Minimal Brain Dysfunction

The world we live in is conceptually organized, and our primary instrument in the construction of a comprehensible universe is language. Children need serviceable verbal tools in order to impose order on their experience. This paper discusses the often severe linguistic processing difficulties of young children who suffer from minimal brain dysfunction. Although such difficulties are frequently precursors of massive learning disorders, they tend to be overlooked. The ability to analyze and organize linguistic input and to generate language is not only essential for learning at all levels, but it is also closely related to ego functions that are crucial for academic functioning, such as impulse control and the capacity to postpone gratification.

At the Pediatric Language Disorder Clinic, which is concerned with children suffering from language and learning disabilities, we see no spastic children and very few from the seizure clinic. These cases are referred to neurology. In other words, we see few youngsters with classical neurological signs.

de Ajuriaguerra (1963) questions the very existence of unilateral, circumscribed damage in the majority of newborns. Instead, he believes that fairly widespread dysfunctions in crucial processes result in disturbances that give rise to a large variety of disorders.

Looking at our children, we are impressed with their process disturbances, their immaturity, and their inability to organize their experience. Their pathology does not resemble that of the aphasic adults with whom I worked at the start of my professional life and who presented structural damage.

Among our youngsters, there are some with frank psychiatric disorders, but the majority are children with a family history of language disorders, a cloudy prenatal and postnatal history, some developmental deviations, and, almost always, delayed speech onset and academic difficulties. Investigation reveals a degree of hyper-

Reprinted with permission from The New York Academy of Sciences, from *Annals of the New York Academy of Sciences* 205:158–163. 1973.

kinesis, hypotonia, global motility patterning and fine motor and graphomotor clumsiness, instability of perceptuomotor experience, difficulty in focusing, and some social dyspraxia. More or less subtle gaps in language processing, semantic limitations, dysnomia, and paucity of syntactical options are present in most of the youngsters. In short, they show what Hertzig and colleagues (1969) call "atypicality" and, one might add, immaturity of central nervous system organization.

Man is an organizing, pattern-making animal. The children I want to discuss have trouble organizing their inner and outer cosmos. Their most striking characteristic is their difficulty with the construction of schemata, from the simplest to the most complex. Whatever happened to central nervous systems of these children happened to organisms in the process of formation, thus interfering with maturation and integration in all areas and on all levels of physiological and psychological functioning. The presenting clinical picture, however, varies from child to child.

In attempting to understand these variations, we find it useful to ask ourselves: what would this youngster be like if he did not present central nervous system dysfunction; what is his genetic potential? Or, given the dysfunction, how would he strike one if he were growing up in a warm, supportive climate, or if his mother had greater tolerance for deviation and frustration (since we know that these children present different stimuli to mothers than do "normal" children)? Above all, what is the youngster's capacity for compensation—a crucial question posed by Birch (1967) some time ago. In other words, what are the child's resources in terms of intelligence and ego strength? Even if we cannot answer these questions, consideration of them helps us at least to look closely at the interaction of forces that have shaped a particular child. I refer to Weil's (1970b) excellent presentation of these dynamics.

In the discussion of youngsters with central nervous system dysfunctions, two characteristics, hyperkinesis and perceptuomotor deviations, have been at the center of interest for the past twenty years. The need for structure has been stressed over and over again. I fully agree with this emphasis, although I have seen highly structured remedial programs that are quite sterile and that do not relate learning to the children's emotional needs.

As regards perceptuomotor training, young children, especially those with atypical central nervous system functioning, can only benefit from it, since touch, smells, sounds, forms, shapes, and textures are the very stuff of living. Body image work is particularly useful as a means of orienting the children in space. However, on the correct assumption that development is by and large a consistent process and that training should therefore proceed from simpler to more highly elaborated levels, special educational personnel and some people in the speech and hearing field have become obsessed even in the case of older children with perceptuomotor aspects of training: with jungle gyms, puzzles, shapes, and a potpourri of seductively packaged commercial materials. They ignore Luria's (1961) teaching that verbalization stabilizes perception, the right kind of verbalization, I may add. Having a youngster trace a square and asking him to say: "This is a square" cannot possibly be meaningful for him. Moreover, the fact that even severe perceptuomotor deficits can be compensated for is often overlooked. I refer to Halpern's (1970) paper, which demonstrates that many bright Johnnies learn to read well in spite of severe visuomotor deficits. Finally, as children proceed through the grades, the demands for perceptual performance decrease rapidly and those for linguistic and conceptual competence increase sharply. Indeed, linguistic and conceptual deficits are at the root of learning and, specifically, reading failure.

It might thus be helpful to briefly discuss some of the ways children learn to process linguistic patterns. The preverbal child probably has some schemata, some means of structuring the world, but these schemata can be assumed to be amorphous (Peller 1966). Friedlander's work (1970) shows that normal infants begin to respond selectively at eleven months to some of the acoustic and linguistic signals that impinge on them from the environment. They attempt to sort out the "buzzing confusion" around them by picking out certain regularities in the input to which they are exposed. This task must be immensely difficult for youngsters who have trouble with all types of schemata and for whom the highly abstract and complex verbal sequences must be entirely confusing. They thus live in a noisy, chaotic world much longer than "normal" children.

How do normal children learn to comprehend language? At first, they simply respond to the intonational configurations that are part of familiar situations. Slowly, phonemic patterns become intertwined with intonational and situational features, until gradually, as further differentiation takes place, phonemic features become dominant, irrespective of the situation (Lewis 1963).

Most young children with mild central nervous system dysfunctions do respond to intonation. Thus, the parents may not suspect that anything is amiss. Developmental milestones may have been grossly normal. The pediatrician may have said: "Give him time, he'll talk all right." But it is not a matter of talking. Input always precedes output, and the deficits on the input side cause the problems. Difficulty with processing of linguistic input between thirty and thirty-six months is a red flag in terms of subsequent, often severe learning disabilities. If one tells such a youngster in the evening: "Go and get your slippers," he will comply. But if one tells him the same thing at 11 o'clock in the morning, he may miss the message. Such children are usually adept at picking up situational and even visual clues. In the framework of a familiar situation, they may understand some nouns and one or the other verb, words that carry the essential information. They may even use stock phrases. Parents often tell us: "Johnny used to talk, but he has stopped." In many cases, however, what he said was not actually language; moreover, all along he had difficulty interpreting verbal sequences. Not only do such children lack refined auditory discriminations and have trouble with complex feedback mechanisms, but above all they cannot cope with temporally distributed patterns of verbal events, and they do not sense how these patterns hang together. As a result, they are unable to deduce even quite simple rules from the linguistic data they receive. Their output mirrors their diffuse reception. In a recent experimental paper, Menyuk (1971) found that linguistically deviant children do not perceive, process, and store language in the same way as do normal children. Their language is not delayed; it is different. They have trouble analyzing the underlying structure of input. When they repeat sentences, their errors are not so much a function of the length of units but of the complexity of sentence structure. Much later, these same youngsters come back to us with difficulties in reading comprehension, even if they have learned the mechanisms of the reading process.

Let me turn to the relationship between linguistic deficits and disorders of ego function that are essential for learning. As Rappaport (1964) said, we never deal solely with the sequelae of the organic insult but also with the resulting disturbances in the epigenesis of the ego. I am not now talking of high order intellectual operations such as classifying, serializing, categorizing. Language is essential for such operations because it frees the child from the here and now. It permits him to discover the common properties of perceptions and events and leads him from learning on an associative to learning on a conceptual level. I am talking rather of more fundamental psychological dimensions of learning, specifically of those related to linguistic deprivation at early ages.

Language, Edelheit states (1969), is an obligatory component of human biological organization and plays a crucial role in the formation of the ego, which is the special human organ for adaptation. Ego development depends largely on an optimal level of verbal expression; conversely, ego defects, of whatever origin, are reflected in disturbances of language. Anna Freud (1936) called our attention to the critical importance of language in ego development, observing that language is inextricably bound to affects and drive processes. Words are needed for impulse control. Postponing gratification is infinitely more difficult without the use of words.

Language permits the child to externalize magical and omnipotent fantasies and thus render them less dangerous (Katan 1961). It makes possible the distinction between fantasies on the one hand and the external world on the other, thus assisting reality functioning, one of the most essential functions of the ego and a prerequisite for learning. Finally, language facilitates the shifting of frames of reference, which is important for social adaptation.

What, then, happens to children with central nervous system disorders who have difficulty processing language and expressing feelings by way of words? Bender (1949) pointed to what has been called their "primary anxiety." The fears of organic children over intactness and bodily injury are probably related to early problems with homeostasis and orientation in space. These fears are all the more threatening if the child cannot express what must occasionally amount to terror.

The assumption that learning difficulties in children must rest on either a neurotic or an organic basis is, of course, simplistic. Neurosis may be part and parcel of the biological dysfunction; it may be the consequence of the dysfunction; finally, the two may exist simultaneously, one reinforcing the other. The presence of organicity does not exempt a child from emotional disturbance. Kurlander and Colodny (1965) speak about the psychopathology of organicity. Inability to comprehend and use language, the instrument for organization in time and space, gives rise to feelings of helplessness in the face of both inner demands for control over drives and reality demands from the environment. Feelings of helplessness in turn result in increased infantile needs. In fact, mothers respond to these needs quite legitimately (We saw this in our prematurely born group.) The two, physiological immaturity and emotional infantilism, go hand in hand. The former has its root in the organic dysfunction, whereas the emotional regression and the resulting internal conflict is neurotic in nature.

Children who do not comprehend words such as *tomorrow* have a harder time tolerating frustration than do others, and they have more severe difficulties in postponing gratification (Peller 1966). Some of these difficulties are greatly alleviated once the children acquire appropriate verbal tools. Similarly, children who have trouble expressing feelings of fear and anger tend to be overwhelmed. If they cannot express rage by means of words, they are bound to act. But acting out gives rise to repercussions both at home and at school; it interferes with learning and leads to delinquency and dropping out.

What does all of this suggest concerning intervention in the case of children with atypical central nervous system functioning?

1. The normal vocal and verbal exchange between the mother and her baby has to be intensified. In the case of youngsters with

cerebral dysfunction, this exchange is often reduced because the children fail to stimulate their mothers. Long before the age of two and a half, the mother must feed the child short, simple phrases much the way she used to feed him food. Wyatt (1969) calls the vocal and affect communication between mothers and their babies a process of mutual feedback.

2. Communication must be heavily invested with affect and must involve the person the child is emotionally tied to. Cognitive teaching in young children has to be infused with the energies derived from their affects and drives; otherwise, teaching will not take. In the process of language learning, cognitive and affective streams must flow together. It is, of course, a mistake to make children repeat words. It may simply turn them off. Moreover, the referential function of language is not the same thing as communication. Giving a youngster a piece of a puzzle that depicts an apple and saying, "This is an apple; it is green," does not provide him with the give and take of communication. Shaping his responses certainly will not do it. It cannot possibly call forth the energy that pushes the child to say *down* if he throws the sister doll from the roof of the dollhouse. (Needless to say, we do *not* interpret his action, but we use the affect behind it to elicit language.) Swinging a two-and-a-half-year-old and saying *up high* incorporates these words in an emotionally heavily charged cluster, which helps retention. The therapy of choice is modeling: describing in the shortest phrases what the child is *doing* when he is engrossed in some favorite activity, expanding what *he* says into the closest short phrase. This is a technique used by mothers instinctively, and it can be adapted to the needs of these children in terms of the length and complexity of the verbal structures they are able to deal with.

3. Linguistic intervention has to be continued for several years, because, as shown by Menyuk (1971), linguistically deviant children quickly arrive at a plateau and must be helped from there on to process and generate more complex verbal material.

4. Most important: linguistic intervention cannot come too early. I know from many years of experience how much better the chances are for success at thirty than at forty months. We need the earliest possible intervention because of the far greater plasticity of the brain at earlier ages and because failure to process and use language has severe repercussions on the ego functions that are essential for learning.

I remember a little boy who was referred to us at age four by the psychiatrist because he did not talk. He was a youngster who presented central nervous system irregularities. After a year and a half, he would occasionally come in and say: "This is one of my days, put that junk away"—meaning the materials set out for him. Having said that, he was able to work. He had used his newly learned language as a way of coping with his drivenness and his tendency to be overwhelmed. But it was a slow process. And we might have spared him and his parents much anguish had we started him earlier.

Let me therefore repeat my plea for the earliest possible linguistic intervention.

Part ***II***

THE CHILD AT RISK

Tests Designed to Discover Potential Reading Difficulties at the Six-Year-Old Level

It is a well-known fact that our schools carry a fairly large percentage of educational and emotional casualties, bright children whose life at school is a burden because they suffer from a more or less severe reading disability. We have only to look at the intake of a pediatric-psychiatric clinic or at a sample of the youngsters referred to our child guidance centers to find a sizable number of intelligent children whose somatic complaints or behavioral disturbances developed only after they had been exposed to the experience of continued failure at school.

Since remedial facilities in our private and public educational institutions are few and far between, we shall have to find ways to prevent the occurrence of reading failure. In order to do this we need tools which enable us to predict with reasonable certainty which youngsters are liable to run into trouble in the first and second grades. Once we select these children we may find that some of them simply need more time in which to mature, but that others might do very well if given specific techniques right from the start. Careful selection and consistent planning on our part might easily prevent a great deal of heartache and frustration later on.

How then can we find out at the end of the kindergarten year, in the five- to six-year-old group—and I stress this time since it is crucial as far as certain maturational processes are concerned—which children are liable to find the going rough?

The remarks offered here are of an entirely tentative nature.

At the Pediatric Language Disorder Clinic, Columbia-Presbyterian Medical Center, we believe that we have evolved some procedures designed to predict future reading performance, and we think that in a fair percentage of cases our prediction has been correct. We have not as yet done a statistical evaluation, but having experimented along certain lines, we are now trying to find out where such experimentation will lead us.

Reprinted with permission from The American Orthopsychiatric Association, Inc., from *American Journal of Orthopsychiatry* 27:566–675. 1957.

We use the well-known intelligence tests as an overall measurement of the child's basic intellectual endowment. Among them the Bellevue-Wechsler Scale for Children seems to be the most satisfactory. However, in a large percentage of cases these tests do not predict future success or failure in reading, spelling, and writing. The better-known reading readiness tests, which we also use, do not seem to us to cover all the facets of behavior which we think are significant. The Metropolitan Readiness test is probably the best since it stresses comprehension not only of single words, but also of more complex verbal units. It does not, however, test ability to use verbal material and it fails to evaluate a variety of aspects which enter into reading performance. We agree with Gillingham's observation (1949) that children with a mental age under six and a half are not ready for the printed word.

Reading readiness is a function of development. We look on development, emotional and neurophysiological, as a progressive increase in complexity of behavioral patterns. Studies on normal development show that psychological functioning and cerebral organization reveal a steady increase in differentiation and integration through adolescence. As the child grows older he has to cope with increasingly more differentiated and highly integrated organizations. Among these more complex skills is the ability to use verbal tools. At the age of six children are supposed to have mastered oral symbols. We expect them to have organized an enormous number of arbitrary phonetic signs into the pattern of language, a formidable achievement which by no means all children have accomplished at this age, as evidenced by the numerous youngsters who still show infantile speech patterns.

Once a child reaches first grade he is expected to cope with a secondary symbolic system, with visual signs which have to be correlated with meaning. In order to read a little word like *hat*, a sequence of letters seen, a sequence in space has to be translated into a sequence of sounds heard, a sequence in time. We feel that without a measure of maturation—perceptual, motor, conceptual, and behavioral maturation, the child will be unable to cope with this task. The youngster whose neurophysiological organization still is primitive, the one whose language equipment is inferior, is the one who will probably run into trouble in the first and second grades. It is this often very intelligent child whom we have to single out before he is exposed to reading failure.

Children between five and one-half and six and one-half usually make dramatic strides in overall maturation, strides so dramatic, in fact, that one occasionally feels one can literally see them blossoming forth. The best time to test them, therefore, is at the end of their year in kindergarten.

Since maturation and development involve the whole child, we observe the youngster's total behavior in order to determine reading readiness.

We usually direct our attention first to those who have trouble with integration of coordination. Movement, like perception, requires patterning. A certain level of motor skills is not only essential for learning to write and print, but it is also indicative of the child's overall maturity.

The youngsters I refer to do not usually show the severe deviations in large muscular control which we find in cerebral palsied children, but they sometimes have trouble throwing a ball, riding a bicycle, skipping rope. We ask our children to throw darts, to walk on their heels, to hop on one foot. We do occasionally find some who not only have difficulty with the execution of these movements, but who also fail, as in ideomotor apraxia, to get the idea of the act itself. Their overall motility is often like that of younger children, and it is of interest that Bender and Yarnell (1941) have commented on motility disturbances in children suffering from various forms of language disabilities.

Some have not attained the neurological maturation which enables them to execute movements of specific muscle groups. They retain some of the characteristics of the global, total motor response which is typical for the very young child. For instance, they turn the whole head when asked to flex the tongue.

Lags in integration and patterning of finer muscular control and a degree of dyspraxia, as described by Orton (1937), are observed relatively frequently, though occasionally this dyspraxia is confined to graphic activities. Oseretsky's tests (Doll 1940) provide an extensive survey of muscular skills and have been standardized in terms of normal development. They are thus useful in determining in which areas a child's performance lags. Unfortunately, these tests are difficult to administer and for practical purposes we have to rely on our own observations. We give our children identical tasks to perform in order to get a basis for comparison. We watch for jerkiness and arrhythmicity in the smaller muscles of the hand and tongue. The way in which a child handles construction toys will not only reveal his manual dexterity and the fluidity of his movements, but it also provides opportunities for observing many other facets of his behavior: his span of attention, his frustration threshold, his curiosity, and his zest.

Research of the last ten years, especially Werner's work (1952), has revealed the close relationship between perceptual and motor functioning. Basic to reading, of course, is the child's ability to cope with perceptual organization.

The very young child normally has difficulty in breaking up the totality of a pattern; his perceptual organization is somewhat diffuse;

single parts are poorly differentiated. However, the differentiation of small details and the understanding of the essential relationship between the parts and the whole are *sine qua non* in reading.

In the Metropolitan Readiness test we find a few items which require the child to discriminate between small visual details. In fact, much of the reading readiness work done in kindergarten and in the earlier part of the first grade is dedicated to the training of such discrimination, and any of the books used in this readiness work can be used for testing.

The Bender Gestalt test (1938), designed for evaluation of visuomotor functioning, is one of the most important in our battery. Visually perceived configurations are offered to children with the request that they be copied. Obviously the infant does not experience perception as the adult does. But the child who is expected to read and write must have visuomotor experiences similar to those of the adult.

Bender says the evolution of visuomotor gestalten is a maturational, not an educative process. It is true that the average six-year-old does not usually copy all the figures correctly. Developmentally there is a progression in the performance of the copied patterns from a controlled scribble at age three to all figures clearly perceived and reproduced at age eleven. However, as Silver (1950) points out, it is of interest that many of our highly intelligent dyslexic children are unable to cope with this task even at twelve or thirteen. They are unable to grasp or retain visual patterns made up of discrete elements. In our children we not only observe difficulty with the handling of the pencil and trouble with manual control, but we also see immature forms (loops, perhaps, instead of dots) which are characteristic for the ages of four and five. We note verticalization of horizontally-oriented figures. We find, in other words, inability to perceive and reproduce given configurations correctly, functions required in the reading process.

Many of our youngsters have great difficulty spacing these figures on paper. The ability to cope with spatial relationships is of primary importance since in reading and writing the child has to deal with a pattern laid out in space. A developmental lag in this area will thus show up in the youngster's reading performance.

Notions of space originally derive from the child's consciousness of his own body. We use the Goodenough Draw-a-Man test (1950), not as an intelligence measurement, nor as a way to evaluate the child's image of self in the emotional sense, though both are of interest. We use it primarily as a relatively reliable indicator of the child's body image, a concept which refers to his awareness of parts of his own body and their relationship to each other. This image is closely related to spatial concepts and is often strikingly immature and primitive in the type of child we are discussing here.

Awareness of left and right, of course, is a significant aspect of the child's notion of space. Since the ability to cope with the specific directional discipline of left to right progression is required for reading in our culture, this aspect deserves further discussion.

As described earlier, we carefully watch the child while we test his finer muscular coordination. Since most of the activities in which he is engaged are untrained and are not influenced by early conditioning, they are useful in determining the degree to which a youngster has established a functional superiority of one hand over the other. Failure to establish such superiority may be related to familial factors; it may also indicate physiological immaturity and thus tend to show up in reading. We take note of early attempts to switch handedness, as well as of the family history with regard to laterality. In testing we evaluate strength, precision, and speed. We carefully note eye dominance since crossed laterality may adversely influence reading performance.

In the small child, awareness of concepts of right and left progresses slowly. The average child of six can demonstrate right and left on his own body, usually with the help of gestural (motor) responses, but not on anybody else's. That is why Head's finger-to-eye test (1926) (originally devised for brain-injured individuals and first used with children by Simon [1954]), which calls for mirror imitation of the examiner's movements, had to be discarded in this form. It seemed to us that the test requires a level of abstraction which the six-year-old has not yet attained. The child of six, however, should be able to imitate one's movements when sitting alongside one and watching one's gestures in a mirror. We have observed that a good many children who fail in this respect later develop reading difficulties.

The Horst's tests (Simon 1954), which we include in our battery, are useful because they give us a clue as to whether or not the youngster is able to discriminate between identical shapes when they are presented in correct and in reversed form.

Spatial and directional concepts are not the only ones which are pertinent in reading. Language, spoken or printed, is laid out in a time-space pattern. Thus we have to investigate not only spatial but also temporal organization.

It is of interest that a number of workers, like Stambak (1951) and Mottier (1951), have consistently found rhythmic difficulties in children suffering from reading disabilities, especially in those whose oral language is already somewhat insecure.

We ask our youngsters to imitate tapped-out patterns of varying difficulty and have observed that a goodly percentage of them fail in the repetition of even short and simple sequences. Rhythm is a configuration in time, and fundamentally our children have trouble with all types of configurations.

We further require that our children repeat a series of nonsense syllables and find in the large majority of cases that they have strikingly short auditory memory spans. The correlation of this feature with language disability seems especially high. The child of six should be able to repeat at least four or five syllables, but most of our youngsters manage just three.

There is another area which has so far received little attention and which is closely related to perceptual organization. We know that brain injury, and in fact any lowering of integrative efficiency, brings about an impairment in figure-background relationships. Weaknesses in figure-ground relationships have not been systematically explored in children with severe reading disabilities. However, the indications are that these youngsters, though to a lesser degree than do brain-injured ones, have difficulties in this area.

In order to cope with spoken or printed language the child must be able to pick out the figure from the background. For one to interpret a sentence heard (the spoken configuration), the message (like the tapped-out pattern) must stand out clearly. For one to decipher a printed sentence, the configuration must be well defined and sharply delineated against the page. I have seen innumerable youngsters look at printed material as if it represented a meaningless design. Only if the figure does stand out will the sentence or the phrase have structure, or, in other words, meaning. Some of our children have trouble separating figure from background. They do not discover, for instance, the significant design in one of the puzzles when asked to find the lion in the jungle. If one gives them raised geometric figures to reproduce graphically from touch, one often finds that they are drawn to the background, to the roughness of the cloth, for instance. The Marble Board test, which was originally designed to evaluate figure background relationships in brain-injured children, is difficult to administer. At the clinic we therefore use an adaptation of the Figure Background cards presented in Strauss and Lehtinen's book on brain-injured children (1947).

It has been established by Goldstein's work (1948) that a certain measure of abstract functioning is a requisite of language performance. The question then arises, what does abstract functioning mean at this early age?

We know that the formation of abstract relationships is a developmental process which starts with perceptual and configurational relationships and develops in the direction of conceptual classification. This applies to both nonverbal and verbal behavior.

The small child who tries to use the toy toilet for his own use while playing with it has not yet understood that a toy only represents the real thing. This experience, a nonverbal one, comes later. It is a tremendous step forward when the child first pretends to be a nurse or a pilot. Some children are relatively concrete at the age of six. Practically all brain-injured children are. But we find the group which has difficulties with various aspects of language function to be similarly concrete, if to a lesser degree, and this concreteness is by no means restricted to the verbal area.

In order to test abstract behavior on a nonverbal level, we give our youngsters block designs to copy, observing whether they are able to analyze wholes into parts and, as the next step, to synthesize these parts into wholes. Guided by the Goldstein-Scherer tests (1941), we give them a variety of objects to sort out, noting whether they are able to isolate eating utensils, things to eat with, so as to find out whether they have some form of categorical behavior, at least on a perceptual level.

The testing discussed up to this point has been confined to nonverbal tasks; we go from these to verbal ones. The ability to handle verbal tools is basic to reading. In order to cope with visual symbols the child must have mastered auditory ones, oral language. Careful testing in this area often reveals significant gaps which are frequently overlooked. Authors like Orton (1937), McCarthy (1954), and Borell-Maisonny (1951a) have long stressed the close relationships between reading efficiency and oral language skills.

First of all we have to make sure that the youngster fully understands spoken material. Units like *in front of*, *inside*, *beneath*, which are fairly abstract concepts, are by no means always as securely established as we are inclined to think. We place the child in front of the dollhouse and suggest he put the baby *next* to the bathtub and so on. Carrying out complex directions is not always easy for our children; many are unable to interpret a somewhat involved story; as matter of fact, a few are not ready to listen at all. Some do not catch on when presented with an absurdity couched in verbal terms, although they are easily able to see the point if the absurd is presented in pictorial form.

Comprehension of language is one thing; use of language, another. We carefully check on articulatory patterns; we note length of units and listen for difficulties in word finding. There are children who have a relatively good use of the idiom on an auditory perceptual basis; they *sound* as though they have a large vocabulary, but some of them fail when asked to give a word on being presented with a picture.

We are interested in vocal patterns; an unusual degree of monotony may reflect a difficulty with structuralization, perhaps a figure-background problem.

The child's ability to form correct grammatical constructions is of importance. Grammar is an expression of structure, and the child who leaves out small connectives in the sentence may have difficulties with the temporal, spatial, and causal relationships expressed by these words.

We further want to know whether the youngster is able to tell a simple story and to bring out its salient features. Some children's organization of verbal material is so poor that they never get their point across; they get so involved in the intricacies of the Three Little Pigs that they ramble on indefinitely.

In the beginning the child's spoken language is on a very concrete level. A three-year-old who says *brush* does not refer to the category *brush*, to the object whose essential qualities are unchanging from situation to situation. *Brush* to him might mean one time, "Brush my hair;" another time, "The brush is on the table." He does not use the word in a categorical sense.

In testing abstract functioning on a verbal level we look for the youngster's ability to classify and categorize. We ask him to name all dining-room furniture. If he includes the wallpaper or the silver dishes on the sideboard, he shows thereby that he has not yet understood the category "furniture." Werner (1940) cites the example of the boy who includes bread and a pipe with the bench, the saw, and the hammer when asked to list tools, explaining, "When you have finished working at the bench you want to eat and smoke a pipe." In other words, he grouped objects according to a concrete situation and not according to the more abstract category "tools." We use the Columbia Mental Maturity Scale to test categorical behavior. The intelligent boy who, when shown a picture of a hen, a stove, a pot, and an egg, says that the egg and the pot belong together, "because you cook an egg in the pot," indicates that he is unable to free himself from the concrete and is not yet ready for classifications.

We test the child's ability to give definitions. At the age of six children define objects in terms of function. A six-year-old who says, "You hold it up here," when asked what a violin is, behaves in a very concrete way, which, if persisting, is a poor prognosis in terms of academic functioning.

If one asks a number of six-year-old children what a policeman is, one is apt to receive a variety of answers from: "He wears a blue suit," or "He stands at the corner," which are concrete responses, to "He directs traffic." In the last response the child tries to cope with function, while in the first ones he limits himself to description. It is usually the child with a language difficulty who is more concrete than others are.

Most children who later develop reading disabilities seem to have trouble with patterning the units of words and sentences in spoken speech. Orton (1937) has shown how frequently these youngsters tend to reverse both oral and printed symbols. The same boy who says *Crice Ripsies* for *Rice Crispies* is the one who later on reads *was* for *saw* and *now* for *won*.

Reversal and confusion in the order of sequences, which are closely related to temporal organization in the sense in which it has been discussed, are usually not confined to syllables and words. The whole sentence is often jumbled, showing again that it is in the area of organization and structuralization of both short and long units that children with language deficits have outstanding difficulties.

Most of our tests are designed to measure the child's ability to pattern, structuralize, and adequately respond to the endless stream of stimuli to which he is exposed at every moment. However, organization of perceptual and motor patterns is not the only area which presents difficulties for our children. Many of them have trouble with integration of behavior. The result is hyperkinesis and lack of control. Most children suffering from developmental language lags are enormously hyperactive. Their trouble with inhibition and channeling of impulses seems to be but another aspect of their inability to organize stimuli (arising from inside as well as from outside) into behavioral configurations. Hence they find it difficult to sit still several hours a day. Such children (they may or may not be emotionally disturbed) are bound to have trouble concentrating. Since they are unable to exclude a variety of stimuli, they are incapable of focusing their attention on a specific gestalt, or an assigned task.

Children in kindergarten are usually given a good many motor outlets, but once they get into first grade they find it difficult to cope with a more structured framework, since their frustration tolerance is low and their need for large muscular activity considerable.

Among the children whom we have tested during the last few years we have found a fairly steady, though small, number of youngsters whose perceptual deviations, trouble with figure-background relationships, outstanding poor motor performance, and limitation in abstract behavior seem far more severe than is usual for the child who suffers from a developmental language disability. Careful investigation of these cases has sometimes revealed a positive history, for instance, anoxia at birth. These youngsters do not necessarily show the usual positive signs of the classical neurological examination. However, more refined testing procedures show that they have difficulties at various levels of integration. Watching these children copy the Bender gestalt figures, one often finds a marked tendency to disinhibition, accompanied by compensatory rigidity. We find perseveration in various areas and a tendency to go to pieces when the number of stimuli becomes too great. Many of these relatively subtle signs go undiscovered until the time when these children are confronted with a task which is a complex as is the mastering of oral and printed symbols.

I do not want to give the impression that our testing takes a great deal of time. After some experimenting we have brought the time down to between 40 and 45 minutes. The tests are usually administered during one session or, preferably, two. Careful observation of the child as he functions in kindergarten, moreover, will eliminate many of the more formal procedures.

In conclusion I should like to sum up a few points: Maturation is largely a process of integration and differentiation. The child of six and older whose perceptual, motor, visuomotor, and conceptual per-formance is still relatively primitive, the child who has trouble with structuralization of behavioral patterns, is the one who is liable to run into difficulties when he is exposed to reading, which requires the smooth interplay of many facets of behavior.

Some of these children need more time in which to mature. Postponing formal training and discipline for six to twelve months may prevent future regrading with its attending experience of failure and humiliation which might easily spoil the youngster's entire learning pattern.

But our testing should do more than simply pick out the children who are not as yet ready for first grade. It should assist us in deter-mining what type of help would be suitable for those youngsters who we feel are able to make the grade if given specific assistance and support.

The hyperactive child, for instance, needs a teacher who has some tolerance for the child's specific difficulty. He needs, if possible, a setting which allows him a good many motor outlets while at the same time providing a somewhat structured environment which protects him from an excess of environmental stimuli. Such a youngster would fare better if seated in the front of the room where he sees only the teacher and not his classmates.

The child with an oral language disability, on the other hand, whose lags are confined to specific areas, might do all right if he were referred to a speech therapist and helped to establish more adequate motor speech patterns and a more extensive vocabulary. Another youngster might need assistance with straightening out his confusion in cerebral dominance and help in establishing left-to-right progression.

Most of these children, as Orton (1937) has pointed out, usually do better with a phonetic approach to reading than with the whole-word attack. There are good reasons for this fact and they lie precisely in the direction we have discussed. The child who has trouble with the organization of visual patterns is naturally bewildered and confused if he is confronted with what to him seem to be diffuse and un-differentiated configurations. He will benefit immensely if words are broken up into small phonetic units. This breaking-up process actually represents a transposal of spatial sequences into temporal ones. In this manner many youngsters are able to cope with single sounds, short auditory configurations which they slowly learn to fuse into larger entities. This procedure facilitates the structuralization of, for them, undifferentiated wholes and thus gives them a larger measure of security.

There are, of course, exceptions. There are children who fail to respond to the phonetic method. These particular children fall into three categories. The hyperactive child does not always possess the span of attention required for the laborious sounding out of words. The process is too slow for him and he tends to get discouraged and frustrated. Into the second category fall the youngsters who have trouble with abstract behavior. The process of analyzing a word into its parts and then synthesizing the parts requires a certain level of abstraction. Moreover, the very concept that a letter seen represents a speech sound heard is difficult for the brain-injured child (who is usually hyperactive as well) to grasp. In the third category falls the youngster who shows obsessive tendencies. He will stick compulsively to single sounds; he will be too anxious to blend them successfully into words or to integrate them into meaningful sentences.

Thus the tests for prediction of future reading disabilities are not only designed to discover the child who is liable to run into trouble with reading, but are also meant to indicate the areas in which a child's performance lags. The tests should actually do more: they should provide a lead as to what specific techniques could be used to advantage in future training.

Precious time is thus saved, and some children, at least, are spared the humiliating experience of failure in reading, writing, and spelling (which are all important in the earlier grades), a failure which will often carry over into other learning experiences.

Not all children suffering from potential reading difficulties are primarily emotionally disturbed. However, their basic developmental lag in physiological-psychological functioning makes them especially susceptible to adverse educational experiences and as a result they often develop secondary emotional difficulties very early.

We hope to discover some of these youngsters before they become educational and emotional casualties.

Early Prediction of Reading, Writing and Spelling Ability

with Jeannette Jefferson Jansky

Twenty years of experience with intelligent and educationally disabled children whose learning drive was often severely damaged has convinced us that a sizeable number of these youngsters need not have required remedial help had their difficulties been recognized before first grade entrance. Early identification would in many instances have obviated the need for later remediation. Prediction of reading, writing, and spelling disorders—that is to say, early identification of a specific pattern of disfunctions—was the purpose of this investigation which was supported by the Health Research Council of the City of New York and carried out in the department of William S. Langford, M.D., under the auspices of Columbia University.

Prediction of reading success or failure has been the objective of a number of both clinical and more formal studies. Among the statistical investigations, some have taken single variables, such as auditory discrimination (Thompson 1963), visuomotor competence (Koppitz 1964), anxiety level (Cohen 1963), or self-concept as measured in kindergarten or early first grade (Wattenberg and Clifford 1964), in order to predict reading competence nine to twelve months later. A few have constructed a battery of predictive tests (Petty 1939); one of the earliest and best was Monroe's (1935).

The present investigation differs from others in three important respects. It explores a far larger section of the child's perceptuomotor and linguistic organization than do other studies, it predicts spelling and writing in addition to reading achievement, and finally the interval between prediction and outcome is more than twice as long as it is in most other investigations.

Schools have, of course, informally assessed children's readiness for years (Austin and Morrison 1963) and they have by and large relied

Reprinted with permission from The College of Speech Therapists, from *The British Journal of Disorders of Communication* 1:99–107. 1966.

on three types of evaluation: on reading-readiness tests, on determination of IQ, and on informal sizing-up of the child by the kindergarten teacher. All of these techniques are legitimate, but all have certain disadvantages: reading-readiness tests do not always reveal enough about a child's specific weakness and strength to assist the teacher in the planning of educational strategies; most, moreover, fail to predict for writing and spelling. Reliance on intelligence tests has been challenged first because severe reading disabilities are known to occur on practically all intellectual levels, secondly because an intelligence quotient represents at best a global rather than a differentiated evaluation of a child's potential, and finally because IQ does not sufficiently take into account important perceptual factors which, we feel, are significant for reading success and failure. The developmentally-oriented teacher's assessment of a child, finally, though often remarkably accurate (Henig 1949), cannot be easily duplicated. Such a teacher will often say that a given child is immature without being able to state what went into her judgment.

Our own attempts at prediction in the Pediatric Language Disorder Clinic, Columbia-Presbyterian Medical Center, New York City, go back over twenty years. They were largely informal and stemmed from our experience with preschool children referred for a variety of oral language deficits. An extraordinarily large proportion of these children developed reading, writing, and spelling difficulties several years later. The clinical impression of these youngsters was one of striking immaturity. In spite of adequate or better intelligence their performance on a variety of perceptuomotor and language tasks resembled that of chronologically younger subjects. Our original predictions were based primarily on a clinical evaluation of the child's developmental level and only secondarily on his performance on a battery of tests which we had assembled over the years. By and large our predictions were successful (de Hirsch 1957), but they raised a number of new questions. We were dealing with a language defective, that is to say with a clinical, group, and we were by no means sure that our predictions would hold also for an unselected group of children. We did not know, furthermore, how far our predictions relied on clinical judgment and how far on the children's objective scores on tests. In any case, it became clear that whatever it was we based our clinical judgment on could not be handed on to someone else.

Thus, we became convinced that we would have to use statistical tools. In order to shape an instrument for the schools which would enable them to identify at early ages what we call *academic high risk* children, we felt we would have to (1) use an instrument relatively untainted by subjective clinical judgment and (2) use, in addition to a clinical group, a group that would be representative of a school population.

A sample of 53 children from the general population and a sample of 53 prematurely born children then were the subjects studied. The investigation of the children from the general sample was designed to assist us in our practical goal: to shape a predictive instrument for the use of schools. The study of the prematurely born youngsters, who can be assumed to have started life with neurophysiological lags would, we hoped, teach us something about the relationship between neurophysiological immaturity and language disabilities. Criteria for excluding certain children were: bilingual home, sensory deficit severe enough to interfere with learning, IQ beyond the range of one standard deviation above and below 100, and significant psychopathology, as judged clinically.

The heart of the investigation consisted of an attempt to determine which of 37 perceptuomotor and linguistic tests would prove to be potential predictors of reading, writing, and spelling two and a half years later. A further goal was to combine the best potential predictors in a way which would yield an instrument of widespread applicability.

We fully realize that a multiplicity of social, environmental, and psychological factors enter significantly into the acquisition of reading skills, and we believe as does Fabian (1951) that learning to read requires the developmental timing of both neurophysiological and psychological aspects of readiness. If, nevertheless, we limited ourselves to perceptuomotor and linguistic facets of readiness, it was not only because we are impressed with their significance, but also because until recently they have been largely neglected.

Development proceeds from a state of relative globality and undifferentiation in the direction of increasing articulation and hierarchic organizations (Werner 1957). Our tests, some of them of a standardized variety, some adapted by us, some fashioned by ourselves, reflect our theoretical position derived from Piaget (1952), Gesell (1945), and Werner (1957) who postulate evolving states in sensory motor and linguistic functioning. Since development is by and large a consistent and lawful process, we assumed that a kindergarten child's perceptuomotor and oral language level would forecast his performance on such highly integrated tasks as reading, writing, and spelling. The tests administered covered several broad aspects of development: behavior and motility patterning, large and fine motor coordination, figure-ground discrimination, visuomotor organization, auditory and visual perceptual competence, ability to comprehend and use language, and, more specifically, reading readiness. After the administration of the large test battery we wrote a short profile on each child in which we summarized our impression of his overall functioning, of his learning style, as well as of his specific weakness and strength.

Administered two and a half years later at the end of second grade were standardized reading, writing, and spelling tests. We also visited each school to get the teacher's assessment of the children and an impression of the teaching methods used in each classroom.

Computation of a coefficient of association between the 37 tests, on the one hand, and end of second grade performance scores, on the other, provided a basis for ascertaining which kindergarten tests might be strongly enough associated with end-of-second grade reading, spelling, and writing achievement to have predictive value. Those tests for which the coefficient of association with subsequent performance scores were statistically significant at the 0.05 level of confidence or less were considered potential predictors.

Using these criteria we found that 20 out of the 37 tests administered at kindergarten age had predictive possibilities.

To begin with, a marked degree of hyperactivity, distractibility, and disinhibition appeared to be a poor prognostic sign, since at kindergarten age it denoted a lack of behavioral control which was bound to interfere with academic functioning later on.

It was of interest that pegboard speed which is a relatively sensitive test of finer motor control was significantly associated not only with writing, which could have been expected, but with spelling as well. This lends support to various statements by Orton (1937) who drew attention to psychomotor lags in children with difficulties in the language area. Graphomotor control, the way a child held the pencil at kindergarten age, showed a high correlation not only with writing, but with reading and spelling as well, probably because in addition to motoric factors, verbal symbolic behavior is involved in the handling of the pencil.

A child's ability to draw a human figure showed a weak, but statistically significant, association with reading and spelling thirty months later. It did not correlate with writing which means that motor competence plays a relatively small role in the ability to project graphically the image of the human body. This image is a gestalt, determined by laws of growth and development (Bender 1951); it reflects the degree to which a child has integrated information about his body, its parts, and their relationships to each other. Appreciation of these relationships is basic to the child's orientation in space and enters into his awareness of right and left. It is this awareness, according to recent research, rather than the establishing of hand dominance, that discriminates between good and poor readers. (Coleman and Deutsch 1964; Birch and Belmont 1965).

The Bender Visual Motor Gestalt Test, which better than most others measures spatial organization and integrative competence, ranked near the top of the predictive tests in that its correlation with end-of-second grade achievement was very high, indeed. It is a particularly sensitive test at this age because certain of its features, such as crossing wavy lines and the drawing of a diamond, seem to mature at the very time the child enters first grade.

We administered a heavy battery of oral language tests, 14 of them. The literature is filled with statements referring to the close relationship between organization in *time*, as reflected in oral language, and organization in *space*, as reflected in printed and written language. Lashley (1954) says the two are interchangeable and, in fact, in reading, space is used to express time, the printed word is a time chart of sounds (Diack 1960). When we inquired into the extent to which auditory sequencing *predicts* scholastic performance several years later, we found, for instance, that the ability to imitate tapped-out patterns, the ability, in other words, to retain and reproduce a nonverbal auditory gestalt, was a surprisingly good predictor of later reading achievement. This was true also for auditory discrimination, not surprising when one considers the large number of poor spellers whose auditory discrimination is extremely diffuse. Among the *expressive* language tests, the number of words used by a child in the telling of a story was by far the best predictor; in telling the story of the Three Bears, the number of words used ranged from 54 to 594. Beyond factors related to environmental stimulation, the richness of a child's verbal output undoubtedly reflects his inherent linguistic endowment.

Organization of a story which requires ability to integrate details into a meaningful whole was another test that showed a statistically significant association with end-of-second-grade reading, as did the capacity to group objects or events verbally in terms of their common denominator.

As could be expected, a number of specific reading readiness tests were significantly associated with later achievement. A reversal test was one of them, parts of the Gates Matching Test was another; Name Writing and Letter Naming have long been known to be predictive, but they are, of course, largely dependent on previous training. Three tests which involved the practice teaching of words were others considered to be reliable predictors.

In summary, 20 out of 37 tests administered at kindergarten age showed significant correlations of varying degree with second-grade reading, writing, and spelling scores.

We furthermore correlated IQ as evaluated at kindergarten age and, treating it as one among other possible predictors, found that it was associated to a statistically significant degree with second grade performance. However, IQ ranked only twelfth as a predictor; in other words, eleven other tests in our battery were better predictors than was IQ Moreover, the correlation between intelligence quotients as measured at kindergarten age and end-of-second-grade spelling was nonsignificant, which confirmed our clinical impression that spelling disabilities are highly specific and cannot be compensated for by intelligence.

Ambiguous lateralization at ages between five and one half and six and one half years, on the other hand, was not significantly correlated with end-of-second-grade performance. Two thirds of our children had settled on a preferred hand in kindergarten; but those who had did not read or spell better than those whose handedness had been undetermined. At this early age, and probably considerably later, ill-defined laterality does not discriminate between good and poor readers. It probably is, in combination with other phenomena, nevertheless a pathognomonic sign in children over eleven years because it seems to denote ambiguous cerebral dominance which, in turn, may point to a generalized lag in central nervous system maturation. We refer to Subirana's (1961) findings which show that the electroencephalograms (EEGs) of strongly right-handed children are more mature than those of ambidexterous or left-handed ones.

Not even in our group of Failing Readers who had not scored at all at end of second grade was failure to establish a functional superiority of one hand over the other a distinguishing feature. If one would summarize the characteristics of these eight failing children, whose IQ's were comparable to those of the remaining youngsters in the study and ranged from 94–116, one would say the following: as a group, for what it is worth, they were unusually small in size, they were largely boys, they were disorganized, hyperkinetic, impulsive, and infantile. Their motoric ability was inferior, their Bender gestalten primitive and spatially deviating, their human figure drawings were crude and undifferentiated, and their language tools were very poor. They missed out on comprehension of time concepts. The stories they told were barren and did not hang together, they had severe difficulties with word-finding, and they were nowhere on reading readiness tests. It was, however, not failure on *single* performances which characterized this group (the superior readers in the sample also showed one or the other dysfunction); it was the *accumulation* of deficits and their severity, the pervasive diffuseness and primitivity of their performance which in these failing children pointed to a profound and basic maturational deficit, a deficit, so severe in a few cases that it seemed rooted in the very biological matrix of the child.

We feel that certain clinical aspects of our investigation throw an interesting light on the concept of maturational lag and on its relationship to developmental language disturbances.

1) When we compared three groups of kindergarten children in our general population, the Failing Readers, the Slow Starters, and the High Achievers on six tests–the Bender Gestalt, the

Drawing of a human figure, Auditory Discrimination, Categories, a Reversal and a Word Recognition test–we found a progression from diffuse and primitive to differentiated and highly integrated responses. In all six areas the Failing Readers functioned at levels characteristic of children of lower chronological ages.

2) When we compared the prematurely born subjects, the children in other words, who had started life with physiological lags, to the full-term children, we found that as a group their performance on 36 out of 37 tests was weaker than that of their maturely born peers. These prematurely born subjects' behavior and performance looked strikingly like that of our Failing Readers and also resembled that of chronologically younger subjects.

The third argument in favor of the maturational bias was of a statistical nature; Gesell (1940) maintains that maturation is by and large a function of age, rather than of experience and training; Piaget (1952) states that the development of organizational schemes is age-linked.

We therefore classified all 37 kindergarten tests according to the degree to which they discriminated between the oldest and the youngest kindergarten children. Those tests on which the oldest subjects did best and the youngest did least well, we considered to be *maturation sensitive*. According to this criterion 25 out of the 37 kindergarten tests administered were considered to be maturation sensitive. The expectation that these particular tests would be better predictors of performance than the not-maturation sensitive ones, those that did not discriminate between the oldest and the youngest kindergarten children, was upheld by the findings. Of the maturation sensitive tests, 76 percent were significantly correlated with second grade scores as against 17 percent of the not-maturation sensitive ones.

School admission procedures are, of course, based on chronological age, and, to the degree that chronological age reflects maturational level, it is in fact a fairly good predictor of subsequent achievement.

However, the focus in our study was on those intelligent children in whom chronological age does *not* reflect maturational level, the children who suffer from maturational lags and who therefore present a high risk of academic failure. For these children chronological age is misleading as a predictor. There were 18 children in our study who were six and a half years or older at time of first grade entrance. On the basis of chronological age and IQ they should have done well. However, four of them failed in both reading and spelling at end of second grade. Our predictive tests which assessed developmental level, on the other hand, identified at kindergarten age, three out of these four children; the data on the fourth were incomplete. The findings thus support our contention that there is indeed a close link between a child's maturational status at kindergarten age and his reading and spelling achievement several years later.

Since the administration of 20 separate tests would be far too cumbersome a procedure to use in schools, we decided to construct a Predictive Index, consisting of those single predictors which, in combination, would most effectively identify high risk children. To begin with, we established that the intercorrelations between reading and spelling at the end of second grade were very high, which enabled us to use the same index for both reading and spelling. Those of the original 20 kindergarten tests that exhibited relatively high and significant correlations with achievement at the end of second grade, and that thus seemed promising, were then put together for trial indices. Over one hundred of them were tried out and compared in order to determine which combination would best single out those children in our sample who subsequently failed. The index we selected—consisting of 10 tests—five of them in the visual-perceptual, three of them in the oral-language area, one concerned with visuomotor organization and one with pencil grasp—was finally chosen as the instrument which identified at kindergarten level 91 percent, that is to say, 10 out of 11 students who failed all reading and spelling tests thirty months later. An investigation designed to validate this index on a large number of children, 450 to 500 of them, is under way in New York City. Before this is done, we are not justified to rely heavily on our findings. In the process of validation we might add two or three tests to the original ten to see whether we can better our results.

It is, of course, important to report also on those cases in which the Predictive Index did *not* work out. The Predictive Index failed to pick out one boy whose performance at kindergarten level, though not outstanding, had at least been acceptable. The index, moreover, picked up as prospective failures four children who did, in fact, make the grade. Two of them had been slow starters and had failed all tests at the end of the first grade. One of the two had barely passed at the end of the second year. The vision of the second child had been poor and she had been fitted for glasses the day before the kindergarten tests were administered. This clearly interfered with prediction. A third subject, a boy, had quite obviously made dramatic developmental spurts in the interim between kindergarten and end of second grade; his initial performance had been very immature, indeed. Such sudden spurts are probably the pitfalls in this type of prediction. The fourth, another boy, had been quite disturbed at kindergarten age; he had vomited each day before going to school and when we saw him again at age eight he was pulling his hair to a degree which left him with a bald spot; nevertheless he did well.

It goes without saying that in the interval between kindergarten and end of second grade a number of variables, the quality of teaching, illness, frequent change of schools, major upheavals in the home, all enter into academic achievement and are bound to influence prediction. Limitations in time and funds did not permit us to take these important variables into account. It is, therefore, impressive that in spite of these limitations the Predictive Index reported here effectively identified at kindergarten age the overwhelming majority of failing subjects.

Our tests should, however, do more than simply pick out the children destined to do poorly; they should reveal also in which particular area a given child is lagging, what kind of help he needs, and what to do about it. Educational diagnosis is productive only if it can be translated into specific educational strategies. Comparing a given kindergarten child's performance in the auditory and in the visual perceptual areas makes it possible to assess his specific strength and weakness and to determine which particular pathways facilitate learning. In our study, the majority of children did *not* show what we call erratic modality patterning. They did either well or poorly, both auditorally and visually, their integrative competence or lack of it cut through all modalities. On the other hand, 19 percent of our children showed erratic modality patterning, striking deficits on the four visual-perceptual tests administered, and superior competence on the four auditory perceptual performances. Seven children belonged to this group; three others showed the opposite picture, excellent visual perceptual ability and failure in the entire auditory perceptual realm. The three children with superior *visual* competence did very well in reading in spite of their auditory lags; they even made the grade in spelling. Reading, is after all primarily a visual perceptual task and thus, the usual procedures offered at school were entirely adequate. The seven youngsters with *visual* perceptual deficits clearly needed phonics, and, in fact, the five youngsters who were exposed to heavy doses of it did well, while two, who were not, failed.

It should be said once and for all that one method of teaching is not necessarily per se better than another. The child who does well in both auditory and visual perception will benefit from the usual methods offered; the one who does poorly in both will need heavy reinforcement and the activation of as many pathways as possible. The poor visualizer needs phonics. However, to the brain-injured child, for instance, phonic teaching often presents overwhelming difficulties. Such a child, with his frequently severe integrational defects, is often totally unable to analyze or synthesize, and his failure to cope with phonics may lead to a catastrophic reaction, the disorganized response of the organism that is exposed to a task with which it is unable to cope.

The point we want to make is this: teaching methods must be determined in terms of the individual child's inherent strength and weakness and both can be determined at kindergarten age.

Roughly twenty percent of our children from lower middle class homes showed a kind of performance at kindergarten age which clearly revealed that they would meet with total failure in second grade, an experience which may have seriously damaging effects on their self image and may adversely affect their attitudes to learning in general.

We therefore suggest that the school system introduce transition classes between kindergarten and first grade for those children who according to the Predictive Index are found to be immature.

The index is, of course, only a formula and it would be unfortunate if it were to draw the teacher's attention away from the child's actual behavior and performance. Rather than being a substitute for observation, the Index should assist the teacher in translating her often excellent but impressionistic judgment of the youngster's readiness into a more specific assessment of his perceptuomotor and linguistic status.

Saying that a child is not ready or is immature does not mean that one can afford to sit back and let maturation take its course. Schilder (1964) said that training plays a significant part even in those functions in which maturation of the central nervous system is of primary importance. The question is only what kind of training and above all at what level. What is desirable is a match between a child's developmental readiness and the type of teaching offered him. It is this need for a match which must be met in what we call transition and the Swedes call maturity classes (Malmquist 1963).

Immature children's developmental timing is atypical. At kindergarten age they are unable to benefit from prereading programs. Repeating the kindergarten year would give them an additional year to mature in and would thus have certain advantages. However, it would not provide the intensive and specific training they need. Promotion into first grade would not solve their problems either, since the pace is usually too fast for the child who is ready to learn but is as yet unable to cope with organized reading and writing instruction at the conventional age.

The transition class, on the other hand, would start on the ground floor. It would aim at stabilizing the child's perceptuomotor world and would take him, in slow motion, as it were, through a program in which each step is carefully planned. Teaching methods in such a class, unlike those in first grade which provide fairly uniform training for all children, would be tailored to the child's individual needs. Needless to say, the teacher in such a transition class would have to have special qualifications, since immature children require a greater than usual degree of tolerance and empathy.

The transition class would, finally, provide an opportunity to translate into educational practice the insights gained from a careful study of the child's weakness and strength in the various modalities. Instruction would be geared differentially to children with auditory-perceptual deficits and to those with gaps in visual perception. During certain times of the day children with receptive and expressive language deficits would receive specific language training. Others would get assistance with visual discrimination and configurational techniques, a third group would work on directional and graphomotor patterning. In short, this instruction would be geared to fill in specific gaps in some areas and to utilize assets in others.

Marie van Hoosan (1965) has called the interval between kindergarten and first grade the "twilight zone" of learning. It is this twilight period which would be served by the transition class.

A few children in such a class would be integrated into the regular first grade after a few weeks or months of intensive training. Most others would be ready to cope with first grade a year later. A small number of children suffering from severe and persisting lags might require continuing help for at least two or three years.

At present most schools do not provide remedial help until the end of the third grade. This is unfortunate because the development of perceptual and language functions probably follows a sequence analogous to that in organic morphological development. There are according to McGraw (1943) specific critical times in the child's life when he is especially susceptible to certain kinds of stimulation. The basic perceptuomotor functions that underlie reading may be harder to train at the end of third grade than they are earlier. By the end of third grade, moreover, emotional problems and phobic responses may have so complicated the original problems that they may no longer be reversible.

The earliest possible identification of high risk children was the goal of our study. Identification is, however, only a first step towards reversing a situation that now results in an unjustifiable waste of educational opportunities. A second step is equally essential: high risk children must be provided with teaching techniques that will enable them to realize their potential and to become productive members of the community.

Summary

This paper describes an investigation that is concerned with early prediction of reading, spelling, and writing competence.

Subjects were 53 full-term children from the general population and 53 prematurely born children, all with I.Q.'s in the average range. At kindergarten level the authors administered 37 perceptuomotor, oral language, and reading readiness tests to all subjects and correlated the performance of the children from the general population with their reading, writing, and spelling achievement at the end of the second grade. Computation of a coefficient of association between the 37 kindergarten tests and subsequent achievement measures provided a basis for ascertaining which of the kindergarten tests might have predictive value. Those tests for which the coefficient of association with later performance were significant at the 0.05 level of confidence or less were considered to be potential predictors. From the 20 tests which showed predictive possibilities, the authors then constructed a Predictive Index for the use of school, consisting of those ten tests which in combination identified at kindergarten age the overwhelming majority, 10 out of 11, children who failed all reading and spelling tests at the end of the second grade.

These failing children, 20 percent of the sample studied, presented at kindergarten age a specific constellation of dysfunctions reflecting a maturational lag. A separate section of the report deals with these particular children and makes specific recommendations as to early intervention. Another section discusses the children's overall approach to learning and their weakness and strength in the visual and auditory modalities.

Comparisons of the perceptuomotor, oral language, and reading and spelling achievement of the prematurely and the maturely born subjects revealed that the performance of over half of the prematurely born children was inferior to that of their maturely born peers. The prematures, thus, may constitute a significant segment of the group here called academic high-risk children.

Studies in Tachyphemia:

Diagnosis of Developmental Language Disorders

Clinical Background

Over the past nineteen years we have seen, at the Pediatric Language Disorder Clinic, Columbia Presbyterian Medical Center, a large number of children who by and large fell into two groups: one group of adequately intelligent youngsters aged between three and six years who had been referred for delayed speech development or some other kind of functional speech disorder; and a second group of equally bright children, aged between seven and twelve years, who were sent to us for evaluation of a more or less severe reading, spelling, and writing disability.

As the years went by we found that we were able to predict future reading disabilities in a large percentage of the group under age six, and we found that in the older group not only were there many youngsters who had a history of earlier speech disturbance, but a good many who still showed residual signs of a language deficiency.

Eventually we learned to recognize clinically that the performance of these children fell into a distinct pattern, and it is this pattern which I shall try to describe.

Theoretical Assumptions

An examiner's theoretical position largely determines his diagnostic procedures. It is this position which causes him to focus attention on certain phenomena and makes him ask specific kinds of questions.

The following are a number of assumptions, all of them distilled from our clinical experience and observation, which underlie our diagnostic approach.

Reprinted with permission from the author, from *Logos* 4:3–9. 1961.

1. Language is a complex tool for shaping and expressing concepts. It is a tool which the growing child has to learn to master as he develops, a tool, moreover, which is more difficult to handle for some than for others (Orton 1937; Rabinovitch 1939). Language is also a means of self-expression and a bridge to another human being. Language dysfunctions thus might reflect a disturbance of self, a difficulty with interpersonal relationships, or trouble with the instrumentalities of verbal communication. In evaluating language disturbances we have to take both instrumental and interpersonal aspects into account and determine not only their relative significance but the dynamic interrelation between them.

2. We believe with Orton that the syndrome we call developmental language disability has a significant familial constitutional element (Orton 1930; Hallgren 1950; Luchsinger 1959).

3. We look on language as a continuum embracing all aspects of verbal communication: speaking, writing, reading, spelling, and composition. Although emphasis varies, our diagnostic procedures are basically the same for all types of language disorders, be it dyslalia, word-deafness, cluttering, or reading and spelling disabilities. We believe that a more or less marked degree of neurophysiological immaturity underlies these difficulties and prefer with Bender to consider these disturbances as "developmental lags" (Bender 1950; de Hirsch 1957).

4. We believe, moreover, that these lags are in no way confined to verbal performance. Language in all its aspects is a highly complex activity. In investigating language disturbances we have to go beyond overt verbal manifestations and carefully evaluate neurophysiological phenomena underlying linguistic behavior. We therefore test all children referred to us for overall motility, body image, motor and neuro-motor patterning, competence in dealing with auditory and spatial configurations, and figure-ground discrimination. All of these are, we feel, highly pertinent in terms of verbal performance and it is competences and weaknesses in these areas which we are trying to assess.

5. The ability to perceive and respond in terms of gestalten is basic to cortical functioning (Katz 1951; Köhler 1933; Koffka 1953; Goldstein 1939). We believe that children suffering from language disabilities have trouble responding to the meaningful features which determine the various types of gestalten. Speech defective youngsters usually show defective auditory and motor gestalten; dyslexic youngsters and those with severe spelling disabilities demonstrate weakness predominantly in the patterning of visual and spatial ones (Bender 1958; Drew 1956; de Hirsch 1954). However, in most cases of severe language dysfunction we find a combination of poor visuomotor and motor patterning as well as trouble with both auditory and spatial configurations.

6. The presence and absence of physiological immaturity, some-times demonstrable on the electroencephalogram (EEG) as well (Kling-man 1956; Silver 1951), helps us in the differentiation between specific language disability and one which is emotionally determined. We do by no means want to deny that many difficulties with verbal communi-cation are on a psychogenic basis. In the phobic stutterer (Froeschels 1942–3), for instance, and in the child with a massive learning disability (Fabian 1951), dysfunction may be related to hostility, to emotional infantilism, to severe compulsive mechanisms—in some cases to psychotic pathology. However, the phobic stutterer or the youngster whose learning disability is on a psychological basis does not neces-sarily demonstrate the gestalt difficulties and the trouble with pat-terning which are typical for the clutterer (Arnold 1960; Freund 1952; de Hirsch and Langford 1950; Weiss 1935) or the child suffering from a specific reading difficulty (de Hirsch 1952).

Diagnostic Procedures

The following are our diagnostic procedures outlined in an abbre-viated form.

History: There is the preliminary interview with the parents which serves to evaluate grossly dynamic emotional factors in the family set-up. Our interview includes a detailed family history of speech, reading, writing, and spelling disabilities of near relatives and also a family history of motor competence. In numerous instances the parents bring in several of their children—one for trouble with read-ing, the next boy because he stutters, and the youngest because in spite of adequate intelligence he is late in starting to talk.

It goes without saying that we take a careful neonatal, natal, and postnatal history of the child. Many of the youngsters referred to Speech and Reading Clinics nowadays show evidence of en-cephalopathies (Grewel 1959) or of subclinical diffuse organic in-volvement which were not picked up until these children were faced with such complex activities as reading and speaking. Not all of them show deviations on the classical neurological examination or on the EEG. However, their performance on more subtle neurological tests leads us to infer minimal diffuse neurological deficit or at any rate severe neurophysiological immaturity (Bender 1958; Strauss and Leh-tinen 1950).

Motility and Motor Patterning: In the observation of our children we start out with an evaluation of overall motility (Bender and Yarnell 1941). Many youngsters suffering from speech and reading disorders are hyperkinetic, disorganized, and at the mercy of environmental stimuli. The psychiatrist might say, and in many instances he might be right, that the hyperactivity of these children is indicative of the same emotional disturbance which is responsible for their difficulty with verbal communication. The speech therapist or the remedial reading teacher might say, and again he might be right in many cases, that these youngsters are hyperkinetic and restless because they are so tremendously frustrated in their desire to use language and to function effectively at school. However, many mothers tell us that these particular children have been hyperactive since birth, even in utero.

Any experienced kindergarten teacher knows that these youngsters are often reasonably well adjusted but unable to sit still. Their motor patterning is like that of younger children. At age six and older they turn the whole head when asked to flex the tongue. They still cannot separate individual muscle groups and respond instead in a more infantile, more global fashion (de Hirsch 1957). At eight or nine they show associated muscular movements of the uninvolved hand on the finger-to-thumb test. Some, who at the age of ten and eleven struggle with the rudiments of reading, still turn along a longitudinal axis, a sign of immaturity of the central nervous system, which usually disappears at around age seven (Silver 1951, 1952). Children with developmental language disorders frequently show immaturity of reflex behavior, primitivity of posture and tonus which is typical for the chronologically younger child (Teicher 1951).

Gross motor control is sometimes poor; some of our five-year-olds have trouble hopping, skipping, or maintaining balance (Clark 1959; de Hirsch 1957).

Evaluation of finer manual control is the next step. As far back as 1932 Orton (Orton 1932; Luchsinger 1959) commented on the motor awkwardness of these children. We have our youngsters string beads, manipulate wooden clowns, insert pegs, all of which gives us a chance not only to observe handedness in untrained activities, but also to get an idea of the way a child approaches a task—his zest, his ingenuity, his frustration threshold. Many children suffering from language disabilities have trouble with motor patterning, sometimes not only with the actual skills but, as in ideomotor dyspraxia, with the gestalt of the movement itself. There are other youngsters who manage quite well until it comes to handling a pencil. Some very bright children have a difficult time in kindergarten because they cannot draw or color. We see a good many later on, at age eleven or sometimes much older, who are severely handicapped because of writing disabilities.

Body Image: The human figure drawing of these children (Goodenough 1926) is often strikingly primitive and developmentally at least two or more years below their chronological and mental age. It is true that a youngster's ability to draw a person is partly a matter of finer motor coordination and of body image in the psychological sense of the word. However, a child's notions of space originally derive from his awareness of parts of his body and their relationship to each other (Bender 1958; Caplan 1952; Gerstman 1958; de Hirsch 1957; Schilder 1950; Vernon 1952). Thus a child's human figure drawing also reveals his spatial competence which is of pertinence in terms of the visual forms of language since reading, writing, and spelling are patterns laid out in space.

Visuomotor Organization: We give all our youngsters a Bender Gestalt test (Bender 1938). Dyslexic and cluttering children's responses are usually developmentally primitive as are those of children presenting severe dyslexias. Their visuomotor patterning is immature and even if they do respond adequately to the essentials of the gestalt, they practically always show poor spatial organization (de Hirsch 1957; Silver 1952).

Spatial Organization: As mentioned before, we assess lateral dominance by watching our children during untrained activities (Benton 1959; Harris 1958; Orton 1932). We give our older youngsters a bimanual numbering test and one which requires them to discriminate between correctly and reversely presented shapes and letters so as to check on residual ambilaterality. Such ambilaterality is related to difficulty with temporal and spatial sequences. The child who says *crise ripsy* for *rice crispy* and the one who reads *now* for *won* have the same trouble, though in different modalities. We feel that confusion in temporal and spatial orientation is frequently related to familial factors but is at the same time indicative of central nervous system immaturity.

Figure-Ground Organization: Another area we are interested in because we feel it is closely related to gestalt functioning is figure-ground discrimination (Werner and Strauss 1941). We present our children with our adaptation of the Strauss-Lehtinen (1950) cards on which figures are embedded in a strongly structured ground. To differentiate between figure and ground, as is required for this task, is essential for both speech and reading. The word-deaf child who responds to speech as if it represented an undifferentiated, diffuse kind of noise, the dyslexic youngster who looks at the printed page as if it were a meaningless, undifferentiated design have the same difficulty—the former in the auditory, the latter in the spatial area.

Temporal Organization and Receptive Language: We ask our children to reproduce patterns we tap out for them (de Hirsch 1957; Masland 1960) and we are impressed how many have trouble with structuring more or less complex temporal configurations. Most speech therapists are well aware of the fact that the auditory memory span of speech delayed and speech defective children is often very short (Rabinovitch 1959), and since the number of nonsense syllables a youngster should be able to repeat at a specific age has been standardized we have a measure of comparison (Beebe 1944). Speech therapists have also known for the longest time that most of the children they see have a hard time with auditory discrimination (Wepman 1958). I believe that these youngsters experience sound sequences in a diffuse way. However, it is less well known that dyslexic youngsters and above all those suffering from severe spelling disabilities have exactly the same trouble. Thus in severe cases of language disturbance we find marked weakness in differentiation and integration on various levels of performance and in different sensory modalities. One cannot help but feel that these children suffer from a basic and generalized gestalt deficiency (de Hirsch 1954).

Expressive Language: Careful evaluation of all aspects of oral language is, of course, *sine qua non* in our testing (Borel-Maisonny 1954; Werner and Strauss 1941). We are interested in vocal patterns. We feel that a marked degree of monotony is an important feature in children suffering from developmental language disturbances. Literally all of our clutterers, dyslalics, and dyslexics are strikingly monotonous (Weiss 1950). Such monotony might reflect a difficulty with structuralization, perhaps a figure-ground problem. Rhythmic disturbances (Arnold 1960; Borel-Maisonny 1954; Stamback 1957) are not only typical for speech defective children but also for dyslexic ones, as has been shown convincingly by Stamback. We also find rate deviations in these youngsters, most of them speak at a rapid pace (Arnold 1960; Froeschels 1946; Weiss 1950).

Some show excellent use of the vernacular but have trouble word-finding. Their verbal definitions tend to be concrete (Goldstein 1939).

In testing articulation we are not only interested in the way a child produces sounds in isolation or in repetition of a given pattern. We want to know above all whether or not his articulation stands up under the added burden of having to organize complex thought units. Under such pressure articulation often breaks down, since the organizational competence of our children is weak in all areas.

The concept of organization has not been studied nearly closely enough. All of us see numerous youngsters who talk perfectly well in short phrases but who become unintelligible when trying to organize complex material. There is little or nothing wrong with their sounds; what is wrong is something else, another dimension. They have trouble with patterning and structuring of long configurations. If one listens to their rapid, cluttered, dysrhythmic speech (Arnold 1960; Froeschels 1946), and if one then looks at their arrhythmic disorganized handwriting (Roman 1959), one realizes that one deals with the same basic disturbance. The papers these children hand in *look* the way these children *sound*.

Their grammar is often defective, and no wonder, because grammar is an expression of structure and it is in the area of structuring and patterning of movements, of perception, of language, and of behavior that these youngsters fall down.

Conceptualization: These children have weaknesses in other areas as well. One of them is with conceptualization. Rabinovitch (1959, 1960) has emphasized their difficulties—amounting almost to disorientation—with time, space, weight, size concepts. The number of eleven-year-olds who say that Christmas happens in spring and who do not know the dates of their birthdays is impressive.

Residual Language Disabilities in Older Children

In older children many of the earlier perceptual motor and visuomotor deviations tend to disappear. At around the age of twelve many of our severely hyperkinetic children "jell". However, even in these older children we find residual signs of language disability, such as trouble with formulating ideas, poor ability to pull a story together, and difficulty functioning on a high abstract verbal level. Some of the older children might have trouble understanding the difference between the literal and the figurative use of words. They might do better with pictorial than with verbal absurdities. A good many run into trouble with metaphors in literature. We give our adolescents proverbs to define; those who have a history of reading and spelling difficulty are often strikingly concrete.

Much more refined testing is needed to discover residual signs of a language disability in an older child. At this age, moreover, the youngster has suffered so severely from the effects of his communication and learning disability and emotional complications have come so much to the foreground that they often obscure the original problem. However, even in these older children, at any rate up to the age of fourteen or more, it is often possible to find evidence of physiological immaturity.

The adolescents who come to us with a history of severe scholastic difficulties often present complicated problems. In what has been called in other disease entities the "spectrum of causation" many factors play a part: the child's original constitutional endowment; the adjustment he makes to his psychological competences and deficits, and the emotional climate in which he makes the adjustment.

There are undoubtedly children who are grossly immature on all levels of integration, physiologically and psychologically. If the psychiatrist says they lack ego strength he is right; however, he might overlook significant residual neurophysiological immaturities.

The fact is that these children (and many of them *look* strikingly young for their age) mature late in all areas. It sometimes looks as if they suffered from an organismic deficiency in spite of more than adequate intelligence. From way back their infantile needs were greater than those of other children, they were more scattered, less well organized and in no way ready to comply with the demands imposed upon them by their family and by the public school system, which is, after all, tailored to the average child.

Early Diagnosis

Early diagnosis is thus essential, for several reasons:

1. Therapy has to be directed towards the basic organizational weakness in patterning and the child has to be helped early to structure motor, perceptual, and last but not least, behavioral configurations.

2. The youngster has to be protected against often overwhelming anxiety engendered by his disorganization and the failures resulting from it.

3. The child needs help with the repercussions of the environment which stem from his original disabilities and weaknesses.

Ours is a strictly clinical approach. Much remains to be done to test our assumptions and we are now seeing a number of children who show no evidence of language disability in order to find out the constellation of symptoms which determines language disability.

Comparisons Between Prematurely and Maturely Born Children at Three Age Levels

with Jeannette Jefferson Jansky and William S. Langford

The present report arose out of a larger investigation which attempted to predict children's reading, writing, and spelling performance before their entrance into first grade. This larger undertaking had used two groups of subjects, children born at term and children born prematurely. In the course of administering a battery of perceptuomotor, linguistic, and academic tests to these subjects, the writers had been struck by the differences between the two groups. The impression of more erratic perceptuomotor and linguistic maturation in the prematurely born children motivated the writers to scrutinize closely the performance of both groups at three age levels: in kindergarten and at the end of the first and second grades.

Whether prematurely born subjects in general present learning hazards has never been unequivocally established. Researchers such as Hess, Mohr, and Bartelme (1934) have maintained that by kindergarten age prematurely born children whose IQs fall within the average range and who do not present gross neurological sequelae, measure up to children born at term. A number of reports, (Benton 1940; Douglas 1956; Drillien 1964; Kawi and Pasamanick 1958) on the other hand, have commented on the high frequency of reading disabilities in prematurely born subjects. Whether or not deficits observed in young prematures persist into their first years at school cannot, according to Wiener, (1962) be decided on the basis of studies done since 1940. In view of these contradictory findings it seemed desirable to attempt to answer the following questions: (1) How did the prematurely born children in the group investigated compare with those born at term on a large battery of tests administered at kindergarten age? (2) Did the prematurely and maturely born children progress at different rates

Reprinted with permission from The American Orthopsychiatric Association, Inc., from *American Journal of Orthopsychiatry* 36(4):616–626. 1966.

during the years between kindergarten and the end of the second grade? (3) Did the prematures at the end of their first and second grades in school read, write, and spell at the same level as their maturely born peers?

Subjects

The data reported here were obtained from 106 children: 53 born prematurely, the other 53 born at term.

The group of premature children used in the present study was selected from a population of 158 prematures born during 1955 and 1956 and cared for in the premature nursery of Babies Hospital, Columbia-Presbyterian Medical Center, New York City. (According to the definition established by the World Health Organization in 1948, a prematurely born child is one who weighs 2500 grams or less at birth.) These children had previously been studied by Dr. William Silverman in a bilirubin investigation (Shiller and Silverman 1961). From this population were selected subjects who met the following criteria: came from homes in which English was the predominant language, had no significant sensory deficits, rated IQs within one standard deviation above and below 100 (as obtained on Form L of the Stanford-Binet Intelligence Scale, 1937 Revision) and showed no evidence of psycho-pathology as judged clinically. This selection process resulted in a group of 53 subjects. Their birthweight ranged from 980 to 2239 grams; in only six cases had gestation time been longer than thirty-seven weeks.[1]

At age three, these children were evaluated psychometrically and with regard to language development (Kastein and Fowler 1959). Neurological examinations were done at the same time. Of the 49 children then available, five showed definite or probable evidence of neurological deficit, as manifested by squint, abnormal or extraneous ocular movements, hypotonia motor retardation, deviating gait, seizures, or slow developmental history.

The 53 maturely born subjects were drawn from children born in 1955 and 1956 who had participated in the Fetal Life Study carried out at Babies Hospital between 1953 and 1959. (The children in this population originally had been selected at random from admissions to the

---

[1]Children whose birthweight falls below 2500 grams and who are, therefore, by definition, premature, do not necessarily constitute a homogeneous group. Drillien (1964) mentions three categories: one consisting of babies weighing less than five pounds, but born at term, to mothers of small stature; another, of infants born at or near term but markedly underweight as a result of intrauterine malnutrition; the third, of children who are actually premature in terms of both weight and gestation time.

Sloane Ante-Partum Clinic.) The same selection criteria obtained for the maturely born as for the prematurely born group.

Comparison Between Groups
on Background Variables

Although the two groups had been drawn from different populations, an evaluation of their background characteristics failed in most areas to reveal gross differences. Table 1 shows that age distributions were very similar. Slight differences in sex and race favored the prematurely born children; the premature group contained more girls, who are thought to be more mature than boys of the same age (Tanner 1961), and more white children, who are believed to enjoy more cultural advantages than their black peers (Deutsch 1960). The two groups were nearly identical with respect to mother's employment outside the home, the number of times the children were read to each week, and kindergarten attendance.

On the other hand, among the prematures a significantly greater number of mothers had continued their own education beyond high school.[2] The two groups also differed as to IQ: the IQ levels of the prematurely born children were significantly lower than were those of the maturely born. This last fact will be considered later.

Tests Administered

In all, three sets of tests were administered to both groups: one set at kindergarten age and one each at the end of the first and second grades.

Kindergarten Tests

The kindergarten tests were designed to cover several broad aspects of development. In the area of behavioral patterning, observations were directed toward hyperactivity, distractibility, and disinhibition. Motility patterning was judged in terms of the presence or absence of concomitant movements. Three measures of large motor coordination, hopping, throwing and balance, were included. Tests designed to assess finer motor control and laterality consisted of

---

[2]Knobloch and Pasamanick (1960), as well as Wortis and Freedman (1965), believe that mothers' educational status is a more reliable measure of environmental stimulation than is social status.

Table 1
Background Characteristics of Prematurely and Maturely Born Children

Background Characteristic	Percent of Prematures (N = 53)	Percent of Maturely Born (N = 53)	P
Age at time of kindergarten tests			
6 years and older	38%	36%	. . .
5 years, 8 months and younger	34	28	. . .
Sex: Boys	47	59	. . .
Race: Black	32	40	. . .
White	68	60	. . .
Mother's education:			
Post-high school training or college	30	8	≤.01
Mother's employment status:			
Mother works	24	24	. . .
IQ			
113–116	9	25	≤.05
84–94	26	8	≤.05

pegboard speed, knot tying, whittling, and graphic activities. In the area of visual perception the children's ability to differentiate figure from ground was investigated along with their visuomotor competence, as shown on the Bender Visual Motor Gestalt test. Fourteen oral language tests, five in the receptive- and nine in the expressive-language area, were administered. Reading readiness was evaluated by means of six tasks. Finally, the children were rated on their ability to invest effort. A profile summarizing the writers' clinical impressions was written at the time of the first testing and then added to as the child returned for follow-up interviews.

End of Grade I Tests

At the end of Grade I, a writing test, prepared by Freeman and the staff of the Zaner-Bloser Company, (1958) and three standardized reading tests, the Gray Oral and the Gates Primary Sentence and Paragraph Reading Tests, were administered to all the children. A single index[3] of overall reading performance was then constructed and was used as a basis for comparisons between groups.

---

[3]The children's scores on all three tests revealed an unexpected degree of unitariness. Therefore, a combined version of the Gates and the Gray tests—one Index of Overall Reading Performance—seemed both desirable and justified, in accordance with the principles of scaling theory (Stouffer 1950).

End of Grade II Tests

At the end of Grade II, two reading tests (the Gray Oral and the Gates Advanced Primary Reading Tests),[4] one spelling test (the Metropolitan Spelling test) and one writing test (devised by the authors) were administered.

Finally, four kindergarten tests were readministered at this level: Behavioral Control, Hand Preference, Bender Visual Motor Gestalt, and Auditory Discrimination.

Procedures

The procedures described below were used, when applicable, for two types of data: (1) for comparisons *within* the premature group, premature girls being compared to premature boys, and heavyweight prematures to lightweight ones; (2) for comparisons *between* the prematurely born and the maturely born groups.

The Chi-square test, standard test of independence in contingency tables, was used for all comparisons. (Yates' correction of the Chi-square coefficient for small samples was employed where it was deemed appropriate.)

Comparisons were based on that level of performance, called the "critical score level," which yielded the best differentiation.

Findings

Comparisons Within the Premature Group

Sex. Prematurely born girls performed better than prematurely born boys in reading, writing, and spelling at the end of both Grades I and II. These differences reached statistical significance for writing and spelling at the end of second grade (Table 2). This would confirm Blegen's (1952) findings as to the relatively poorer performance of premature boys as compared with that of girls. The findings also support Wortis' and Freedman's (1965) contention that males are particularly susceptible to the effects of prematurity.

Birthweight. Lightweight prematures have been reported in the literature to present greater hazards in terms of learning than those whose weight approaches that of children born at term (Drillien 1964; Freedman et al. 1960; Harper, Fischer, and Rider 1959; Knobloch and Pasamanick 1962). The findings bearing on this point are offered here

---

[4]As were the three reading tests in Grade I, the two second-grade reading tests were combined to form an Overall Reading Performance Index (ORP Index).

Table 2
Performance of Prematurely Born Children on Grade I and Grade II
Achievement Tests According to Sex
(Percent of children attaining critical score level)

Test	Boys (N = 25)	Girls (N = 28)	P
Grade I			
Reading	20%	43%	. . .
Writing	64	86	. . .
Grade II			
Reading	36	57	. . .
Writing	36	79	≤.01
Spelling	36	73	≤.05

with reservations because the prematurely born group in the present study was in effect cut off at both extremes: there was only one child with a birthweight over 2000 grams and only one with a birthweight below 1000 grams. Although the relative homogeneity of the group would tend to reduce the association between weight and performance, the prematurely born children were nevertheless placed in three weight categories: 1500 grams or less, 1501 to 1750 grams, and 1751 or more. Each weight group's performance in reading, writing, and spelling at the end of the first and second grades was then tabulated. No gradient in performance was found with ascending birthweight (except in reading achievement at the end of first grade); however, on four out of five scholastic tests children with birthweights below 1500 grams performed at lower levels than did subjects with higher birthweights (Table 3).

Comparisons Between Prematurely and Maturely Born Groups
Kindergarten Age. Table 4 shows the proportion of prematurely and maturely born children who attained the critical score level on each of the 37 kindergarten tests.

The most striking result was the almost uniformly poorer showing of the prematurely born children. The differences favored the maturely born subjects on 36 out of 37 tests; on 15 of these 36 tests differences in favor of the maturely born subjects reached statistical significance. It is noteworthy that of these 15 tests, 11 were oral language and reading readiness tasks, in other words, tasks that require a relatively high level of integrative competence.

End of Grade I. On both the Overall Reading Performance Index and the Writing Test at the end of Grade I the prematures did significantly less well than did the children born at term (Table 5).

Table 3
Performance of Prematurely Born Children on Grade I and Grade II
Achievement Tests, According to Birthweight
(Percent of children attaining critical score level)

Test	Birthweight		
	1500 grams or less (N = 14)	1501–1750 grams (N = 22)	1751–2500 grams (N = 16)
Grade I			
Reading	14%	27%	37%
Writing	43	32	62
Grade II			
Reading	28	54	37
Writing	14	45	37
Spelling	35	59	56

End of Grade II. At the end of Grade II, the prematures' performance in all three academic areas was significantly inferior to that of maturely born subjects (Table 5).

Rate of Progress Between Kindergarten and End of Grade II

The possibility was next considered that the prematures, in spite of their poor showing on Grade II academic tests, might nevertheless in the interval between kindergarten and the end of second grade show signs of accelerated progress in some areas.

This possibility was explored by readministering at the end of Grade II, four kindergarten tests (Behavioral Control, Hand Preference, Visual Motor Organization and Auditory Discrimination) and then determining whether the prematures had made greater progress in the intervening time than had the children born at term. (The fact that the prematures had started at relatively low levels at kindergarten age and thus had clearly more room for improvement was taken into account in the statistical procedure.) The data do show that except on the Bender Visual Motor Gestalt test the prematurely born children had indeed progressed faster than the maturely born (Table 6).

In *absolute* performance on the same tests, on the other hand, the term children continued to lead; only on the Bender Gestalt test did the differences in favor of the maturely born children reach statistical significance (Table 7).

In summary, the prematurely born subjects functioned considerably less well than did the full-term children. While the former showed signs of "catching up" in some areas between the ages of five and one-half and eight, their academic performance at the end of second grade continued to lag.

Table 4
Performance of Prematurely and Maturely Born Children
on 37 Kindergarten Tests
(Percent of children attaining critical score level)

Test	Prematures (N = 53)	Maturely Born (N = 53)	P
Behavioral Patterning			
Hyperactivity, Distractibility and			
Disinhibition	62%	81%	
Motility Patterning			
Concomitant Movements	35	62	≤.01
Gross Motor Patterning			
Balance	87	91	
Hopping	76	89	
Throwing	80	85	
Fine Motor Patterning			
Pegboard Speed Index	58	81	≤.05
Tying a Knot	87	94	
Pencil Use	61	72	
Body Image			
Human Figure Drawing	76	89	
Laterality			
Hand Preference Index	59	72	
Visual-Perceptual Patterning			
Figure-Ground Organization	39	55	
Bender Visuomotor Gestalt	62	91	≤.01
Auditory-Perceptual Patterning			
Tapped Patterns	61	93	≤.01
Auditory Memory Span	82	89	
Auditory Discrimination (Wepman)	67	81	
Word Recognition (Peabody Picture			
Vocabulary Test)	74	90	≤.05
Language Comprehension	72	94	≤.01
Expressive Language			
Consonant Articulation	15	29	
Articulatory Stability	70	83	
Word Finding	83	98	≤.05
Story Organization	45	71	≤.05
Number of Words	30	47	
Sentence Elaboration	49	55	
Number of Grammatical Errors	27	10	
Definitions (Binet)	35	45	
Categories	35	59	≤.05
Reading Readiness			
Name Writing	70	92	≤.01
Copying of Letters	70	94	≤.01
Letter Naming	47*	78*	≤.05
Reversals (Horst)	33	45	

Table 4 (continued)
Performance of Prematurely and Maturely Born Children
on 37 Kindergarten Tests
(Percent of children attaining critical score level)

Test	Prematures (N = 53)	Maturely Born (N = 53)	P
Word Matching (Gates)	50	79	≤.01
Word Rhyming (Gates)	69	85	≤.05
Word Recognition I (Pack)	37	60	≤.05
Word Recognition II (Table)	38	57	
Word Reproduction	53	72	
Style			
Ego Strength	65	81	
Work Attitude	61	74	

*Based on 32 prematurely and 27 maturely born children.

Consideration of the Findings in the Light of Selected Background Variables

Intelligence. It will be remembered that the prematurely born children performed less well than the children born at term not only on the kindergarten battery, but also on the Stanford-Binet Intelligence Test administered at the same time. However, the kindergarten tests and the Stanford-Binet, which is heavily loaded with verbal items, measure overlapping, although not identical competences. It would, therefore, be inappropriate to try to account for group differences by Stanford Binet scores. Because the competences evaluated by the two sets of tests do overlap, any attempt to account for IQ differences could be expected to reduce the observed disparity between groups.

Table 5
Performance of Prematurely and Maturely Born Children on Grade I and
Grade II Achievement Tests
(Percentage of children attaining critical score level)

Test	Prematures (N = 53)	Maturely Born (N = 53)	P
Grade I			
Reading	34%	57%	≤.05
Writing	13	34	≤.01
Grade II			
Reading	47	79	≤.01
Writing	58	79	≤.05
Spelling	55	77	≤.05

Table 6
Comparison of Prematurely and Maturely Born Children in Rate of
Progress from Kindergarten to Grade II on Four Nonacademic Tests
(Percent of children attaining critical score level)

Test	Prematures (N = 53)	Maturely Born (N = 53)
Laterality Index		
Kindergarten	59%	71%†
Grade II	66%	65%
Net degree of progress or regression*	+ .17	− .08
Bender Visuomotor Gestalt Test		
Kindergarten	46%†	66%†
Grade II	39%†	59%†
Net degree of progress or regression*	− .15	− .11
Auditory Discrimination		
Kindergarten	30%†	55%†
Grade II	81%†	86%†
Net degree of progress or regression*	+ .73	+ .69
Behavioral Index		
Kindergarten	64%	81%
Grade II	71%	77%
Net degree of progress or regression*	+ .19	− .05

*The net degree of progress (+) or regression (−) is the ratio of the actual change in percent attaining the critical score level to the maximum change possible, taking into account the fact that the prematures, starting from a lower level, could achieve greater absolute improvement. The laterality Index illustrates the calculations:

$$\text{Net progress of prematures} = \frac{\text{actual progress}}{\text{maximum progress possible}} = \frac{66\% - 59\%}{100\% - 59\%} = +.17$$

$$\text{Net regression of maturely born children} = \frac{\text{actual regression}}{\text{maximum regression possible}} = \frac{65\% - 71\%}{71\% - 0\%} - .08$$

†Based on 33 prematurely and 29 maturely born children who were born in 1956. The Bender Gestalt and Auditory Discrimination Tests were not readministered to children born in 1955.

It seemed worthwhile, nevertheless, to minimize the effects of intelligence by comparing the 19 prematurely and the 22 maturely born subjects with IQs in the narrow range between 90 and 105 on those 15 kindergarten and academic tests which had originally discriminated significantly between groups. These comparisons showed the same trend reported previously: the prematurely born children did less well than the maturely born on all but one test. On only three tests— Concomitant Movements (related to central nervous system maturation), the Bender Gestalt (related to integrative competence), and

Table 7
Performance of Prematurely and Maturely Born Children on Four
Kindergarten Tests Readministered at Grade II
(Percent of children attaining critical score level)

Test	Prematures (N = 53)	Maturely born (N = 53)	P
Laterality Index	74%	83%	. . .
Bender Gestalt	67*	93*	≤.05
Auditory Discrimination	73*	79*	. . .
Behavioral Index	71	77	. . .

*Based on 33 prematurely and 29 maturely born children who were born in 1956. The Bender Gestalt and Auditory Discrimination Tests were not readministered to children born in 1955.

end-of-second-grade reading—did the differences remain statistically significant.

Socioeconomic Background. Socioeconomic and educational status of the parents are widely regarded as being among the determinants in the reported differences between prematurely and maturely born children.[5] Drillien (1964) as well as Wortis and Freedman (1965) who explored the contributions of both prematurity and social environment, feel that prematurely born children, many of whom show neurological deviations, are more vulnerable to the effects of an impoverished background than are children born at term. This finding would suggest considerable interaction between the sociological and the physiological aspects of prematurity.

In the present study, however, in which the educational achievement of the mothers in the prematurely born group was higher than that of the mothers of the maturely born, it seems highly unlikely that socioeconomic differences would have been determining factors in the poorer performance of prematures.

Uddenberg's findings (1955) point in the same direction. Although the mothers in his prematurely born sample came from a higher social stratum than did the mothers of the controls, the prematurely born showed poorer perceptuomotor and reading performance than did the subjects born at term. Drillien (1964) in her extensive study also found that prematurely born children are more likely to

───────

[5]Rider, Taback, and Knobloch (1955) refer to the fact that in the lower socioeconomic stratum more children are born prematurely (7.3 percent) than in the higher (5.1 percent). (See also Wiener (1962), who stresses the importance of control for social class in the study of prematurity). Douglas (1960) in a nationwide study of the mental ability and primary school progress of prematurely born children found a number of striking handicaps, which later were shown to be of environmental origin. See also Robinson and Robinson (1965).

work at a level below their intellectual capacity than are maturely born children of comparable intelligence and from similar homes.

Early Neurological Status. The relatively poor performance of prematurely born children often has been ascribed to the higher frequency of brain injury (Bradley 1955) in this group, the assumption being that interference with the integrity of the central nervous system would be reflected in widespread developmental and learning disturbances.[6] Burks (1957) feels that reading disabilities may occur as sequelae of brain impairment and are related to difficulties in pattern-making and physiological integration.

The limitations of the present project did not allow for neurological examination of the prematurely born children at the end of second grade. Thus, the effects of possible brain injury on their academic achievement could not be directly assessed. It will be recalled, however, that records were available of the neurological evaluation of these subjects at the age of three. Thus the writers felt that it might be of interest to examine the prematurely born children's scholastic performance at age eight in the light of these early neurological findings.

Five out of 49 children examined at age three presented, "definite or probable evidence of neurological deficit."[7] Of these five, three subjects passed and two failed reading and spelling tests at the end of second grade. It is possible that among the three who passed on-going maturation had resolved most of the original problems; Bradley (1955) refers to a diminution in symptoms as children grow older. Since the number of prematures with positive early neurological signs was so small, however, it was not possible to draw conclusions as to the relationship between positive neurological signs at early ages and subsequent learning difficulties.

On the other hand, of the 44 children who at age three had shown *no* definite or probable neurological deficit, 23 failed reading and spelling tests at age eight, (although it should be added that approximately half of these failing children had impressed the writers as "organic"[8] in the sense described by Birch [1964]). Thus, the findings suggest that absence of demonstrable early neurological deficits in prematurely born children does not necessarily imply a good prognosis for learning at later ages. Subtle dysfunctions seem to persist in

---

[6]See also "Psychoneurological Learning Disorders in Children" by Myklebust and Boshes.

[7]Thelander, Phelps, and Kirk emphasize the fact that electroencephalograms and neurological examinations are not usually sensitive enough to pick up subtle dysfunctions, while psychological, educational and developmental tests might reveal dysfunctions pointing to future learning disabilities.

[8]The term "minimal brain injury" has not been used here, since as Reed (Kasten and Fowler 1959) points out, the diagnosis is clearly inferential and criteria for it vary from one clinical setting to another.

those aspects of the learning process, which, like reading, writing, and spelling, require a high degree of differentiation and integration (Koch 1964; Lubchenco et al. 1963; Pasamanick and Knobloch 1960).

To ask whether the premature's inferior performance is related to actual neurological damage[9] which interferes with the establishing of complex sensorimotor schemata, or to a severe and pervasive maturational lag, would probably fail to do justice to the complexity of the clinical phenomena. The two may be related, since clinically nonfocal brain injury may manifest itself clinically in disruption of or interference with crucial maturational processes.

Clinical Impressions

In view of the investigators' continued contact with the prematurely born children (a contact that extended over a period of two and a half years) some clinical remarks may seem justified.

The writers were struck by the diffuseness of these children and by their difficulty in mobilizing energy in the service of a goal. It is possible, of course, that maternal anxiety played a part here. Kaplan and Mason (1960), as well as Oppé (1960), have made the pertinent observation that the prematures' unusual appearance at birth, the prohibitions against the handling and fondling of these babies,[10] and their slow early development, cannot but arouse profound anxiety in their mothers.[11] The mothers' anxiety may flow over to the children and inhibit their freedom to function in a variety of ways.

It seems likely, finally, that as a result of their early difficulties in homeostasis, motility, perceptuomotor patterning, and spatial orientation, prematurely born children are themselves more anxious and dependent than are their full-term peers.[12] Schilder (1964) believes that a child with disturbed equilibrium needs the help and support of his mother more than do others. It seems probable that prematurely born children pass through the normal stages of infantile dependency at a considerably later age than children born at term.[13] Such continuing dependency may be viewed as one other aspect of their physiological immaturity, which would make it difficult for them to become active participants in the learning situation.

---

[9]See Wiener's et al. (1965) comprehensive and excellent paper which appeared after the conclusion of the present study.

[10]These prohibitions may result in additional sensory deprivation, which in turn, may contribute to these children's relatively slow initial development. The question of whether prematurely born children are able to tolerate as much stimulation as full-term subjects has been dealt with by Oppé (1960) and Koch (1964).

[11]One important question that arises in this context has to do with maternal guilt, since, as Blau et al. (1963) point out, the majority of prematurely born children are unwanted babies.

[12]Greenacre (1953) feels that the premature baby is predisposed to anxiety.

[13]Izmusi (1963) found more "baby wishes" among prematurely than among maturely born subjects.

The prematurely born subjects in the sample investigated here seemed much more vulnerable than the maturely born children.[14] Lawrence (1960) speaks of injury to the ego apparatus as a result of physiological deficits. Perhaps it is because of such deficits that the ability of prematurely born children to tolerate stress of any kind is low.

Clinically, the prematures appeared to be "different" from the children born at term. One of the writers, who had no previous knowledge of which subjects were prematurely born, had no difficulty identifying most of the prematurely born children. This identification was based as much on their general approach to work as on their test scores. The prematures' central nervous system functioning seemed more primitive, their behavioral controls less firmly established,[15] their level of neurological integration lower than that of the maturely born subjects. They presented subtle difficulties in motor, perceptual, vis-uomotor, and linguistic patterning, difficulties that extended into the early academic years and resulted in relatively inferior performance, especially with regard to tasks that required a high level of integration.

Summary

In answer to the question asked at the beginning of this paper, it can now be said that in the present study prematurely born children whose IQ fell within the average range of intelligence did less well than maturely born peers on a large battery of tests administered at kindergarten age. While they showed some indications of "catching up" during the years between kindergarten and end of second grade, significant lags persisted well into the eighth year of life.[16] These children, therefore, have to be regarded as an *academic high risk group*. In view of the fact that at the very least 4 percent of our schoolchildren are prematurely born, (Harper 1964) these findings would seem to have more than theoretical relevance.[17]

---

[14]Reference is again made to the observations of Wortis and Freedman (1965), who feel that infants with defective or vulnerable nervous systems are especially sensitive to environmental stresses and pathology.

[15]In Burks' (1960) hyperkinetic group, there were five times as many prematurely born children as controls.

[16]Koch (1964) speaks of possible ". . . subtle and long time influences . . ." of prematurity even in children who are accepted for normal school programs. It should be pointed out, however, that a number of prematurely born children in the group seem to have compensated for their original deficits. In fact, the investigators' clinical experience seems to show that prematurely born children with genetically high endowment often excel though perhaps at later ages than their peers.

[17]Frisk, Takkunen, and Holmstrom (1964) say that 50 percent of prematurely born children are not ready for first-grade entrance, and recommend for these children a year's postponement of formal education. Howard and Worrell (1952) also recommend delayed school entrance.

Part III
THE LEARNING DISABLED CHILD

Learning Disabilities: An Overview

Children who suffer from learning disabilities do not constitute a homogenous group. Such disabilities cannot be viewed as a single clinical entity. They embrace a variety of dysfunctions, grouped together because the presenting symptom, academic failure, is their most outstanding feature. Children who fail in school do not necessarily present a specific pattern of dysfunction, nor do their difficulties stem from a single root. Psychological and physiological factors, the child's genetic endowment, including his vulnerability to stress, his prenatal, neonatal, and postnatal history, the emotional climate in which he is reared, and the social milieu of which he is part all interact in complex ways. The resulting constellation, which varies from child to child, may or may not be conducive to the assimilation of the values, attitudes, skills, and intellectual operations that enter into academic functioning. Learning requires the integration of a number of physiological and psychological processes and the acceptance of a specific set of values. It also requires of the child the ability to submit himself to the constraints and demands of the classroom.

The literature contains a large number of excellent studies which deal with one or, at most, two or three of the variables that enter into the learning process. Any one variable, however, can be evaluated only in the context of the child's total situation, which differs in each case. A given configuration of deficiencies may or may not result in failure, depending on the child's specific pattern of strength and on the availability of adaptive and compensatory resources.

In attempting to organize learning disorders in what are admittedly crude diagnostic categories, one is forced to admit that this is an unpopular undertaking. There are those who reject educational diagnosis because this approach is based on a model of disease. All that counts, according to this point of view, is behavior and its modifications (Bateman 1973). It does not matter, behaviorists maintain, whether a child fails in school because he has an alcoholic father or

Reprinted with permission from New York Academy of Medicine, from *Bulletin of the New York Academy of Medicine* 50:459–477. 1974.

because he suffers from dysfunction of the central nervous system. The approach is the same: observe the child, see what he does, and plan appropriate remedial measures. An approach, however, which would be effective for the child with an alcoholic father, such as providing him with a male tutor to serve as a model, may be inadequate for the child with a dysfunction of the central nervous system. For him we would have to modify the strategies of teaching. Possibly we might refer him for medication.

Obviously a good deal is wrong with our present diagnostic procedures. Often they fail to provide recommendations specific enough to help the teacher who, unfortunately, is usually not part of the diagnostic team. In spite of such shortcomings, however, I feel that diagnosis is essential. The question is not diagnosis or no diagnosis but what kind of diagnosis.

Four categories of disorders of learning are presented here: psychogenic, neurogenic, those related to developmental language disabilities, and those that stem primarily from environmental conditions. These are gross simplifications. There are no "pure" categories; symptoms overlap. In clinical reality we deal with the interactions among a variety of forces—richness or poverty of cognitive endowment, presence or absence of environmental support, availability or lack of adequate teaching. It is not always possible to unravel the child's inherent deficits, physiological and psychological, the kinds of adaptations which he makes to them, and the effects of the social, cultural, and emotional climate in which he makes his adaptations and which, in turn, condition his scholastic effectiveness.

Psychogenic Learning Disabilities

In discussing psychogenic disorders of learning it is appropriate to start with those of psychotic youngsters. They are not a homogeneous group. Among them are a number of children who have sustained cerebral injury and who present psychotic responses to dysfunction of the central nervous system. One can say in general that psychotic children invest large quantities of psychic energy in the primary process and that the breakthrough of magical modes of experiencing life plays havoc with learning. The lack of boundaries between their inner and outer world and the primitive character of their organizational schemes interfere with logical operations, objective reasoning, and the assessment of reality, all hallmarks of the secondary process and essential for academic success. These children may be so beset by affects and drives belonging to an early developmental stage, their world so fragmented, that they cannot integrate subject matter into an already existing framework. They may be so overwhelmed by terrifying fantasies that they are unable to sift, analyze, or assimilate material. They may invest the subject matter itself with highly idiosyncratic meanings and confuse both symbol and referent. For Ted, an eight-year-old schizophrenic boy who said that he does not like the letter *k* because it has too many spikes, letters and numbers are not symbols; they have a life of their own. In his case they represent archaic feelings of aggression and retaliation and as such acquire magical properties. This does not mean that all schizophrenic children are unable to benefit from educational intervention. While teaching must be flexible and must be greatly modified according to needs of these children, the acquisition of academic skills is assumed to stimulate essential ego functions.

We do see a large number of nonpsychotic children who have psychogenic learning problems (de Hirsch 1963). They are usually referred by guidance clinics and schools because of what are vaguely called learning blocks. The trend nowadays is away from interpretations such as "inhibition of curiosity," "refusal to know," etc., although it is true that occasionally we do see children for whom "knowing," that is, learning, represents a threat. And we do see youngsters in whom learning has become involved in more basic conflicts. There are phobic children who may dislike a specific subject matter (mathematics or reading, for instance) because the content has become attached to a larger cluster, parts of which may be experienced as frightening or disgusting. Some of these children present constitutional difficulties in the area of written and printed langauge which make reading an especially suitable object for a phobic response.

The vast majority of youngsters, however, who suffer from psychogenic disabilities in learning are those in whom crucial ego functions are lagging or have been impaired, children who do not persist, who do not push through, who fail to incorporate values such as pride in achievement, pleasure in solving problems, and delight in discovery and mastery. Such children are unable to invest in subject matter. They do not become excited over some period in history or some laboratory experiment. Nor do they "fall" for a teacher. Their ability to identify is limited, and since their relation to the teacher remains shallow, he cannot fire them with excitement for learning or help them incorporate his own attitudes: involvement in and devotion to a task and the courage to push through even if the going is rough.

We no longer believe that children learn because someone pushes information down their throats. Learning is fundamentally an aggressive act. Passivity may serve some children well, it may keep them out of trouble, but anyone who has worked with passive adolescents knows that if he fails to make the youngster carry the ball he is defeated before he starts. Some children present what one might call a "depletion" syndrome. They literally imagine that effort, any effort, impoverishes them, that they are left poorer when they give of themselves.

Among these children are many who turn away from any task that threatens failure because they dread the attendant pain and discomfort. Such highly perfectionistic youngsters cannot afford to make mistakes, since any shortcoming serves to confirm their doubts about themselves. This is seen clearly in boys entering the first grade of school. Failure at this stage entrains feelings of impotence and extreme helplessness that set the stage for a paralyzing fear of venturing in the future. Since such children have to be perfect, they cannot afford to try.

There are compulsive children who sit down dutifully to their homework and then spend hours sharpening their pencils, making lists, or sorting their papers. Such children are too doubt-ridden and too heavily laden by conflicts to push through to the heart of a problem.

Finally, there are those who are so fantasy-ridden, so preoccupied with daydreams, that they cannot concentrate on work. In many of these cases we find adverse reality situations, divorce in the family, death or crippling illness, rage against a high-achieving sibling, or feelings of guilt which leave the youngster with little psychic energy to invest in academic endeavor.

Neurogenic Learning Disabilities

The second category is that of children with neurogenic learning disabilities, those who are "brain injured" in the sense of minimal brain dysfunction. The term "brain injury," minimal or not, has frequently been used far too loosely. It is dangerous because it implies to the parents and, indirectly, to the child a structural lesion of the kind found occasionally in adults who have lost a previously established function, such as speech, as a result of a cerebral insult.

Apart from youngsters with cerebral palsy and those with seizures, only a small percentage of children have brain injury in this sense. The term should be reserved for those who, along with a history of cerebral injury, present positive signs on the classical neurological examination or the electroencephalogram. In the very young we usually deal with fairly widespread, diffuse, often mild, dysfunctions in central processing that may result directly or indirectly in a large variety of disorders of language and learning. Whatever it was that happened to the central nervous systems of these children in utero, at birth, or postnatally, happened to an organism in the process of formation and may have interfered with maturation and integration in many areas and on different levels of psychological and physiological functioning.

We deal, of course, with a continuum from mild to severe. The children come with a cloudy prenatal and postnatal history, with vague reports, which may or may not be significant, of complications during delivery, and with a history of some developmental deviation. The varied clinical symptoms, singly or in combinations, include difficulty in managing sensory and specifically linguistic information, irritability, various degrees of hyper- or hypoactivity, hypotonia, global motility patterning, perceptual deficits, fine motor and visuomotor weakness, problems with body image, occasional finger agnosia, difficulty in right-left awareness and spatial orientation, uneven patterning, and sometimes severe disorders of attention and a lowered threshold for anxiety (Bender 1956).

What are the forces that interfere with learning in children who have subtle dysfunctions of the central nervous system?

Man is an organizing, pattern-making animal. The outstanding features in these "organic" youngsters is their difficulty in analyzing and constructing even the simplest schemata, that is to say, in structuring themselves as well as their environments.

As a result of early difficulties with homeostasis and orientation in space these children tend to suffer from a pervasive sense of helplessness in the face of inner and outer forces with which they cannot cope. Their need for infantile gratification (and mothers instinctively respond to it) often persists into later years and is in all probability a residue of early inability to be in command of themselves and their surroundings. This was abundantly clear in the prematurely born group that we followed from the age of five to eight (de Hirsch, Jansky, and Langford 1966).

These children are often unable to pattern their primitive motility. They are frequently so preoccupied with the simple task of sitting still that they cannot address themselves to learning. Further, they tend to be extremely impulsive. Even at late ages they continue to be too disinhibited to withhold a response in a problem-solving situation.

The profound concern over bodily intactness that is so frequently found in the protocols of organically-impaired children probably goes back to early trauma. As a result of their perceptuomotor deficiencies, their picture of the world must have been somewhat distorted from the start. This distortion has contributed to their psychological vulnerability and their proneness to anxiety. Further, the irritability and hyperreactivity of these babies may result in a disturbance of the early mother-child response pattern inasmuch as the infant fails to pick up the mother's cue. At the mercy of a thousand stimuli, such youngsters are hard to live with. This places a heavy strain on the parents' interactions with the child, thereby introducing still another variable.

Control of drives is a central problem in organically impaired children. The older ones whose academic tools are usually poor are very prone to act out. This is dangerous because it results in re-percussions from the environment and alienation from the main-stream of the culture. Many of the children referred for behavioral disorders and for failure in school are organic youngsters. It might be asserted that their disruptive behavior is the direct result of academic difficulties. Up to a point this might be correct, but their failure to learn may have been aggravated by early trouble with drive control, thus initiating a vicious cycle. Some children who have difficulty in struc-turing themselves and their environment take refuge in less dangerous but nevertheless counterproductive measures. They employ rigid defenses and compulsive-obsessive-like mechanisms. Unlike those of neurotic youngsters, these defenses are not erected against forbidden impulses, but against a deep-seated fear of disintegration. No matter what their origin, these mechanisms in themselves may constitute a barrier to learning.

Communicative disorders complicate the situation. Early and often severe difficulties with analysis and construction of schemata may make it difficult for organic children to detect the ever-recurring patterns that are embedded in the swiftly flowing stream of language.

Normal babies begin early to respond selectively to many of the acoustic and linguistic signals that impinge on them from the envi-ronment. Friedlander's work (1970) demonstrates that infants attempt to sort out the buzzing confusion that surrounds them far earlier than we had suspected.

Some older children with dysfunctions of the central nervous system may not even separate the stream of speech from the back-ground of noise. They may not recognize the boundaries of phonemes and words. They are bathed in a sea of sounds and do not grasp the underlying schemata and the way they hang together. In the end such children "tune out." At the age of four they may understand most nouns, many verbs, and some adjectives; they may comprehend simple messages in familiar situations; they may use some stock phrases. Therefore the parents may not realize that anything is amiss until the kindergarten teacher complains that the youngster fails to follow any but the simplest directions. Early gaps in the processing of linguistic input provide clear signals of future academic problems. They point to subsequent difficulties in the handling of numerical and verbal systems and to the likelihood of failure to cope with the increas-ing conceptual and linguistic demands of the higher scholastic grades.

Early gaps in the processing of language not only interfere with scholastic functioning; they also constitute almost insurmountable obstacles to the development of ego functions that are essential for learning. Rosen (1966) has discussed the reciprocal relations between the appearance of the ego as a psychic structure and the emergence of language. Language allows the child to externalize magical and omnipotent fantasies and fosters reality testing, one of the most important functions of the ego. Language, which is organized in time, helps children to postpone gratification. For the two-year-old child who does not understand words such as *soon* or *wait a while*, pain and unhappiness last forever. Children who have no tools for labeling feelings of sadness and anger tend to be overwhelmed.

The sometimes striking variability in the performance of organic youngsters, not only from session to session, but also within one session, has usually been interpreted as being related to psychological interference. But this variability often has an organic flavor. In these youngsters the perceptual and linguistic schemata themselves appear to be unstable and shifting. Such children do worse when fatigued or under stress.

Their legitimate handicaps make it hard for organically impaired children to develop a feeling of mastery and a drive toward autonomy. As they grow older, emotional problems resulting from an uninterrupted series of failures may so mask the original organic deficiencies that it is difficult to sort out what is related to the primary organic dysfunction and what is referable to the child's reaction to his inability to cope with the school situation.

The assumption that disorders of learning must rest either on an organic or on a neurotic basis is simplistic. Kurlander and Colodny (1965) speak of the psychodynamics of organicity. The presence of organic features does not, of course, exempt children from emotional conflict. They may exist side by side, one reinforcing the other. The drive to act out may be organic in origin, but the child's inability to reconcile his behavior with an internalized moral code will result in intrapsychic conflict.

In summary, neurosis in children with neurogenic learning disabilities may be part of the biological dysfunction; it may be the consequence of the dysfunction, or it may have originated in conflicts unrelated to organicity but interacting with it.

Within the category of neurogenic learning disabilities there is another group of youngsters who do not suffer from irregularities in the central nervous system. So called soft signs, if they are present at all, are minimal. But this group appears to present neurophysiological lags which often, if not always, tend to disappear with maturation. A number of children from five to eight years of age do not seem to be ready, physiologically or psychologically, for formal education. Among them are bright children; Ilg and Ames (1964) call them the "superior immatures." The majority of them are boys. If one has seen hundreds of them, as we have, one recognizes them at a glance. Their prenatal and postnatal history is not necessarily significant, although we may occasionally receive a report of prematurity or of the "failure-to-thrive" (de Hirsch, Jansky, and Langford 1966) syndrome. Their development did not present dramatic obstacles except that linguistic development is often delayed. These boys often look as if they had not quite crystallized. They hop across the room like three- or four-year-olds. They need an inordinate number of motor outlets. They are not ready for table work and cannot stick to it longer than 10 minutes at a time. Any teacher knows that such youngsters are in no way ready for the first grade of school. Their outstanding characteristic is impulsiveness, inability to inhibit responses.

Some have not established superiority of one hand over the other. Establishing a master hand is normally related to familial and maturational factors. Symptoms, of course, mean different things at different ages (de Hirsch, Jansky, and Lanford 1966). At the age of eleven, switching hands during writing may signal a maturational defect or some irregularity of the central nervous system. What counts is directionality. Progression from left to right is necessary for reading and writing in our culture.

The human figures drawn by these children are not necessarily bizarre but they are usually very primitive, as are their Bender Gestalt copies which reflect difficulties with spatial organization and lack of awareness of the essence of the gestalten. Although the Bender Gestalt test is a good predictor of subsequent reading, this does not mean that the two are casually related, and it certainly does not mean that training children to match and discriminate between geometric figures (nonverbal forms) advances their academic readiness. We have no proof that nonverbal training transfers to reading.

Immature children do present perceptuomotor deficits, but as they advance into the higher grades the importance of such deficits decreases rapidly and what counts in the long run is conceptual and linguistic competence. Thus, it is imperative to check carefully the linguistic performance of kindergarten children. Friedlander (1973) demonstrated that 25 percent of children in kindergarten and first grade are poor listeners. They are unable to follow the line of a story. Most of those who fail in reading produce primitively constructed sentences only. Mason, in Edinburgh, (1967-68) found that, independent of intelligence quotient, 75 percent of children from high-income groups whose linguistic development at the age of four years was at least eighteen months in arrears failed in reading several years later. Ability to perceive, process, store, and retrieve linguistic information is a prerequisite for learning.

The physiological and linguistic immaturity of such children is matched by their emotional infantilism. They continue to live in a somewhat egocentric world. Aggression is crude and mostly nonverbal. Wish-fulfilling and magical solutions are ready to hand. An impressive number are still preoccupied with food, that is, with early infantile gratifications. They have not moved from the pleasure to the reality principle; they retain the infantile expectation that life should provide rewards without corresponding efforts. It is essential to identify these immature children before they are exposed to formal education.[1]

Disorders of Printed and Written Language

A third group of children present disorders of printed and written aspects of language. These so-called dyslexics constitute a distinct but by no means homogeneous group. Orton (1937) first described these youngsters who have specific disabilities in reading, writing, and spelling.

The label dyslexia has been used excessively during recent years. There is a measure of agreement, however, that the term signifies the inability to cope with printed and written language by children who possess average or better-than-average intelligence, who have had adequate educational opportunities, and who do not present evidence of significant psychopathology or positive signs on the classical neurological examination.

Language is a relatively late acquistion. It is highly vulnerable, often slow to develop, and easily disrupted. Difficulties with printed and written language belong in the category of developmental language disorders.

Jansky (1972) has noted that reading is a complex cognitive competence that requires the interplay of several different processes. It is fed by the perceptual systems. It depends on an intact neurological substrate, and it is based on the linguistic and experimental background that the child brings to school. Reading requires a level of emotional maturity that permits the child to postpone immediate gratification in the service of a long-term goal and to invest in the task

---

[1]Jansky's new screening index (Jansky and de Hirsch 1972) is based on her testing of 400 public school children whose intelligence quotients ranged from low to very high and who had a variety of socioeconomic backgrounds. Two instruments are presented in the index, one for the identification of high-risk children, the other for the careful diagnostic investigation of children so identified. The screening index, based on earlier research, has advantages over the battery described in 1966: 1) It takes only 15 to 20 minutes to administer. 2) It can be taught to school personnel and volunteers in two days. 3) It uses as additional information the independent judgment of kindergarten teachers, which was found to be highly predictive.

Once the high-risk children have been identified they are subjected to careful diagnostic assessment. The diagnostic battery was derived from a factor analysis of 20 kindergarten tests: children's scores are presented as a profile of strengths and weaknesses which points directly to remedial measures. In the case of high-risk children, postponing entry into first grade for another year, strengthening the areas of deficits, and exploiting competence will make a world of difference. The first two years of school are decisive for the child's concept of himself as a learner. He must not be allowed to fail.

of learning. It assumes a value system that includes an appreciation of printed information. But while the act of reading rests on a number of different competences, it is nevertheless an autonomous process which represents the integration of many systems.

Failure in reading does not necessarily stem from inability to master one or more subordinate kinds of skills (Jansky 1971). Goodman (1972) says that progress in reading is not a matter of mastery of parts leading to mastery of the whole, but rather a matter of successive approximations to proficient reading. Children, he says, sometimes grasp the subskills only after the process has moved forward. In other words, reading is a new gestalt. Anyone who has worked with severely dyslexic youngsters has observed that there comes a point where the child abruptly takes off. In contrast to earlier painfully slow and laborious efforts, a new gestalt seems to "jump out" (de Hirsch 1963). This is not to say that such children can be left to their own devices; they need intensive and, if at all possible, individual help.

Reading is a linguistic task. Ability to process and generate oral language is necessary for the mastery of printed and written verbal symbols. Difficulties with some or all aspects of language often occur on a familial basis.

Take Martin as an example. He is a boy with whom we have worked for a long time and he is now repeating the second grade. The family history of language difficulty is heavily positive. The father is a terrible speller. Years ago we worked with Martin's much older stepsister on her compositions. Martin's four-year-old brother stutters. There is now a two-year-old baby brother who, his mother swears, is slow at picking up words.

Martin is blond, slight, and has a charming face, but he looks as if he were not quite finished. He is a bright youngster and a psychologically solid little boy, immensely good-natured and highly entertaining. He has many friends. He is incredibly hyperactive and hard to live with at home. Nevertheless, he does work. His oral language is strikingly immature and his vocabulary is limited. He has in no way incorporated the fundamental syntactical rules which most children of his age have mastered. He will say: "I dag clams" because he has a vague feeling that the past tense of *dig* is irregular. Coming from an assembly, he will cheerfully announce "I was a rusher and passed out telegrams," when he wants to say, "I was an usher and passed out programs." His poor retention of spoken verbal sequences is mirrored by his abysmally poor recall of printed verbal sequences. It took him forever to learn to read the word *sit*. Verbal configurations clearly look different to him in different contexts. It is his perception of verbal configuration that is poor; he does perfectly well with puzzles. If he had a feeling for the flow of a sentence, he would compensate for this instability by guessing from the surrounding syntactical configurations just what the options are. Unfortunately he has no feeling for this.

One outstanding feature in disorders of reading is failure to maintain a linguistic gestalt. Word-finding difficulties—inability to retrieve stored verbal symbols, names of common objects, of people or book titles—are usually overlooked. In Jansky's (1972) study, dysnomia proved to be an excellent predictor of reading lags at the end of the second grade. The children who cannot recall the names of colors or the title of a film they have seen the day before are the same youngsters who have trouble recalling not only printed words but also the names of the letters of the alphabet or their sound equivalents. For Martin, who has such difficulties in recalling whole words, a phonics approach seems the logical avenue for the acquisition of reading. However, retaining and evoking the names of sound equivalents is equally hard for him. When sounding out a simple word such as *flop*, he loses the name of the first sound while struggling with the last one. With his relatively poor auditory discrimination, at least where verbal configurations are concerned (he has an unusually good ear for fine shades of sounds in the environment), the short-vowel sounds are, of course, a hurdle.

Another important feature in disorders of spoken, printed, and written language is the child's difficulty in recalling and reproducing verbal events in a given order. In Jansky's screening index, sentence memory is one of the best predictors (1972). Dyslexic children have difficulty not only in the retrieval of separate verbal items but in reconstructing them in correct sequence. Their difficulty in recalling the months of the year and the multiplication tables bears witness to this. Martin, for example, scrambles the order of sounds and words in speech and in reading and spelling. In this case, as in so many others, it is the instability of printed verbal perceptual configurations, combined with severe linguistic deficiences, that makes for reading failure.

Nowadays reading difficulties are called "perceptual disorders." Labeling them in this way seems to obviate further search for causes and to constitute a prescription for treatment. Training a child to draw triangles, however, may produce excellent triangles, but does not result in advanced reading readiness. The vast amounts of seductively packaged materials designed to prepare children for reading are probably the reason why the theory of perceptual deficits is vastly oversold. Nonverbal perceptual deficiencies in young children show a positive but weak correlation with poor reading scores, but this does not mean that there is a causal relation between the two. During the early states of acquisition of reading, perceptual cues are helpful, but it should be added that the very process of perception is assisted by information as to available linguistic options. Verbalization stabilizes perception. Linguistic cues make much of the perceptual information redundant. If one knows instinctively that the construction *I have been* is often followed by either a passive construction or by a word ending with *ing,* one has already excluded any number of perceptual errors.

Many intelligent children, moreover, sometimes compensate for massive perceptual and visuomotor deficiences. Evaluation of the children's difficulties makes sense only if one takes into account important mechanisms of compensation; they cannot possibly be overstressed. We know little about them but we assume that intelligence, ego strength, and environmental support are important determinants.

It is far more difficult to compensate for unstable visual patterning in spelling than in reading. The poor speller may remember a word in a list but may lose it when it is embedded in a sentence. He loses the overall gestalt and its internal design (de Hirsch 1963). Spelling requires not only a sharp memory for the graphemic configuration but also a feeling for the phonology and morphology of English words. Cazden (1972) reports that while good and poor spellers do not differ when a series of nonsense syllables containing non-English combinations of sounds is dictated, good spellers do far better when the nonsense syllables contain phonetically acceptable combinations. Good spellers, in other words, have internalized certain phonological rules and have acquired a degree of sensitivity for those combinations of sounds that the permissible in their mother language. They know clearly, for instance, that *pf* is not acceptable in English, while *pl* is.

Disabilities in spelling can be predicted from disorganized, cluttered speech. The clutterer's rushed, monotonous, jumbled verbal output, (de Hirsch 1964) with his telescoping of words, his tendency to transpose sounds and syllables, and his neglect of phonetic detail (Masland 1967–68), all of which reflect poor auditory discrimination and memory, are closely mirrored by his messy handwriting, his misspellings, and his disorganized compositions. In other words, poor spellers write the way they sound; both reveal an inability to retain sharply outlined verbal configurations.

Instability, Bender (1966a) says, is the characteristic feature of maturational dysfunctions, which Zangwill (1962) feels are genetically determined. While the immature six-year-old children described earlier may evidence a transient delay in maturation, the dysfunction in older children who fail in reading and in related language skills may be so severe that it amounts to a maturational defect.

Some youngsters do not suffer from perceptual deficits, they have learned to decode efficiently, and have mastered the mechanics of the reading process, but they fall down when it comes to reading comprehension by the time they are in the third grade. Such difficulties invariably go back to early trouble with the processing of oral language

and point to the necessity of remedying gaps in linguistic processing before children are exposed to formal education.

Children who have difficulties in comprehension do not form anticipatory schemata of what a sentence is about to say.[2] They are miserable guessers. They have difficulty in drawing inferences, constructing hypotheses, and shifting frames of reference. They often have trouble with metaphors and their definitions of proverbs are abysmally concrete. They manage mathematical symbols but fail when problems are couched in verbal terms. At higher levels they find it difficult to explain the difference between *idleness* and *laziness* on the Stanford Binet test. They are good at recognizing pictorial absurdities, but they often miss the point of a sophisticated joke. Boys of this kind will say, "Yes, I do read but I don't get it," and in the end they just look at the page and think of something interesting, for instance, how to construct a device for catching hijackers on an airplane. Such speculations understandably are much more attractive than the unscrambling of verbal constructions on a page; much of the time such youngsters merely go through the motions. Most of them cannot tell a halfway complex story. While they clearly know what they want to say, they are unable to bring out the salient points. Their excessive use of pronouns makes it impossible to figure out who did what to whom. Some youngsters manage when they dictate their compositions but have great difficulty in putting them down on paper. Apart from their trouble with formal aspects, such as punctuation and capitalization, their output is barren, the essential information does not stand out, and supportive details are lacking. I have seen numbers of such children stare at the blank page in despair. By the time we see them, there often is a phobic quality to their inability to express ideas in writing.

The differential diagnosis of learning disability is much more difficult in older than in younger children. Soft neurological signs tend to disappear in adolescence, although careful clinical investigation may reveal telltale signs of earlier instability of the central nervous system. Maturation may have modified some of the original deficiencies. At the same time, the child's catastrophic scholastic history, with its damaging effect on his self-image and the resulting stresses and strains in the family, have usually exacerbated earlier conflicts and the diagnostic label "psychiatric disturbance" is applied legitimately,

---

[2]Lieberman et al. (1967) found that normal children can hear 15 phonemes per second but that they take in as many as 30 because they anticipate those that will fit into what follows. Something of the kind assuredly happens in reading. The reader forms anticipatory sentence schemata that help him to guess successfully at the available options.

often, however, without taking specific disabilities into account. On the other side of the fence, the label "learning disorder" may be insisted on while phobic attitudes and important ego impairment, going way back, are denied.

Take two adolescents; both are underachievers in terms of their superior intellectual potential (de Hirsch 1963). In the first, failure to master printed and written language has spread into other educational experiences, and by the time he is referred for treatment he has adopted an "I don't care" attitude. He has given up. Anna Freud (1936) says that in the theory of education the importance of the ego's determination to avoid pain has not been appreciated sufficiently. The first boy is not willing to expose himself to additional defeats. He is angry, defiant, and somewhat phobic, but in his case psychological difficulties are the result rather than the cause of his failure to learn. He is able to invest energy in nonacademic pursuits; thus there are areas to which he has recourse. Probably he will need not only intensive educational help from a tutor with whom he can identify, but will also need assistance with his rage and despair.

The second adolescent has not done badly in the early years at school despite a tendency to daydream. In the higher grades, however, when the demands for active involvement with learning increase, he has lagged farther and farther behind. His passivity, his inability to identify, his difficulties in investing affect in either subject matter or human models, in other words, impaired ego functioning, is the cause and not the result of his learning failure.

In calling a child dyslexic we must make certain that we are not dealing with a brain-injured child, or with one who presents a primary emotional disturbance, or with a deprived child. Symmes and Rapoport (1972) used an uncontaminated group of children who, they felt, presented dyslexia in pure form. They found two outstanding traits: difficulties with verbal sequencing and familial occurrence. The latter factor is impressive and confirms not only the findings of Orton (1930) and his pupiils and those of most Scandinavian workers (Hallgren 1950) but also the recent investigations by Owen et al. (1971), who tested siblings and parents of children with reading difficulties.

What happens to dyslexic children in their later careers in school and college? Many compensate for their difficulty in reading but continue to have a hard time with spelling and writing. Much depends on the support which they obtain from home, on the kind of remedial help they have received, on their cognitive endowment, their ego strength, and their willingness to work. Many manage because, in contrast to youngsters with psychogenic difficulties in learning, they become interested in other areas: science or mathematics, baseball, or some hobby. They are fortunate if they have superior gifts in the nonverbal areas and if they possess a powerful drive toward mastery. Among successful surgeons and engineers there are quite a few dyslexics.

Learning Disorders Related to Environmental Deprivation

There remains a fourth group of children whose massive difficulties in learning are based primarily on environmental deprivation. Birch (1972) pointed out that their physical health and intellectual potential are at risk even before birth and that their failure is virtually foreordained. Malnourishment, illness, and poverty going back for two or three generations result in reproductive risks that may mimic poor genetic endowment. It may be worthwhile to mention that among preschool children anemia rates as high as 80 percent were reported from Alabama and Mississippi (Merrimann 1966).

In the discussion of learning failure among deprived children, moreover, the prevalence of subtle or not-so-subtle neurological deficits is stressed insufficiently. Kappelman (1970) found that varying degrees of such deficits are the main cause of reading failure in more than half the urban children. Not only is the incidence of prematurity in the slums, for instance, 17 percent as against 7 percent in the middle class, but the resulting physiological deficits are bound up inextricably with the life experiences of these children. Deprived youngsters who have neurological dysfunctions compensate far less effectively for their lag than do their middle-class peers, since they lack the nurture, both in the literal and the figurative sense, to make up for their physiological vulnerability.

Deprived children are not necessarily understimulated. On the contrary, they are often swamped at an early age by an array of stimuli which they are entirely unable to sort out. These children live in a continually shifting world. The pervasive instinctualization of the milieu, the crude sexual stimulation to which they are often exposed, the absence of stable love objects, and lack of models for identification do not help these children to curb impulsivity, to delay gratification, or to sustain effort. In other words, they receive no assistance in developing ego functions that are essential for learning.

Some environments are not oriented toward achievement, but it should be added that this orientation is not solely a matter of social class. Among three-year-old Puerto Rican and white American children from middle-class backgrounds, Hertiz (1968) suggests that in the former group the emphasis was on social relations rather than on achievement. Steward and Steward (1973) found that children from a variety of ethnic groups are exposed to different early learning environments and to different standards of performance before they enter school. This tends to result in different skills and expectations brought by the children into the classroom. Their value systems differ according to social and ethnic background. The middle-class tendency to look at the world in terms of a temporal succession of events does not necessarily prevail in all sections of society. Leshan (1952) said that temporal orientation varies with social class, perhaps because deprived individuals have no future literally and figuratively. However, goal-oriented behavior and a stake in achievement are closely linked to the ordering of life in terms of temporal sequences. Learning requires the sacrifice of present gratification for the attainment of a distant goal.

Attitudes toward achievement are laid down in infancy and are mediated through the social group in which the child lives. Children are exposed to distinct patterns of learning long before they start their formal education. Years before they enter school, children must have mastered the basic phonological and syntactical rules of their language. Linguistic deficits are especially glaring in deprived youngsters. Their frequent difficulties in processing complex verbal input, their restricted choice of syntactical options, and their limited ability to shift frames of reference are massive obstacles to academic performance, which is concerned primarily with the manipulation of verbal symbols. The meaning of deprivation, Hess and Shipman (1965) say, is the deprivation of meaning.

It is, of course, essential not to confuse linguistic differences with linguistic deficits (Cazden 1966a). We have no right to apply developmental norms standardized on English-speaking, middle-class children to youngsters who use nonstandard dialects or have a foreign-language background. Houston (1970) maintains that nonfluency, foreshortened utterances, simplified syntax, and one-word responses to questions occur in situations in which deprived children interact with adults outside their own culture. Their communication with friends and family is characterized by greater ease and fluency. This may be true, but is also true that disadvantaged children do not exploit the full potential of language, perhaps also because childrearing practices are usually authoritarian; children are told to carry out orders and there is relatively little discussion, exploration, or ventilation of issue or feelings. It has been said that at the age of five disadvantaged children are one or two years retarded linguistically (Jervchimowitz, Costello, and Bagur 1971). Training in language almost always comes too late. Our experience has shown that training is far more successful at the age of three than at four or five. This applies especially to delay in the processing of linguistic input. At the age of five many children who enter school have learned *not* to listen.

In view of all of this, it is impressive that many deprived children *do* learn. The deprived are, of course, not a homogeneous group. And among the mothers there are those whose "teaching style" to use Hess's expression, is extraordinarily effective. This teaching style heavily influences linguistic development and orientation toward tasks. In fortunate cases, there is a gifted teacher whose attitude toward black dialect is positive, who encourages the child to communicate in his code while exposing him to her own, a teacher who is not easily frustrated or shocked, above all, a teacher who does not feel guilty or scared.

The interactions among race, sex, socioeconomic condition, and adequacy of teaching are extremely complex. It is often helpful to ask what a youngster would look like without the organic dysfunction; how, given the dysfunction, he would manage if he had been embedded in a nurturing environment. It is interesting to speculate about his genetic endowment, his vulnerability to stress, his ego strength, and his drive toward growth. Such speculations may help one to look at the interaction of forces that shape the individual learner (Weil 1970).

We now see a succession of deprived young children destined to fail at school. At the age of four they are referred to a specialist because of failure to speak. They probably have subtle neurological damage; they are neglected, overwhelmed, and exposed to frightening situations. They lack a stable framework to which they might relate, and they are expected to decode and encode in two different linguistic systems, although they cannot cope with either.

To sum up: A child's learning disability may be psychogenic, neurogenic, based on developmental language disorders, or related to environmental causes. It is in no way helpful to describe the deficiencies of a child without taking into account significant compensatory and adaptational resources. Diagnostic labels are artificial at best. In reality we deal with a large variety of forces that interact in complex ways. Hence different interventional and therapeutic approaches are needed for every single child.

Specific Dyslexia or Strephosymbolia

It was Kussmaul who as far back as 1877 first used the term *word blindness* to describe patients who although not blind were yet unable to read letters or words. *Coecitas syllabaris et verbalis* is, according to Kussmaul, the result of disease or lesion in the left angular gyrus in right-handed people and can be met with as an isolated condition even in cases where the powers of speech are preserved.

Badal (1886) in Paris and a number of British ophthalmologists and school physicians—among them Hinshelwood (1895a,b, 1896 a,b, 1898) Kerr (1897), and Nettleship (1905)—became interested in the symptom, and in 1896 Pringle Morgan reported the first case of congenital word blindness. The patient was a fourteen-year-old intelligent lad who read numbers fluently but could not recognize printed words no matter how often they were presented to him, and in spite of the fact that his memory and his understanding of auditory material were good. In 1900 Hinshelwood analyzed and published two cases of congential word blindness. A little later he and Fisher (1905) drew attention to the fact that the condition is frequently encountered in given families. It was also recognized that congential word blindness is observed more frequently in boys than in girls, and some authors thought it likely that a number of children were diagnosed as feeble-minded who actually were suffering from this condition. As early as 1908 Thomas commented on the tendency of these children to transpose letters and syllables. He discussed the relative merits of different teaching methods: phonics versus whole word techniques.

All interested authors followed Hinshelwood (1904) in his assumption that congential word blindness is the result of a congenital deficiency in or faulty development of the visual centers located in the left angular gyrus, and up to 1924 these theories dominated medical thinking on the subject.

In 1924 and 1925 Apert (1924) in Paris and above all Orton (1925) in the United States reviewed the problem. Orton rejected Hin-

Reprinted with permission from S. Karger, from *Folia Phoniatrica* 4:231–248. 1952.

shelwood's theory that congenital word blindness is based on focal agenesis. Orton maintained that in reading disabilities we deal with a physiological variant and thus opened the way for new theoretical insights and therapeutic procedures. These are still under discussion.

Although the statistics on reading difficulties in this country vary, most people agree that from 8 to 14 percent of all school children—more than three times as many boys as girls—have difficulties in mastering the printed word. This is not really surprising when one considers that reading is one of the most abstract forms of learning. Activities, feelings, and experience come first. Spoken words, the arbitrary phonetic symbols for such experiences, come next. Through auditory pathways the child stores up the meaning of an increasingly large number of words. In a relatively short period he organizes an enormous system of auditory symbols into the pattern of language.

When he subsequently enters school he has numberless new adjustments to make, new patterns of behavior to work out, new values to accept; and on top of it all, having only recently mastered auditory symbols, he is exposed to a secondary set of visual symbols still further removed from concrete experience.

Learning to read requires the formation of new associations between the printed letter and the sound it represents. Reading, according to Orton (1928b) calls for "a new set of reflexes between visual and auditory spheres on the associative level of cerebral elaboration." The child is asked to respond in an organized way to visual signs. In order to read a little word like *mat* a sequence of sounds heard—a sequence in time—has to be translated into a sequence of letters seen—a sequence in space. A visual image has to be correlated with oral language. Inability to form such associations or their blocking is at the root of every reading difficulty (Bachman 1927).

Reading disabilities are frequently confounded with learning disabilities, and as a result theoretical thinking as well as therapeutic procedures suffer.

A learning disability, as distinct from a reading difficulty, may have at its root a number of causes. It might be the result of inferior intelligence. Obviously a dull youngster will have trouble with reading, but he will have trouble with other subjects as well. Such a child's reading disability is, therefore, of a secondary nature. It is nonspecific.

Emotional disturbance may lie at the bottom of a learning disability. There is the youngster who lives in a fantasy world of his own and does poorly at school because he has little psychic energy left to meet academic requirements. There is the child who in all of his behavior reveals that he does not really want to grow up, for whom the world of adults is terrifying and dangerous, and who will not try to learn because he feels safer at the more infantile level. There is the youngster who is too hostile to learn and resists passively because he knows no other way to express hostility. There is the boy whose obsessive behavior blocks his performance; he cannot read primarily because he sticks to single words so compulsively that he cannot take his cues from context.

Learning means reaching out (Liss 1950). Many a youngster is too fearful to reach out. At some time or other in the past the acquisition of some vital bit of knowledge has proved too distressing. Curiosity may have been inhibited when the child was very young. Passivity might have served his particular psychological needs better. A child of this type in all probability represents a learning and not a reading disability. The chances are that he will do poorly in all subjects, not in reading only; his difficulties with reading are of a secondary nature. They are nonspecific.

A secondary reading difficulty might be the result of a variety of causes: physical illness, poor teaching, frequent change of schools, environmental pathology. None of these should be confused with the primary variety of the disorder.

The educational profile of primary dyslexia is shown in Figure 1 (Monroe 1928).

It reveals an arresting discrepancy between the youngster's reasoning ability, his intellectual endowment, his performance in arithmetic on the one hand and on the other his performance in reading, spelling, and English composition.

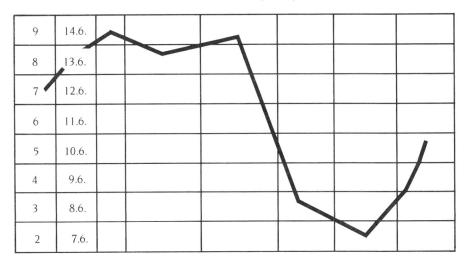

Figure 1

It is easy to see where the confusion between learning and reading difficulty arises. A youngster who has consistently failed in reading is apt to turn into a learning disability for two reasons: in the first place, reading becomes more important as the child progresses through the grades; being unable to read, he is bound to fail in social studies and other subjects as well; in the second place, the youngster is liable to develop secondary emotional difficulties because of his inability to meet his own and his parents' expectations. Failure in reading extends to other learning experiences, and by the time the youngster is in the fourth grade, he may have begun to bite his nails and may have become restless, aggressive, and difficult to handle. Or he may have become depressed and discouraged. In the best of circumstances and even when there is little or no parental pressure he is likely to be a confused child.

But the youngster who suffers from specific dyslexia, the child Orton calls strephosymbolic, is, theoretically at least, bright and reasonably well adjusted. He is the one who runs into trouble when he is first exposed to the printed word.

What we call reading readiness (Gates 1936) in the six-year-old is probably a fairly complex phenomenon that has both maturational and constitutional aspects. It is significant that children who have, at least grossly, the same intelligence quotient vary strikingly in their ability to cope with both oral and printed symbols. It goes without saying, yet it is easily overlooked, that the same overall IQ in two different individuals may have an entirely different significance in terms of qualitative performance. One youngster will start talking at fifteen months, while another who seems just as bright—may be bright only in a more concrete sense—does not start before he is over two years old. One boy might be ready for reading at five, while another who is good at almost everything else is not ready till he is seven.

There is, however, an impressive feature about specific dyslexia. When we investigate the family history of the children who have severe difficulties of this kind, we find in seven cases out of ten evidence of what Weiss (1950) calls "central imbalance" in the language area. We may find one sibling who was late in starting to talk, another who has a severe lisp, an uncle who is a clutterer, a father who himself has trouble with reading and spelling. It is Orton (1930) who first drew our attention to the familial constitutional chararacter of language disorder.

The *Acta Psychiatrica et Neurologica* published in 1950 an interesting study on congenital word blindness done in Sweden. Hallgren took his material from the Child Guidance Clinic in Stockholm and from a secondary school which has special classes for intelligent dyslexic children. He investigated all parents and siblings in his group as to past and present performance in reading, writing, and spelling. His results were striking: in 88 percent of his cases one or several members of the immediate family had a history of dyslexia or were still suffering from the same difficulty. The author subjected his group to a genetic statistical analysis, and he believes that specific dyslexia follows "a dominant autosomal monohybrid mode of inheritance." Whether Hallgren's material is statistically large enough to permit of such detailed conclusions is open to question. However, it is quite evident that a very careful family history of language functions is important in the case of all children suffering from reading disabilities, and it is desirable that such a history include not only performance in reading and spelling but ability to handle all types of verbal symbols—spoken, written, or printed.

Reading difficulties range in degree from the extreme to the relatively slight. Occasionally we meet some which closely approximate those seen in individuals with verifiable brain lesions. While in the brain-injured patient dyslexia is usually only one feature of a more generalized condition, we have so far assumed that developmental reading disabilities occur as an isolated syndrome. This assumption is based on the fact that many of our youngsters do not show gross deviations in the receptive and expressive aspects of oral language, that they often do well on the standard psychological tests, and that the classical neurological examination, which tests gross functions only, does not reveal any deviations.

Only when one observes severely strephosymbolic youngsters over a period of time does one discover that their emotional, their motor, and their perceptual behavior falls into a distinct pattern. It is this pattern which I wish now to consider.

In the examination of these children we start, of course, with a check on their sensory equipment. Obviously, any significant hearing loss will interfere with reading if only for the reason that the child's oral language is deficient. However, a great many strephosymbolic youngsters who have perfectly adequate hearing fail to differentiate between finer shades of sound in the same way as do speech-defective children. Many dyslalic and dyslexic youngsters have strikingly short auditory memory spans. Occasionally their sense of rhythm is inferior. In testing a number of youngsters I found that they do very poorly indeed when required to imitate a tapped-out sequence. The question whether in such instances we are dealing with an auditory phenomenon at all will be discussed later.

Comparable difficulties are sometimes encountered in visual perception or recall. Many of our strephosymbolic youngsters, in spite of excellent visual acuity, have difficulty in recalling small visual details and in reproducing spatial configurations.

Since the question of vision arises whenever reading disabilities are considered, I would like to refer to Orton's (1943) and Tinker's

(1936) publications on the subject and the 1940 report of the ophthalmological section of the Los Angeles County Medical Association, which states:

> If visual acuity is reduced 50 percent or more the child will have trouble with interpretation of symbols he cannot see well. Except in farsightedness of a marked degree the child's power of focusing is sufficient to give adequate though not perfect vision. A small amount of myopia might be an advantage rather than a disadvantage. Crossed eye with normal vision in one eye has no special value when looking at a flat surface. Compensated muscle balance such as phorias of a marked degree do not affect interpretation of symbols. But effort expended to see binocularly discourages reading.
>
> Eye muscle coordination is a function of vision, vision is not a function of eye muscle coordination. So-called faulty eye movements as judged by regressions depend primarily on poor understanding of subject matter, not on incoordinated eye muscles. Not the eye, but the brain learns to read.

In order to determine whether or not a child suffers from specific dyslexia we need a base line. An intensive psychological study of the child is *sine qua non*. Such a study should give us information not only about the youngster's intellectual potential but also about the way he uses his capacities. A qualitative analysis of his performance in several areas is essential.

Children with severe language disabilities may do significantly better on the performance section of a given test than they do in the verbal area. Such discrepancies are often striking, but they need further elaboration. It is important to know on which subtests the youngster does poorly. Weak performance on the section which tests ability to give abstract defintions, for instance, would mean quite a different thing from inferior memory for digits.

Projective techniques are essential because they help in the differentiation between a learning and a reading disability.

We also need an evaluation of the youngster's motor capacity. Some of our children have a history of delay in neuromotor development and are reported to have been slow in walking, running, hopping, and skipping. Others do very well with large muscle groups but fall down when it comes to finer muscular coordination. Orton (1932) has shown how frequently we find dyspraxic features in the speech-defective and strephosymbolic child. Kopp (1943), who used Oseretsky (1931) tests (he estimated the motor age of his children and compared it with their chronological age), has confirmed Orton's findings. Our children with severe graphic difficulties belong in this dyspraxic group (Orton and Gillingham 1933).

Dyslexic children seen at the Pediatric Language Disorder Clinic are given a Bender Gestalt test (Bender 1938) which requires the child to reproduce a series of geometric figures. Deviations on this test reveal specific lags in visuomotor performance, and a study done at Bellevue Hospital has proved not only that severely dyslexic children show a tendency to verticalization and difficulty with angulation, but also that their maturational level on this test is substantially below their chronological age. These results have been confirmed by our testing, and it would be of interest to investigate whether the same findings are true for children who have difficulties with oral speech.

A Goodenough test (Goodenough 1926) is desirable. Bender (1951) feels that this test can be used not only as a measure of intelligence or as a projective technique but also to reveal the individual's specific apperception of his body image. A significant discrepancy in maturation between the Goodenough and other tests, as we find it so frequently in youngsters with severe disturbances in the language area, would indicate not only poor eye-hand coordination, difficulty with three-dimensional space, and defective manual skill, but also an immature body image.

There is another aspect in the study of these children which has hardly been touched. Werner and Strauss (1941) have found disturbances in figure-background relationships in the case of brain-injured youngsters and they have devised a number of tests—the Klapp Marble Board test above all—which reveal deficiencies in this area. Goldstein (1939) has conceived of foreground-background configurations as one of the fundamental principles of neurophysiological organization. If we study children with severe disabilities in the language area, we find extreme difficulties above all with sequence building, with auditory sequences in the case of the dyslalic child, with visual sequences in the case of the dyslexic one, and, as Orton has pointed out (1937), with the organization of movements in the case of the dyspraxic youngster. We should, therefore, ask ourselves whether this difficulty with structuralization of sequences is not related to a more basic disturbance in figure-background relationships. In the imitation of tapped patterns, for instance, the youngster has to pick out a figure from a background and recognize and reconstruct a specific configuration. Failure to accomplish this may be indicative not so much of an auditory deficiency as of a more fundamental one in the organization of a gestalt.

Another area is of interest: Goldstein (1939) in his work on the aphasic individual has shown that difficulty with language, spoken or printed, is closely related to limitations in abstract behavior. The

Goldstein-Scheerer test, (Goldstein-Scheerer 1941) specifically designed to bring out differences in concrete and abstract performance,
would be of great interest in the case of our children, since some of our
more dramatic cases seem to have trouble with categorical behavior.
Categorical behavior, Scheerer (1944) suggests, is essential for functioning on the highly symbolic level requisite for the use of language.

So much for general testing. In the more specific area we need all
possible information pertaining to the youngster's oral langauge: its
receptive as well as its expressive aspect. Borel-Maisonny (1951b) has
described some of her testing in *Folia Phoniatrica,* and other authors
also have stressed the importance of such investigations (Mottier
1951). Are we sure that the dyslexic child always understands fairly
complex spoken material? Many youngsters with a mild residual word
deafness are not discovered until they turn up with a reading disability. Gaps in the receptive aspect of language are frequently overlooked, while expressive deficiencies, which are easier to spot, are
rarely neglected. Chess (1944) mentions reading and writing disabilities in her group of sensory aphasias. Expressive speech disorders in
dyslexic children are observed very frequently. They not only embrace
difficulties with motor speech patterns, limited vocabulary, and
trouble with word finding and grammatical construction, but include
also the entire groups of speech disorders we call cluttering (Weiss
1950). In the Pediatric Lanaguage Disorder Clinic we can predict at
least 30 to 35 percent of future reading disabilities among the youngsters who are referred at the age of three, four, and five because of
motor speech delay or dyslalia.

Laterality is another factor of importance. Many of our speech-
defective and strephosymbolic children are late in establishing a functional superiority of one hand over the other—substantially later than
other children, that is, since establishing such superiority is also a
matter of maturation. Orton (1937) relates this delay and also the
tendency of some of our youngsters to mirror reading and writing to
the individual's failure to establish a physiological habit of working
exclusively from engrams of the dominant hemisphere. His observations concerning their difficulties with left-to-right progression,
essential for reading at least in our culture, are certainly borne out for
the majority of strephosymbolic children. In learning to read the
youngster has to establish a specific directional discipline, and our
dsylexic children fall down in this respect. They have a marked tendency to static and kinetic reversals—they read *b* for *d*, *p* for *q*, and *was*
for *saw*. One can observe their difficulties with spatial relationships
even in their drawings. Some youngsters not only confuse left and
right but also up and down; for instance, they write *m* for *w*. Some
transpose not only letters but also numbers.

Whenever we are confronted with a dyslexic child we need as a matter of course to inquire into his academic experience. Did he encounter difficulties in the first transition from home to school? Did he like his first classroom teacher? Was he emotionally very immature? Did he always do substantially better in arithmetic than in reading or spelling? For only if his performance in reading and spelling is out of harmony with his performance in other academic areas are we entitled to say that he suffers from specific dyslexia.

Has the youngster changed schools too frequently? What about parental attitudes? Are standards at home excessively high? Above all, which are the teaching techniques which have failed so far? Has the child been taught by the old-fashioned spelling method? Has he been taught by the progressive "look and say" technique? The picture of a rose is pasted on the blackboard and the word *rose* printed underneath. Repeated exposure to this gestalt will help the majority of youngsters to remember the word as a whole. Some do quite well with a word like *rose* but not so well with a configuration like *redistribution*. For about 10 percent of the children who have trouble with the organization of visual patterns this method does not work at all; it is, as a matter of fact, one of the causes of their difficulty (Fabian 1951).

We need to analyze carefully where the trouble lies for the strephosymbolic child, so as to provide him with the links he has failed to establish; we must utilize the discriminations he is able to make and employ all sensory channels available for reinforcement associations. As in the re-education of aphasics we have to provide secondary kinesthetic, auditory, and visual bonds and choose nervous pathways according to the child's particular psychological type (Bachman 1927). Since every individual recognizes printed symbols in different ways, different methods may have to be used with different individuals. The child who has trouble correlating visual images with meaning because his visual recall is poor has to capitalize on his auditory competence (Gillingham 1946). For him words are broken up into their smallest phonetic units. The units *m-a-t* in the word *mat* are taught him one by one and the youngster later learns how to blend them into words, finding out in this way what it is the word "says." This is of major importance in spelling, generally a greater hurdle than reading. If the child's word picture is not exact enough to serve as a basis for recognition in reading, it will certainly not be precise enough to serve as a basis for the reproduction required in spelling (Orton 1931). The youngster with a spelling difficulty needs phonics more than others do. Since he is confused as to spatial sequences and reads *from* for *form*, it will help him if he can rely on a temporal sequence by sounding out the word. To most strephosymbolic youngsters, phonetic techniques provide a feeling of mastery and security where in the past they have relied on guessing only.

For some children auditory and visual stimuli need to be reinforced by kinesthetic ones. We make use of movement in order to fix the association between the sound and the properly oriented letter form. Children are made to *feel* letters; we make them out of sandpaper and plywood; they are made to trace them both in the air and on paper. The use of motor response serves as secondary link. Moving the finger from left to right while the voice slides simultaneously from one sound to the other helps in blending and in synthesizing sound components into an organized whole.

Obviously not all English words can be taught in this way. A good many of them have to be taught by sight. Moreover, we occasionally come upon a youngster who does not respond to either the phonetic or the kinesthetic approach or a combination of both.

One severely dyslexic boy we have worked with exhibits in a dramatic way certain of the features which are typical for the strephosymbolic child.

Billy was eight years old when first seen. He rated an intelligence quotient of 103 on the Stanford Binet, but the examiner felt at the time that this was a minimal estimate and that his potential was at least high average. In reasoning and arithmetical concepts he scored considerably above his chronological age. Billy's hearing was adequate, but his auditory recall was strikingly poor. His Bender Gestalt was very inferior, as was his ability to reproduce any kind of visual perceptual pattern.

Family history revealed that both Billy's father and his second sister were slow readers and very poor spellers. The father incidentally was ambidexterous. One sister was left-handed. There was left-handedness also on the maternal side of the family. Billy himself used his right hand practically exclusively. He was right-footed; eye dominance was inconsistent.

Although the child sat up and walked at the appropriate time, speech development was substantially delayed. He had shown little of the babbling activities usually observed in infants, and he was nearly three years old before he used an appreciable number of words. Sentences appeared quite late. At the time he was first seen he understood fairly complex spoken material, but talked in short sentences only. His speech was muffled and indistinct, and he was unable to concoct a story from a number of pictures I showed him. It is of interest to add that he had difficulty with what Goldstein calls "abstract behavior" and even now at the age of eleven failed to give me the category "vegetable" when I showed him a cauliflower, a tomato, and a lettuce or to give me the category "tools" when he was presented with the pictures of a saw, a hammer, and a nail.

The boy was extremely hyperkinetic and constantly in motion. He was also very clumsy in his finer muscular coordination.

Billy had repeated first grade and was entering the third when he first came to the clinic. He developed a number of somatic symptoms every time he went back to school after the holidays, all of which invariably cleared up during the vacation months.

When he was first seen he did not know all the letters of the alphabet and knew none of the sound equivalents for the letters. When writing down the few letters he did now, he wrote most of them in the reversed direction. He did the same thing with numbers, but he added and subtracted nicely. He guessed wildly when whole words were exposed.

For training purposes we began with the phonetic approach. However, after several weeks it became apparent that the boy was, and still is, totally unable to remember the sound equivalent of printed symbols. He apparently hears words as only vaguely structuralized and incompletely organized auditory sequences and simply cannot isolate their components. Goldstein and Scheerer (1941), in their monograph, Abstract and Concrete Behavior, suggest that the ability to break up a given whole into its parts and the synthesizing of these parts are features of abstract performance. Some of their brain-injured patients were able to recognize words as wholes but could not name the letters of which they were made up. This is true for Billy. Not only is he practically unable to isolate sounds but also he cannot blend them once they are presented separately. Having assimilated the word *am* he does not see that it contains the sounds *a* and *m*. Bachmann (1927) also has commented on the difficulty which some of his patients have in isolating word elements.

Billy actually fails to grasp the underlying concept that a letter, a printed symbol, represents a heard speech sound. He does a little better with the gestalt approach (although he has enormous difficulties with this technique as well), and in this way he has learned a number of words. His associations, however, are quite unstable, and he tends to lose a word like *you* even after he has recognized it many times before. Like an aphasic he will have a hazy idea as to the general area to which a word belongs and for instance will read *father* for *mother* although the words do not at all look alike.

Billy tends to exhibit what Goldstein calls "catastrophic behavior" (1948), a total disorganization of response in the organism faced with a task which it is unable to tackle.

After working with Billy for a few months we were of course wondering whether or not we were really dealing with a genuine dyslexia and referred the boy for an electroencephalogram and a neurological evaluation. The former was technically unsatisfactory because of the boy's hyperkinetic behavior. The neurological report reads: "An anxious boy with a short attention span and poorly patterned behavior. No neurological signs, all findings within normal limits. In view of his hyperactivity he should be seen in Psychiatric Clinic."

Most children with severe language disabilities are hyperactive. Not unlike brain-injured youngsters, they are, as Strauss and Lehtinen (1948) have shown, distractable, uninhibited, and disorganized. Billy was no exception. He more or less conformed at school, but he was wild and uncontrollable at home. His mother complained, "He never sits still; he gets into everything." The question then arose whether Billy's motor restlessness was an outgrowth of pressures and tensions, whether a severe anxiety was blocking his performance, and whether his inability to read and his hyperactivity were manifestations of the same severely neurotic pattern. Billy's Rorschach, though it showed difficulty with control and overly impulsive behavior, was not that of a profoundly disturbed child. Nor did the psychiatrist who worked with him for a couple of months uncover any real psychopathology. It is true that Billy benefited from psychotherapy in a general way. Up to a point he accepted himself and his handicap better than he had done before. Treatment, however, did not improve his reading performance nor his disorganized motor behavior.

Even before they have built up a neurotic superstructure, these youngsters (and this is true also for those who suffer from other types of language disability) show a specific kind of motility. To the clinical observer there is somehow a definite feel to the motor restlessness of dyslexic, dyslalic, and cluttering children. It is not quite like that of the neurotic child; it has, as Bender calls it, in the strephosymbolic young-ster an *organic flavor* and resembles the *organic* brain *driveness* we find in some brain-injured youngsters (Thomson 1947).

Very few cases are as severe as Billy's. The majority can be helped. The first step toward such help is to give both parent and child a clear simple explanation of the nature of the difficulty. If we can make them appreciate that they are not alone, that there are scores of other youngsters, neither stupid nor lazy, who have the same kind of trouble, then we have succeeded in laying the foundation for later remedial work.

Motivation of the child is the next step. Such motivation must be strong enough to overcome indifference and antagonism. Choice of the right teaching materials is important. It is obviously foolish to give a bright thirteen-year-old a primer to read. We must present him with exciting and meaningful material that he can handle technically. Help-ing a child face the fact that he has difficulty in school, dissipating anxiety stemming from the experience of failure, combating attitudes of defeat are important parts of this work. Needless to say that, as in all remedial work, a strong transference from pupil to teacher is absolutely essential. If the transference is good enough, then a variety of technical approaches can produce good results.

This does not mean that the large majority of dyslexias are psychogenic in origin, a statement we find in some of the psychiatric literature of today. Blanchard (1946), in her psychoanalytical contribution to the problem of reading disabilities, states that such problems are the results of severe limitations in instinctual drives and closely related to earlier forbidden peeping activities. Reversals, according to her, represent the symbolic expression of hostility and aggression, and reading content is associated directly and symbolically with unconscious emotional conflict. Fabian (1951) feels that reading disabilities are fundamental ego disabilities and a symptom of individual and familial psychopathology. Gann (1945) reports that poor readers are fearful of emotionally challenging situations. None of these authors, however, have accounted for the discrepancies between the reading performance of these children and their achievement, for instance, in arithmetic. It seems likely that some of them have confused learning with reading disabilities, secondary with primary dyslexia. Undoubtedly there does exist a large group of youngsters whose difficulty with reading is entirely on an emotional basis and part and parcel of their learning inhibition. There are, moreover, hundreds of youngsters who have a language difficulty and suffer from a psychological disturbance as well, children who require help in both areas.

Many of our strephosymbolic children are, of course, emotionally upset. It would be strange indeed if they were not. However, in a large number of these cases this disturbance is the direct result of conflict stemming from environmental repercussion.

In this country excellent work has been done in the area of reading disabilities, but the emphasis, except for Orton, has been on the psychiatric and educational rather than on the neurological and developmental aspect. However, in 1950 Archie Silver, going back to earlier studies done by Schilder and Bender in 1935, investigated neurological and perceptual deviations of fifty severely dyslexic children. Their intelligence rating ranged from 81 to 123, and none showed any significant findings on the classical neurological examination. When Silver (1951) studied the posture, motility, and tonus of these children more closely, he found that they showed a persistence of earlier patterns such as are generally found in much younger children. He found a tendency to whirl along a longitudinal axis which mostly disappears in children over five. Their postural reflexes were less well organized, more primitive, and more plastic than could be expected at their age. Laterality was mixed in the large majority of cases. Electroencephalograms showed dysrhythmia, slow waves indicating immaturity rather than pathology, in all but three cases. The Goodenough revealed difficulty with body image. Many of the youngsters were unable to name their fingers, a competence generally attained around the age of eight. Visual perception as tested by the Bender Gestalt was inferior. Testing with the Marble Board showed specific difficulty in figure-background relationships.

One can conclude from these studies that severely dyslexic youngsters show immaturity in neurophysiological, in motor, in perceptual, and in conceptual behavior. They show, in fact, a developmental lag which is reflected in their failure to cope with as complex a function as is the interpretation of printed symbols. This immaturity, moreover, is noticeable also in their striking lack of integration in social and emotional behavior. It would be of great interest to pursue this line of study in the case of dyslalic and cluttering children.

Conclusions

1.   The syndrome we call specific dyslexia or strephosymbolia is a clinical entity and should be differentiated from reading disabilities of a secondary nature which might have resulted from a variety of causes: physical illness, environmental pathology, poor teaching. Specific dyslexia, above all, should not be confused with a learning disability. In the latter, difficulties with reading are the result of a personality disturbance. It should, however, be borne in mind that a dyslexic child when not helped early enough may develop a learning inhibition.

2.   Specific dyslexia constitutes a developmental lag belonging in the general category of developmental language disturbances and as such often has significant familial aspects. Both the strephosymbolic and the speech-defective child, as well as other members of his family, frequently reveal difficulty with handling of all verbal symbols, spoken, written, or printed.

3.   Both dyslexic children and those with severe speech defects tend to show immaturity of the central nervous system. They are often clumsy and awkward in their finer muscular coordination. They are frequently late in establishing cerebral dominance and usually have trouble with organization of spatial relationships, above all with left to right progression. Their perceptual organization is sometimes primitive, their visuomotor gestalt immature. They find patterning of any kind difficult. The question is raised whether the dyslalic youngster's difficulty in imitating auditory sequences and the dyslexic youngster's trouble in interpreting visual sequences are not related to some more basic difficulty in differentiating foreground from background.

4.   A great many children with severe language disabilities are hyperkinetic, disinhibited, and somewhat disorganized. While this kind of behavior is often secondary to the basic condition, one might ask whether the difficulty of the child in organizing and patterning his

impulses is not itself one of the diagnostic signs, another indication of physiological-psychological immaturity.

5.   Treatment in specific dyslexia, like the treatment of aphasias, aims at the reinforcement of associations. To this end all nervous pathways are mobilized in order to help link the visual to the auditory structure of the word and relate both to meaning. It remains for further studies to determine whether there are special ways and means of helping a child to better structuralization and organization of perceptual patterns of all kinds.

6.   Our present-day knowledge is sufficient to clear the way for preventive work. We are undoubtedly able to pick out those youngsters in kindergarten who are liable to turn into dyslexic children. Exposing these particular youngsters to a different educational approach would eliminate much of the later-developing frustrations and disabilities.

7.   Prognosis in specific dyslexia depends on the severity of the condition, on time when training is begun, and on the intellectual and emotional development of the child. Our educational system severely penalizes the youngster who has difficulties with reading and spelling in the first three grades. It cannot be emphasized enough that early diagnosis and long-term remedial work are essential to prevent the child from becoming an educational casualty.

Gestalt Psychology as Applied to Language Disturbances

The idea that specific and basic dysfunctions are at the root of a variety of language disturbances grew out of our experience at the Language Disorder Clinic at the Columbia-Presbyterian Medical Center in New York, where we found that we were able to predict a large percentage of future dyslexias among the three-, four- and five-year-olds who had originally been referred because of speech delay or severe dyslalia.

Time and again we were confronted with the same clinical picture: a succession of bright youngsters who had been late in starting to talk and who at the age of five were practically unintelligible, whose motor speech patterns were extremely poor, whose grammar was deficient, who omitted parts of words, who condensed and reversed sequences of sounds. On closer observation we found that these children were clumsy in finer muscular coordination, that their auditory memory span was inferior, that they were hyperactive and somewhat uncontrolled. The very same youngsters were later brought back to us at the age of nine or ten because of failure to catch on to reading. They still were hyperkinetic, their auditory memory spans still were under par, they were still awkward when it came to finer muscular control. In their attempts to read, they reversed sequences of sounds, condensed and omitted parts of words in exactly the same way they used to reverse and condense auditory symbols earlier.

At first we assumed that their difficulty with the printed word was the direct result of inadequate language background, that their inability to discriminate between sounds heard accounted for their difficulty with discrimination of letters seen. This assumption, however, when further tested, proved to be valid for only a limited number of cases. The large majority of our dyslexic children had actually acquired a good oral language background, their motor speech patterns had become thoroughly acceptable by the time they were ex-

Reprinted with permission from Williams and Wilkins, from *The Journal of Nervous and Mental Disease* 120(3,4):257–261. 1954.

posed to printed material. The question then was why do a large number of formerly speech-delayed and dyslalic youngsters run into trouble when they are confronted with reading?

Orton (1937) was the first who maintained that there is a close relationship among all aspects of language function in children, that the difficulties with oral speech as manifested by the speech-delayed and dyslalic youngster and the trouble with printed language as shown by the dyslexic one are symptoms only of a generalized language disability. Borel-Maisonny (1951a) in her excellent contributions has emphasized receptive and expressive oral deficiencies in dyslexic youngsters. Weiss (1950) has recently confirmed this hypothesis when he speaks of "central language imbalance."

Starting out then from the hypothesis of such a generalized disability we asked ourselves what does "central language imbalance" actually mean? What does it involve? We believe that a closer investigation into the perceptual, motor, and emotional status of children suffering from severe language dysfunctions may shed some additional light on this question.

All our youngsters at the clinic—and for the purpose of this discussion I limit myself to those of at least average intelligence—are routinely subjected to extensive psychological examination. As a result we have found over the years that a large number of them show a distinct pattern of performance on a given series of tests. Our children sometimes rate up to twenty or thirty points higher on the performance than they do on the verbal part of a scale like the Bellevue Wechsler. Not only is their vocabulary and their information more limited than that of the control group (which could have been expected), but their ability to form abstract concepts is decidedly inferior. If tested for instance for similarities and opposites these children do poorly when compared with other youngsters of the same age. It is of interest that they perform poorly in coding as well, a task which is generally assumed to belong to what is called concrete performance. Coding, however, requires handling of symbols and it seems that in these children all types of symbols, not only verbal ones, present difficulties. Goldstein's (1939) work on disturbances of symbolic behavior in the brain-injured individual is of interest in this context. Again, as a rule, these children score below expectation in finer muscular coordination. Bender and Yarnell (1941) have commented on motility disturbances in children suffering from language disabilities, and Orton (1933) is undoubtedly right when he says that we frequently find dyspraxic individuals—among them those with severe difficulties in penmanship—in the speech defective and dyslexic group. Oseretsky's (1931) investigations point in the same direction.

Another characteristic of our particular group is confusion in motor leads. Establishing a functional superiority of one side over the other is, of course, also a matter of maturation and is seldom firmly achieved before the ages of three or four. However, our youngsters do not generally show a clear cut superiority till much later and in the dyslexic group, which ranges from seven years upward, we find ample evidence of crossed laterality, residual ambidexterity, and difficulty with establishing left-to-right progression, the specific directional discipline essential to reading in our culture.

There are other areas in which our children deviate:

The Bender Gestalt test (1938), which evaluates visuomotor functioning, reveals a striking immaturity of gestalt functioning in dyslexic youngsters. This has been demonstrated in a study made on fifty cases at Bellevue Hospital in New York City. Our own investigations confirm these observations for dyslalic and speech delayed children. Their motor gestalten also are extremely primitive. Not only do they show a tendency to verticalization, a typical phenomenon in chronologically younger children, but they also have great difficulties when asked to copy interlocking figures. They seem to have trouble synthesizing configurations and show what Goldstein (1953) calls "concreteness in motor performance." Their ability to experience gestalten in terms of spatial and temporal relationships is undoubtedly under par.

The Goodenough (1926) test is well known as a measure for evaluating intelligence. Galiferet-Granjou (1951) uses it for grading ability to organize spatial relationships and finds that dyslexic children, are on the average, two years and seven months retarded when compared with a control group. We use this test in our speech-defective group not only for determining hand-eye coordination, capacity to handle three-dimensional space, and manual dexterity, but above all to evaluate maturity of body image, a concept which refers to the image of self derived from parts of the body and their relationships to each other. This body image seems to be consistently primitive in children suffering from severe language deficiencies.

There are a number of interesting studies showing that brain injury, and in fact any lowering of integrative efficiency, brings about an impairment in figure-background relationships (Werner and Strauss 1941). Such figure-ground disturbances are now considered among the diagnostic features in the brain-injured child who does not necessarily present any gross neurological symptoms. These figure-ground disturbances have not yet been systematically explored in children who suffer from language dysfunctions. Our own findings, though limited in scope, show the same tendency if to a lesser degree. Time and again our children fail to find the relevant figure if shown a pattern melting into the background. In many instances they make a poor showing on the Marble Board test because of their incoherent and fragmentary approach and because of their abnormal preoccupation with the background which interferes with the figure.

While little work has been done in the investigation of visuomotor and perceptuomotor disturbances in our children, many observers have commented on their hyperactivity and their lack of control. Interpretation frequently has been along psychiatric lines. The psychiatrist says that the difficulty in the language area and the hypermotility of these youngsters are both symptoms of a psychological disorder. The speech therapist, on the other hand, insists that these children are hyperactive because they lack the tools for effective expression and communication. Both interpretations are undoubtedly correct in a number of cases. In reviewing a large number of family histories taken over a period of years, however, we find reports of early hyperkinesis and disorganization in children under eighteen months, long before speech could have developed. As a matter of fact, some of the mothers offer the comment that their children have been unusually active even in utero. Many of them show no indication of psychopathology, but their driveness, their difficulty with inhibition of motor and emotional responses, seems to fit in with the rest of their behavior.

To sum up, the emotional, the perceptual, and motor performance of our speech-delayed, dyslalic, and dyslexic youngsters seems to fall into a distinct pattern. They apparently have trouble at every level of integration. They appear, and this is our hypothesis, to have difficulty with structuralization and organization of gestalten. We feel in other words that it is gestalt psychology as originally conceived by Wertheimer which will throw light on some of our most baffling language dysfunctions. As formulated by Wertheimer (1941), gestalt function is defined as that function of the organism which responds to a given constellation of stimuli as to a whole, as to a figure, to a sequence of musical tones, for instance, to a tune (even if it is transposed into another key), to a constellation of pencil strokes as to a square (even if it is presented at a different angle). Our contention is that the ability to experience and to respond in terms of gestalten is one of the basic conditions in the successful handling of language phenomena.

Gestalt psychology (Katz 1951) says that any form is characterized by being separated, by standing out in relief. The word-deaf child undoubtedly perceives sequences of sounds, but the figure is not sharply differentiated from the background; he responds to speech as if it were noise; he responds to the background rather than the foreground.

Form, according to Wertheimer (1941), depends on the relationships between the whole and its parts which mutually determine each other. Speech is not a succession of separate units. We believe that the dyslalic child perceives sequences of sounds in a relatively unstructured way. Interpretation of organized language depends not on single sounds but on their relationship to each other. It is likely that the dyslalic youngster misses out in the organization of these relationships. Without the ability to retain and evoke well-organized auditory patterns, motor speech is bound to be defective, since we agree with Kohler (1933), who maintains that the sensory and motor should be thought of not as two different systems connected by communicating pathways, but rather as two parts of a comprehensive mechanism. No wonder, then, that the dyslalic child's own speech, representing in itself a definite constellation, a motor gestalt, is defective. His tendency to reverse sounds, to condense words, to omit syllables, reflects his difficulty with recognition and production of sharp configurations which are clearly organized in terms of parts and whole. The very monotony of dyslalic speech—Weiss (1950) has commented on the same phenomenon in the cluttering youngster—is symptomatic of the fact that he lacks insight into significant relationships, both phonetically and grammatically, since grammar is an expression of structure. The dyslalic child's words, like those of the clutterer, run together. His sentences are poorly organized; the figure does not stand out clearly in relief.

The dyslexic child does perceive printed letters, but his recognition of separate units will not in itself result in meaningful interpretation. The total form quality, according to Wertheimer, determines the quality of the separate units. A sentence read is more than a series of letters; it represents a scheme of organization, a scheme which has to be experienced as a totality and which has to be fitted into a meaningful context. Orton (1937) has found that the child suffering from language disabilities has trouble with the orderly recall of sequences: with temporal ones in the case of the dyslalic, with spatial ones in the case of the dyslexic, and with sequences of movements in the case of the dyspraxic youngster. It seems to us, however, that this difficulty with picturing and building of sequences of sound and letter units is only part of the child's inability to recognize and reproduce the dimensional and organizational details of perception which determine the structural coherence of the gestalt. Viewed in this light, much of our children's behavior, above all their inferior performance on the Marble Board and the Bender Gestalt, takes on added significance. Why do our youngsters so often have trouble with form, size, and space? Why do they so often show tactile defects? Why do they do poorly in digit repetition and in the imitation of tapped-out sequences? Fundamentally because in the recognition and reproduction of such patterns they have to pick out a configuration, have to reject certain stimuli so as to be able to attend to the figure. Not only must the constellation be sharply delineated against the background, but the spoken sentence, exactly as the tapped-out pattern, must be clearly organized in terms of temporal relationships. We agree with Stamback (1951) who says that rhythmic disturbances of dyslexic children are really deficiencies in temporal structuralization. It should be added that in the organization of perceptual configurations certain analytical and synthetical processes are involved. Goldstein maintains that for successful performance "the abstract attitude" is already required on the perceptual level. The perceptual and the symbolic processes cannot be actually separated from each other and in this light our children's poor abstract performance, on both the verbal and nonverbal levels, is of particular interest.

Finer motor coordination also requires patterning. Movement, exactly as is the case with perception, has to be experienced as an entity. A summation of small units will never result in smooth, fluid performance. One cannot compare the successive beats of a metronome, in which one stroke follows another, with living rhythm underlying acts like speaking and writing. The most careful execution of single movements will not produce a flowing hand. A succession of correct sounds will not result in speech. All of us have been in despair over the severely dyslalic child whose speech output is jerky and staccato in spite of the fact that he has mastered all individual sounds.

Our children's difficulty with patterning, however, appears not only in their perceptual and motor performance but also in integration and organization of behavior. Their trouble with inhibiting and channeling of impulses seems to be but another aspect of their inability to organize the endless stream of stimuli into behavioral configurations. The result is hyperkinesis and lack of control. In this framework, we cannot thoroughly discuss the question whether or not our youngsters' relatively primitive gestalt organization is to be considered in terms of a physiological variant or whether it indicates a developmental lag. Studies done at the Bellevue Hospital, where Silver (1951) investigated the postural reflexes, tonus, and motility of fifty severely dyslexic children, point to maturational delay. The encephalograms of these youngsters reveal dysrhythmia, slow waves indicating immaturity rather than pathology.

The studies done by Zazzo (1951) and his collaborators in Paris also stress developmental lag in terms of temporal and spatial organization. Our own clinical observation of children suffering from severe language disability confirm the impression of an overall delay in maturation. Further studies would have to investigate whether Silver's findings hold true also for severely dyslalic and word-deaf youngsters.

It would be of interest from the speech therapist's point of view to evaluate our therapeutic successes and failures in these terms. We should try to find out whether those of our youngsters who respond to speech therapy show simultaneous signs of maturation in their perceptual and motor gestalten, a maturation going beyond that generally expected in normal development. Is it possible that we sometimes succeed dramatically with our cases because our techniques—the cutting down of the flow of speech into shorter and less complex configurations—enable the youngster to acquire some sort of mastery? Are we not more effective, on the other hand, when we practice short phrases, closed figures in other words, rather than isolated units, single sounds? Does verbal training facilitate gestalt organization in other areas, or would our children actually do better if first helped with patterning of motor, perceptual, and behavioral responses before being exposed to speech work proper? We will need much patient observation before we even begin to answer any of these questions.

Summary

Clinical observation shows that it is possible to predict future dyslexias in a fairly large percentage of three-, four-, and five-year-olds who are originally referred on account of motor-speech delay, developmental word-deafness, and severe dyslalia.

According to Orton, certain children suffer from a generalized language disability which manifests itself in disorders of oral or printed language or both. Weiss affirms the existence of such a generalized factor and calls it "central language imbalance."

For the purpose of investigating the nature of this language disability we have examined the motor, perceptual, and emotional performance of our children and have found a number of basic and specific dysfunctions which seem to underlie a variety of language disturbances.

A number of tests show that these youngsters often do relatively poorly in abstract performance in spite of good intelligence. They frequently have difficulty in finer muscular control; some of them show a degree of dyspraxia. Many are late in establishing cerebral dominance and have trouble with right-left pregression. Bender Gestalt tests show striking immaturity of visuomotor functioning. Body image is usually very primitive. These children show disturbances in figure-background relationships, they are often hyperactive and have difficulty with patterning of motor and behavioral responses. They have, in fact, trouble at every level of integration.

According to gestalt psychology the ability to experience and to respond in terms of gestalten is a fundamental principle of psychophysiological functioning. It is our hypothesis that deficiencies in this area are responsible not only for our children's inferior performance on certain nonverbal tasks, but that they are also at the root of a number of language deviations. We feel that the crucial factor in central language imbalance is difficulty with structuralization and organization of perceptual and motor configurations. Differentiation between foreground and background is often faulty. These children have trouble recognizing and reproducing the dimensional and organizational details which make for the structural coherence of the gestalt.

Research done at Bellevue Hospital in New York City, the investigations of Professor Zazzo and his collaborators in Paris, and our own clinical observations point to maturational delay as a significant factor in language disorders. These theoretical considerations bring up certain practical problems for speech therapy which are discussed in the paper.

Two Categories of Learning Difficulties in Adolescents

At the Pediatric Language Disorder Clinic, we have seen over the past twenty years large numbers of young children referred for functional speech disorders. Psychiatric evaluation of these youngsters did not always point to environmental or clinical psychopathology; however, many children showed striking evidence of neurophysiological immaturity.

Along with these children, we have investigated a number of adolescents presenting severe scholastic dysfunction despite high intellectual potential, most of whom were referred from outside sources, with a diagnosis of psychogenic learning disability.

As a group, these adolescents, most of them boys, showed these presenting symptoms: their responses to academic demands were infantile; they were underachievers in terms of their intellectual endowment, little interested in school work, and anxious; some of them were quite hostile.

In spite of superficial similarity in symptomatology, however, these adolescents did not, on close investigation, appear to be a homogenous group. Instead, they fell into two main categories. One, Group A, seemed primarily and severely disturbed psychologically. In the other, Group B, emotional disturbance was secondary and reactive. In fact, some of the boys in Group B were the very same children whom we had originally seen years ago when they had been referred for oral speech deficiencies and who had not then shown symptoms of significant emotional disturbance.

No attempt is made to discuss the psychodynamics of these cases nor relate observation to a specific pattern on the Wechsler Intelligence Scale for Children. However, it seems important nevertheless, to differentiate phenomenologically between these two groups, since failure to do so frequently results not only in faulty therapeutic and remedial procedures, but also in the wrong kind of educational planning.

Reprinted with permission from The American Orthopsychiatric Association, Inc., from *American Journal of Orthopsychiatry* 33(1):87–89. 1963.

Group A

Group A consists of often very charming boys who not only look young but are often actually physically small. Their intellectual potential tends to be very high judging by psychometric tests. The psychological report usually describes these boys as difficult to reach and erratic in performance, as well as strikingly infantile and passive. Their poor academic function is said to be related to more or less severe psychological disturbance.

Usually these boys do rather well in school during the earlier years, as long as they can get by with intelligence alone, despite some early daydreaming and a tendency to withdraw from group activities. Many are avid readers but they sometimes do poorly on reading comprehension tests, not because of poor reading ability but because they are too phantasy-ridden, too phobically preoccupied, and sometimes too depressed to be able to focus attention.

Again, many are highly articulate; their verbal definitions are usually excellent. At age twelve they might be able to explain the difference between *character* and *reputation*. Their abstract competence is often very good indeed.

However, they suffer from what Rubinstein (1959) calls "learning impotence." As they advance into the higher grades in school, they do poorly in practically all subjects: English, grammar, history, and especially mathematics, which seems to be particularly sensitive to anxiety. Their math papers are shot through with careless mistakes, although they have little trouble understanding the fundamental processes. In long additions they lose the thread; they seem to have difficulties "holding the set;" above all, they seem to lack that aggressiveness and tension requisite for learning.

Essentially boys in Group A are passive and infantile individuals with little or no psychic energy to invest. Although nothing points to disturbed thought processes or to bizarre responses, one nevertheless has the impression that they are disoriented and lack a feeling of being in control. Pearson (1954) says of such children that "primary processes" interfere with utilizing learning content. Being divorced from their own feelings, perhaps because they are afraid of being overwhelmed by anger, fear, or despair, learning, which, as Liss (1950) emphasizes, is a "libidinal phenomenon," becomes a meaningless and fragmented experience.

It should be added that these children find it difficult to invest in any area, not in learning only. They are unable to commit themselves, since commitment tends to arouse strong anxiety, perhaps because in the past it has been experienced as dangerous.

Two impressive traits are their striking lack of ego strength and their physiological immaturity. It seems that from earliest childhood their infantile needs were greater than those of other children. Their plasticity, their delayed physical maturation, and their diffuse ego organization seem to be different aspects of the same phenomenon.

If such boys are referred for psychotherapy, which must be intensive, gains are not easily translatable into better academic functioning. Their passivity and difficulty with transference make any modification of behavior patterns a long, drawn-out process. Frequently they fail to achieve a therapeutic relationship sufficiently strong and sustaining to enable them to make drastic changes in approach either to people or to life experiences, of which learning is only a part.

One's hopes for remedial results are usually high because one is seduced by the charm of these children and their superficial cooperation. Actually, it is much easier for them to comply than to resist, and, as one should expect from a severe disorder in ego function, the results of tutoring are disappointing. True, these youngsters undoubtedly do better in a two-way situation than in a group, where they invariably get lost; the very presence of the tutor tends to reduce daydreaming and makes focusing easier.

The aim of remedial work is twofold: to achieve a degree of identification with the teacher and to find some area of interest, no matter what. Since so much of the learning of such children is fragmented, another goal is to integrate specific subject matter into a larger and more meaningful framework in order to reduce disorientation. However, these boys are usually so diffuse that learning remains fragmented. As a result, the discrepancy between potential and performance persists. Prognosis is not good.

Group B

The psychological evaluation of the boys in Group B reads not too differently from that of Group A except that the boys in Group B often do less well on the verbal than on the performance scale on the WISC, and their hostility is far more overt.

In adolescence, many of the perceptual, motor, and visuomotor immaturities we had observed when these children were much younger (de Hirsch 1961a) have disappeared (de Hirsch 1957,1961a). Severe hyperkinesis, a complaint of teachers and parents in the earlier years, has markedly improved. As a result of their altogether adequate intelligence, they have compensated for earlier difficulties and often read very well indeed. However, on closer investigation, they still show signs of a residual language disability. In the main, they are fairly inarticulate youngsters for whom language is not a convenient tool. Some do fairly well in science, but their spelling is usually appalling, since, in contrast to reading, intelligence does not help them compensate for their severe difficulty with retention of verbal visual configurations, which tend to remain unstable. Perceptual, visuomotor, and motor patterning often remain inferior. Their auditory discrimination is often poor, their Bender Gestalt (1938) relatively primitive. Their handwriting is arrhythmic and messy. The papers they hand in are badly organized (de Hirsch 1961b). Organizational weakness seems to be one of the features of the language syndrome, though in some instances there is evidence of compulsive fussiness, perhaps as a defense against earlier disorganization.

Usually these children do better with multiple-choice tests than with essays. Their ability to formulate is strikingly inferior. Their compositions are barren and stiff, especially if the subject matter is not limited to concrete experience. As one boy put it, "I can describe a submarine, but when I have to write a composition on 'To Be or Not To Be,' that's when I get stuck." These same boys find it hard to give samples of the literal and the figurative use of words. They are at sea when it comes to metaphors in literature and do poorly with poetry. The Greek word for metaphor is *transfer* and these literal children have trouble transferring meaning from one area to the other. When asked to define proverbs, they produce concrete responses, quite different from the often concrete but at the same time egocentric and loose definitions of schizophrenics (Kasanin 1944). The boys in Group B will say, for instance, "Of course new brooms sweep cleaner because the bristles are stiffer."

Success in school is highly correlated with verbal intelligence. Words are the very material of thought and greatly increase the efficiency of abstract functioning. Thus, a linguistic handicap is bound to have a detrimental effect on many areas of scholastic performance.

What happens, unfortunately, to the youngsters in Group B is that their original failure in language tends to spill over into other learning experiences. What begins with a reading disorder turns into a learning disability. In an attempt to protect themselves from failure these boys withdraw from learning altogether. To quote Anna Freud: "In the theory of education the importance of the ego's determination to avoid pain has not been sufficiently appreciated" (1946). For Group B children the original painful experience in the Oedipal situation is confirmed by their learning difficulty, which has a basis in reality. Most learning in our culture deals in some way with verbal symbols. In order to avoid defeat, a defeat that we believe is related to an inherent deficiency in language potential—and Pearson (1952) admits that individual children's specific endowment does vary independently of their life experience—these boys retreat and adopt an "I don't care" attitude.

On the other hand, and in contrast to Group A, the boys in Group B are able and often eager to make a personal investment in areas other than the academic one, in mechanical pursuits, in sports and in other fields where they sometimes do a very good job, indeed. Psychologically, practically all youngsters in Group B are explosive and have an extremely low frustration threshold and poor tolerance for tension, which in themselves interfere with learning. They are sometimes openly defiant, very defensive, and usually very angry. Their anger is often conscious, as is their anxiety, which one can literally see rise when they try to cope with an academic task that they find distasteful. They are far closer to their anxiety than are the boys in Group A, who presumably must push their anxiety so far down because they have no tolerance for it.

The two groups do merge, of course; they do have certain features in common. Bender (1958) regards both developmental language disabilities and childhood schizophrenia (and some of the children in Group A have been described, if not as schizophrenic, at any rate as borderline cases) as maturational lags. According to her, schizophrenic children and those with language lags retain primitive and plastic responses, show instability of perceptual experiences and difficulty in giving up more infantile modes of behavior. However, in Group A, plasticity, unevenness of growth, and difficulty with self percept, and boundaries all involve the total personality with resulting ego disorganization, whereas, in Group B, plasticity is far more specific, manifesting itself primarily in instability of verbal gestalten.

In spite of apparent similarities, it is not justifiable to treat all adolescents who fail in school as if they were a homogeneous group, as do Sperry et al. (1958) in their paper on renunciation and denial in learning disabilities. Overemphasis on intrapsychic processes leads to neglect of neurophysiological and maturational factors that might be highly significant. Thus, the bizarre spelling of familiar words so characteristic of the children in Group B is not always and necessarily a symptom of a severe character disorder. Nor is it always associated with some early traumatic event or with faulty identification. We feel that inferior spelling may be related to severe instability of spatial and temporal gestalten (de Hirsch 1954). For Group A children, printed words never acquire a physiognomy, they never become familiar. In Group B, difficulty with verbal formulation is not always a sign of basic unwillingness to communicate, since communicative intent is often clearly evident.

What Pearson (1952) calls "the painful conditioning experience" of the learning process, with its attendant feelings of shame, guilt, and embarrassment, is bound to leave scars. However, in Group B, psychological difficulties are the result, rather than the cause of learning failure.

Early diagnosis is essential, since we feel sure that remedial measures and prognosis are very different for the two categories. The boys in Group B need supportive psychotherapy, help with their anger, and insight into the nature of their difficulty. If the right kind of tutoring is instigated early enough, that is, before the academic gaps have become irreversible, it might make the difference between failing and coping. At best, the going in high school is difficult. Much depends on attitudes in the home. When these are critical rather than supportive, self image may become permanently damaged. Those boys who get into technical colleges or into business sometimes do well.

Summary

This paper describes two categories of intelligent adolescents with severe scholastic difficulties who are usually considered to belong to a homogeneous group. Reasons are given for believing that they form at least two groups. In Group A the academic difficulty is related to ego impairment and a manifestation of a severe character disorder, indicating primary learning disabilities. In Group B scholastic dysfunction is secondary to residual language deficiencies, and psychological problems as well as difficulties in school are the result, rather than the cause, of the original disability.

The Concept of Plasticity
and Language Disabilities

In our work with children suffering from severe speech, reading, writing, and spelling disabilities, we have found Bender's (1953) concept of plasticity extremely helpful, since, more than any other, it seems to do justice to the observed clinical phenomena. The purpose of this paper, then, is to attempt to demonstrate by means of a report on three children suffering from severe developmental language lags that youngsters with disabilities in the verbal area may show some of the plastic behavior Bender describes as characteristic of schizophrenic youngsters.

Developmental processes in general are characterized by progression from unstable, in the immature, to more stable configurations in the more mature organism. Some immature children seem to find it difficult to stabilize various types of configurations, behavioral, perceptual, and motor ones, and it is in this sense that they are plastic.

Plasticity might be observed along a continuum. There are at one end children in whom plasticity is pervasive, ego organization is diffuse, ego boundaries are fluid, and there is trouble with reality testing. At the other end there are those youngsters who are in no way bizarre or deviating, who are able to form meaningful relationships, and whose plasticity shows mainly in inability to stabilize perceptual experiences and to maintain a linguistic gestalt.

The three boys I want to describe here are plastic and immature. All three show retention of primitive central nervous system patterning, fluid motility, unstable perceptual experiences, and immature modes of physiological and psychological response.

Ego organization was assessed in each case by the psychiatrist and ranged from tight to loose to fragmented. Each of these three boys suffers from a different type of language disability.

Frank, the first case, an eight-year-old boy and the middle of three children, was referred because two years in public school had made

Reprinted with permission from The College of Speech Therapists, from *Speech Pathology and Therapy* 8:12–17. 1965.

131

little or no impression on him as far as reading was concerned. Family history of language revealed, as it so often does, that Frank's father, a very successful business man, also had had trouble in learning to read and that two of Frank's cousins had clung to infantile speech patterns until the seventh and eighth year of life.

Frank's home is a lively one. He and his brothers are active and bouncy children, but the mother says that it is Frank who is "explosive." He apparently gets along with his peers but he cannot cope with more than one at a time. In a larger group, "he goes to pieces," becomes completely disorganized, starts running around and in general loses control.

Frank passed all developmental milestones at a normal time. He rated an IQ of 112 on the Stanford Binet. Clinically, the psychologist found him an emotionally solid boy, but she was impressed with the fact that on the Rorschach he seemed to "fall apart." The analyst who evaluated him did not feel that Frank presented significant psychopathology.

What struck one first about Frank was his tiny size. He looked like a five- rather than an eight-year-old boy and physiologically this was the level on which he performed in many areas. In reaching out, for instance, he moved his whole body. During hopping he clenched his fists, his motor behavior was primitive and global. Finer manual control was abysmally poor. The whole child was plastic, that is to say, he was hypotonic, loosely put together, and insufficiently stabilized in striking contrast to the fact that psychologically, and, in spite of some anxiety, he was, indeed, a solid enough youngster.

Frank enjoyed himself hugely during the initial interview. He tended at first to deny his difficulties since they made him anxious, but after a while he was ready to discuss them. In spite of much restlessness he worked hard and at times enthusiastically.

Graphic activities presented a tremendous hurdle. Frank's Bender Gestalt (1938) gave evidence of a severe visuomotor lag. His copies were primitive and crude approximations of the gestalten. "Plasticity," Silver (1950) says, "is an attribute of the primitive gestalt."

Body image as judged by Frank's human figure drawing was in no way bizarre, but it was undifferentiated, and Frank had to verbalize the separate parts of the body before drawing them, indicating that the various sensory, proprioceptive, emotional, and social experiences that make up body image still had not been integrated.

Frank's laterality also was, as yet, ill-defined. He used his right hand for many trained activities but was apt to switch to the left when the right hand as he put it "got tired."

Frank's maturational lag was a pervasive one and extended to all modalities. His auditory impressions were plastic, unsharp, and unstable, which was clearly evident from his performance on the Wepman's Auditory Discrimination Test (1958). His visual perceptual experiences were equally diffuse. To Frank the printed page looked like an undifferentiated meaningless design, nothing stood out. He was, moreover, confused spatially and so fluid that he had trouble holding to the printed line. Letters like *p–q*, *d–q*, *n–w*, *w–m* seemed to pivot. If one exposed the words *tap* and *pat*, he was unable to see a difference. Left to right progression still was an arbitrary matter. Not only did the spatial orientation of letters present difficulties but the very letters and words seemed to shift. He could maintain the visual verbal gestalt only for seconds, then he lost it again. Working with Frank gave one the feeling that the whole child was slithering and sliding; teaching him to read was like trying to embed something in very loose sand. He simply could not remember letter shapes. These difficulties would have been troublesome enough for any child, but they were nearly insurmountable for this very immature youngster whose frustration threshhold was extremely low. His lessons were punctured by a series of catastrophic reactions, and it was only with the help of innumerable lollipops (his oral needs also were those of a much younger child) that he managed not to explode.

It was thus not entirely surprising that the psychologist looking at his Rorschach protocol wondered whether Frank did not, after all, suffer from some underlying psychopathology. The amorphous nature of the projective stimuli was bound to arouse disorganized and chaotic responses and made it difficult for Frank to reject aggressive and primitive phantasies. However, if one considered that Frank whose mental age was consistent with chronological age but who functioned nevertheless in the perceptual realm like a five-year-old, one was hardly surprised to find that his Rorschach, which requires patterning of perceptual configurations, was diffuse and disinhibited. Actually, one could not but be impressed with this boy's ego strength, his willingness and ability to work against fairly heavy odds, and with his capacity to enjoy relationships.

One might, of course, say that this hyperkinetic youngster who was so much at the mercy of environmental stimuli belongs in the organic group, that he is, in fact, a brain-injured child. He might well be. However, diffuse brain injury can only be inferred from performance, while plasticity and primitivity of patterning can be observed clinically. The question arises, furthermore, whether immaturity of gestalt functioning and difficulty with central nervous system patterning is not, in fact, the characteristic and outstanding feature in what we call nonfocal brain injury.

Frank has a long and arduous road in front of him. The chances are that between the age of twelve and fourteen he will "jell." Many of the earlier signs of perceptual and motor immaturity will disappear, though in all probability he will be left with specific gaps. Prognosis is favorable only if Frank gets intensive and skilled remedial help and enough psychological support to prevent serious damage to his self image.

Bruno, my second case, was referred for unintelligible speech at the age of nearly ten years. He is a much more vulnerable youngster than Frank is. He is the oldest of three children from a somewhat overprotective but warm supportive home. On the WISC Bruno rated an IQ of 119 on the Verbal and 100 on the Performance section. Neurological and psychiatric investigation did not reveal any gross dysfunction. Bruno is a friendly, very anxious, transparent, and slightly disoriented-looking boy who is, however, able to form warm, if somewhat dependent, relationships to adults. In spite of his vagueness he draws satisfactions from play and from the world around him. He has a friend or two but is slightly afraid of groups because it is hard for him to cope with aggression.

Bruno's reflex behavior, his tonus, and his posture are immature and plastic. He still turns readily along a longitudinal axis, and in the waiting room he seems to melt into the couch. He tends to lean against one during work. Laterality still is ambiguous. Although Bruno's Bender does not show trouble with conceptualization of gestalten, spatial organization is fluid and there is a tendency to verticalization of horizontally exposed figures. There is a whirling quality about his protocol that seems to reflect the unstable nature of this boy's perceptual world. Bruno's human figure drawing is not deviating but lines are faint; the boy he produced does not look solid and the drawing is placed at a slant.

Only on close observation does one realize that Bruno has some trouble with the receptive aspect of language. He has no sensory deficit, but auditory discrimination is unsharp and he confuses words like *cold* and *coal* which to him sound vaguely alike. He is apt to lose the gist when one talks to him in long and involved sentences. Bruno's trouble with interpretation is not a matter of inattention, since he gives entirely appropriate answers if one cuts the material down into shorter units.

Bruno's expressive language clearly mirrors his diffuse reception. He has some minor articulatory inaccuracies, but he does fairly well when tested on single sounds, on individual words, and on very short phrases. As soon as he tries to express himself in longer units his speech deteriorates. Under the stress of having to formulate complex conceptual material the organizational load becomes too heavy, rate of speech increases, rhythm becomes markedly jerky, he omits parts of sentences, he reverses sounds within words and words within phrases, articulation becomes mushy and in the end breaks down altogether. Bruno's severe difficulties with patterning of long verbal configurations is fairly typical for the cluttering individual (Weiss 1950;

Arnold 1960; de Hirsch 1961d). What strikes one most forcibly in his speech is his disorganization, the lack of structure, the monotonous voice quality, the fluctuation in rate, and the tendency to articulatory disintegration, all of which reflect instability of auditory-motor gestalten. Bruno is at all times anxious to make himself understood; thus his articulatory inconsistency is not a function of poor communicative intent, but a symptom of organizational weakness.

Formal characteristics of speech are not the only deviating features in Bruno's communication. Content also is poorly structured and fluid. The stories he tells hang only loosely together. He is so easily pulled by associations that much of what he produces is random. There is little framework; the logical thread is thin and his fluidity leads him from one thing to the other. Combined with poor intelligibility, his stories might give one the impression of bizarreness, which is misleading. Once one succeeds in unravelling what the boy says, one finds nothing deviating, and if one structures content for him, he manages very well.

His plasticity and inability to structure himself and his environment must of necessity arouse intense anxiety in this boy. His poor spatial organization as evidenced by his Bender and his marked confusion as to time (his references to the past and future are quite vague) are bound to increase his disorientation.

It is of interest that Bruno's anxiety decreased markedly during speech therapy and by no means solely as a result of his warm relationship to the therapist. Relatively little work was done on sounds per se. The emphasis was on sharper reception, on control of rate, on rhythm, and on organization. After ten months of twice weekly therapeutic sessions Bruno's connected speech is still far from perfect. I doubt it ever will be as he is essentially a clutterer. He is, however, intelligible at all times, rate of speech is more normal, articulation crisper.

Bruno's dependency needs, which we feel with Bender (1953) are greater in children with early difficulty in homeostasis than in others, have decreased. The home has contributed to progress by setting more clearly defined limits which helped this loosely organized and vulnerable boy to strengthen his defences, since he had a tighter framework to relate to.

The third case, Charles, a fourteen-year-old boy, was referred for severe difficulties with spelling and writing which, according to the psychological report, were psychogenic in origin. The examining psychiatrist felt, as we did, that Charles was a severely disturbed youngster with evidence of ego fragmentation. Thus this case was a good way further along the continuum discussed previously.

Charles is the older of two adopted children in a home which, to put it mildly, is not conducive to mental health. On the WISC he scored in the high average range on both Performance and Verbal sections. He had always been clumsy motorically and he had been very late in starting to talk. When we first saw him, language did not seem to be a comfortable tool. He did well on multiple choice types of tests, but oral and written communication were inferior. He had originally been tutored in reading, but by the time we saw him reading comprehension was entirely adequate. His spelling was bizarre for several reasons: Charles had little or no "physionomic ability." While he recognized words from crude cues in reading because context provided essential information, the general outline and the precise internal design of the printed words were so unstable that these configurations never became familiar or stable enough for purposes of recall as it is required in spelling. He was able to memorize words and remember them for a while; however, he could not carry the gestalt into another setting and misspelled the same words when they were embedded in context. Not only were the links between the auditory and the visual structure of the word very weak (Schilder [1944] discussed this phenomenon which is typical for dyslexic individuals) but Charles' very auditory impressions were diffuse. He heard words as only vaguely structured wholes. The word *felicity* for instance he would hear as *felsty* and in the transfer from the auditory to the visual-spatial and motor configuration he would lose more of the essential features of the word and write down *fizy*. Charles' incredibly poor penmanship complicated matters. At this late stage he still showed the residuals of an originally severe ideomotor dysgraphia (Herman 1961), inability to remember the precise letter shapes, combined with actual difficulty in producing the proper writing motions. His movements were jerky and disinhibited, and when he wrote for longer than a few minutes, his writing deteriorated to a point where he himself was no longer able to decipher what he had put down.

By the time we saw him the boy's responses to writing and spelling had, of course, a phobic flavor. Charles had little investment in scholastic performance. Unlike Frank who formed warm and lasting relationships and Bruno who identified well enough to help him with learning, Charles related only thinly and fleetingly. He constantly slipped through one's fingers. Thus it might seem that his abysmally poor writing and spelling was on the basis of damaged ego functioning. On the other hand, Charles was not a case of what Rubinstein (1959) calls "learning impotence;" he did relatively well in math and science and he worked hard, if somewhat obsessively, on mechanical pursuits. Moreover, during the past twenty years we have observed a number of children far less disturbed than is Charles with spelling disabilities similar to his that were by no means always reversible. Bizarre spelling is not always and necessarily proof of severe psychopathology. We see this type of syndrome in brain-injured youngsters, but we also find it, as Orton (1937) did way back in the twenties and thirties, on a familial basis. Zangwill (1962), Bender (1938), and Subirana (1961a) think in terms of a genetically determined maturational deficit, and our own clinical observations point in this direction.

The three boys discussed here differ in important aspects—in ego organization, in relatedness, and in self image. However, all three are plastic. They have in common immature central nervous system patterning, unstable temporal and spatial organization, ambiguous laterality, difficulty with finer motor acts and with sharply outlined perceptual experiences. All three are unable to maintain verbal gestalten. In these children plasticity must have engendered anxiety early, and their failure to achieve must of necessity have confirmed very early and basic doubts any questions about themselves. Plasticity is not a diagnosis; it is a description which seems to fit the performance of a good many youngsters suffering from severe language disability.

Summary

Presented are observations on three children who show severe deviations in various aspects of language function. Their ego organization ranges from intact, to loose, to almost fragmented. The three boys have in common instability of perceptuomotor experiences and immature central nervous system patterning. This places them in a continuous stress situation, since despite good intellectual endowment, maturation is delayed in areas essential for the organism's orientation in his environment. If viewed in terms of the concept of plasticity, many of the correlates of severe language disability become comprehensible.

Clinical Spectrum of Reading Disabilities: Diagnosis and Treatment

Reading is the successful response to the visual forms of language. In analyzing the process, one finds a number of partial performances: there is the perceptual grasping of letters and word configurations; there is their evocation in inner speech; there is the comprehension of syntactical relations, the construction of anticipatory schemata of what the sentence is going to say; and, finally, there is the assimilation of content into a contextual framework of ideas and experiences. All of this constitutes a *unitas multiplex,* an integrated performance, each part influencing the other.

Single or several aspects of this process may be disturbed and for a variety of reasons. Children whose intellectual endowment is limited may have trouble with some or most of the partial performances involved in reading. The perceptual competence of some of these youngsters may be adequate; they may master the mechanics of the reading process, but their conceptual level may be so low that they do not comprehend what they read. But the conceptual deficits of such children are likely to depress performance in all academic subjects; their difficulty in reading is *non*specific.

Some children fail in reading because much of their psychic energy is blocked off and is not available for learning. Overwhelming anxiety may immobilize the child. Inability to postpone gratification in the service of a learning goal may interfere with his scholastic functioning. There are youngsters who are so phantasy-ridden that they have little investment in academic pursuits. Schizophrenic children's view of the world may be so fragmented that they are unable to integrate what they read into a meaningful framework. Occasionally words or letters do not serve as referents, but are experienced as if they were the things themselves. Letters and words may be subject to what Freud called "primary process distortion." One eight-year-old schizophrenic boy who came to me for help with his reading told me: "there is no

Reprinted with permission from the New York Academy of Medicine, from *Bulletin of the New York Academy of Medicine* 44:470–477. 1968.

point learning this letter (it was a *k*), it is not sympathetic, it has too many spikes." For Ted the letter *k* had no conventional symbolic significance; it embodied his archaic fears of aggression and retaliation. In children of this type, difficulties with reading are simply one aspect of a generalized and severe disturbance of learning.

At the Pediatric Language Disorder Clinic of Columbia-Presbyterian Medical Center we see a number of asphasic youngsters, some of whom show evidence of structural damage to the central nervous system, who have difficulties in perceiving, processing, storing, and retrieving information relayed through auditory pathways. Such children usually have trouble also with reading, which requires the decoding of input signals received through visual channels. Printed language is a symbolic system superimposed on oral language. Aphasic youngsters usually have difficulties not only with the decoding and encoding of verbal symbols, but with other semiotic systems as well; with mathematics, for instance; these difficulties also are *non*specific.

Children may be retarded in reading because of gross defects in the peripheral sensory apparatus, because of frequent change of schools, inadequate teaching, intermittent illness, or because of environmental deprivation or pathology. But such youngsters usually fail in all academic areas; theirs is not a specific reading disability either.

Specific reading disability (some call it specific language disorder) is not, as is reading retardation, related to limited intellectual endowment, significant sensory deficit, or to a host of extraneous factors. Reading disability is specific only when the child's reading and spelling achievement is substantially below his intellectual potential and his performance in other areas of academic functioning.

You will have noted that I have not, so far, used the word *dyslexia*. This term, like the famous Golem, seems to have taken on a life of its own; it now covers a multitude of meanings. It is used unfortunately as a stick with which to frighten parents; worse, it has become a cloak that shelters all sorts of cults and quick cures. The Interdisciplinary Committee on Reading Disorders has therefore suggested limiting the term dyslexia to those cases of specific reading disability that present positive signs on the classical neurological examination, the electroencephalogram (EEG), or a verifiable history of brain injury.

However, not all reading and spelling disorders are related to encephalopathies. We see large numbers of intelligent youngsters whose severe difficulties in this area appear to be familial. Orton (1930), and after him most Scandinavian researchers postulate that a tendency to disorders in spoken and printed language is prevalent in given families. The large number of reports on families with several affected members certainly bears out this assumption. In such families the oldest boy (the majority of such children are males) may be referred to the clinic because of a massive disorder in spelling; his six-year-old brother may be brought in because of stuttering; and the mother may report that the two-and-a-half-year-old baby does not as yet attempt to put words together.

Regardless of etiology, children with severe reading and spelling disabilities present on close investigation a distinct pattern of dys-functions, and while it is true that not all of these dysfunctions are necessarily present in a given youngster, the investigation of hundreds of such children reveals more or less subtle integrational deficits on many levels of central nervous system organization.

On a fairly primitive level the central nervous system patterning of these children seems to be more immature, more global than one would expect from their chronological and mental age. They tend to be restless and disorganized. They usually need many gross motor out-lets, but tend to do poorly in games requiring coordination of hand and eye. Their manual control is often awkward. Some boys who are exceptionally skillful when it comes to building model planes or tying flies for fishing, handle the pencil in a clumsy fashion, and grapho-motor difficulties are the rule rather than the exception.

A child's drawing of the human figure usually reflects his aware-ness of his body, its parts, and the relation of these parts to one another. Drawings of the human figure by children with specific reading and spelling disorders are frequently at least two years below their mental age; they show deficits in body schema and praxis and a degree of spatial disorganization. Reading is a pattern laid out in space. Inability to discriminate between right and left on one's own body and on that of the other person may be part of the child's difficulty in spatial orientation, and is fairly characteristic of a child who has trouble in learning to read.

Much has been written about ill-defined laterality as a cause of reading failure. Laterality is usually assessed through observation of the hand used in untrained activities, of the eye used for sighting, and of the foot used for kicking. However, we do not really know whether lateral dominance as tested peripherally really reflects cortical domi-nance. We have mounting evidence (Birch [1964] has shown it for his ten-year-old group) that ambiguous lateralization, as tested peripher-ally, is not related to failure in reading. Those of our kindergarten children who had not established a clear-cut functional dominance of one hand over the other did not read better or worse two and a half years later than did the ones who had.

Identical phenomena have, of course, different meanings at different ages. It is well known that functional dominance increases with age and is thus partly a matter of maturation. I do believe, in fact, that ambilaterality in youngsters of fourteen years and over bespeaks a degree of central nervous system immaturity and that it is this immaturity, rather than the mixed dominance, that may be related to difficulties in reading.

Over the years we have become convinced that our failing children perform like younger subjects in a wide variety of perceptuomotor and linguistic tasks. Their copies of the Bender Gestalt tests (1938) are often fragmented and crude, and they reveal the tendency to rotation and verticalization typical of younger children.

Birch's discussion of visual perception and its developmental course (1964) is so exhaustive that nothing further could well be added to it. In the daily remedial work with some of the severely affected younger children one notes that nothing in the printed page stands out; for them printed signs look like a jumble of meaningless designs. One eight-year-old girl told me angrily: "It looks as if ants were running around the page." While this is, of course, a phobic response, it was quite evident that for this child printed configurations did not fall into organized patterns, and that, as the word "running" denotes, these symbols seemed to shift.

Our youngsters appear to have trouble in recognizing the critical features in letters and words: those features that distinguish an *f* from a *t*, or a word such as *fill* from the word *fling*. They will occasionally recognize the word when it is printed in bold black letters on a white card, but they will lose the configuration when the very same word is embedded in context.

The most essential single feature about language is the sequencing of spatial and temporal events. A child, for instance, who reads *now* instead of *won* has trouble with *spatial sequences*.

It is important to remember, however, that *auditory* sequencing is often equally difficult for children with language disabilities. The youngster who substitutes *Crice Ripsies* for *Rice Crispies* may also confuse the spatial order of letters as well. Temporal and spatial organization, according to Lashley (1954), are nearly interchangeable. In order to read a little word like *mat*, the child has to translate a series of letters seen, a sequence in space, into a sequence of sounds heard, a sequence in time. The printed page is a time chart of sounds and words.

Birch (1964) has shown that older children who suffer from disabilities in reading have trouble with *inter*sensory integration, with the integration of visual and auditory input signals. In our younger failing readers we have first to assess *intra*sensory integration carefully; i.e., both visual and auditory verbal competences. Deficits in auditory verbal organization—in other words, oral language deficits—primitive sentence construction, faulty syntax, word-finding difficulties, articulatory defects, trouble with the formulation of thought content are frequent in poor readers. The auditory discrimination of most youngsters with severe difficulties in spelling is inferior. Their spelling errors reflect their diffuse reception of words and their diffuse disorganized output. Most cases of massive spelling disabilities are, moreover, complicated by disorders in writing. The papers these youngsters hand in must be seen to be believed. Their jerky, dysrhythmic handwriting, their omission of sounds, their telescoping of words, their transposition of letters and syllables tend to mirror their rapid disorganized cluttered manner of speaking. This kind of clinical evidence leads us to believe that in such youngsters we deal with a deficit that embraces all forms of verbal communication: speech, reading, writing, and spelling. What characterizes the children who have trouble in all of these areas is an inability to maintain a linguistic gestalt.

An intelligent older subject whose self-image has not been severely damaged as a result of failure may in the end become a fairly adequate and sometimes quite effective reader. His intelligent use of contextual clues will enable him to compensate for his earlier perceptual instability. But he invariably remains a poor speller. Spelling, unlike reading, requires not only recognition but reproduction of the configuration of the word. The youngster has to remember not only the overall gestalt of the word, but also its intricate internal design. In spelling, intelligence is of little help; intelligence does not enable an individual to compensate for what one might call his physiognomic deficit. Both bizarre spelling and illegible and messy handwriting complicate the task of writing compositions, and it is in this area that bright older children fail, even if they more or less make the grade in reading.

Specific disabilities in reading range from slight to severe. While there are youngsters who overcome their early perceptual instability in the normal course of development, and while there are others who manage up to a point with intensive remedial help, there are some who have trouble all through their school and college years.

Bender (1958) maintains that perceptual instability is the typical dysfunction in maturational lags. The term maturational lags implies, of course, that these youngsters catch up at some point and, in fact, many do so, at least in reading. But there are a few in whom these lags are so severe that one might speak of a maturational defect so deeply rooted in the biological matrix that it constitutes a type of cerebral dysfunction.

Diagnosis of specific reading disability, then, entails a familial history of language, that is to say, of disabilities of speech, reading, writing, and spelling among close relatives; a medical history including prenatal, natal, and postnatal data; an appraisal of neurological and sensory status, in our case provided by the referring physician; a careful developmental and academic history; and some assessment of the youngster's potential. Diagnosis involves not only a detailed analysis of the child's actual functioning in reading, spelling, and composition and a sophisticated investigation of his oral language tools, but also some information as to the perceptuomotor and integrative competences that underlie performances as complex as reading and spelling. It is important in every single case, further, to understand what failure in school means to both the parent and the child and to distinguish between a specific reading disorder and a generalized disturbance in learning.

The purpose of the diagnostic procedure is to pinpoint specific lags. The resulting profile of weakness and strength in the various modalities will serve as guidelines for the appropriate remedial program.

If, for instance, the child has inferior physiognomic ability, if he cannot cope with perceptual wholes, he will need techniques of revisualization to help him with his deficit. If a youngster's disability in spelling is related to weakness in auditory discrimination, if, for instance, he perceives the word *monastery* as *monstery* he will require help with syllabification and with techniques enabling him to get a more sharply defined picture of the auditory gestalt of words. If a child has trouble with spatial sequencing and reverses the spatial orders of letters, an attempt must be made to substitute auditory for visual sequencing; emphasis must be on phonics.

I hold no brief for any particular method. While phonics is helpful in a great many cases, many brain-injured youngsters, for instance, cannot be taught by phonics because their often severe difficulties with analysis and synthesis may make this approach so burdensome that some of these children respond with a catastrophic reaction—the disorganized response of the organism that is faced with a task with which it cannot cope. A few children must be taught entirely by touch, by using three-dimensional models of letters; they are made to close their eyes if the visual input proves to be disturbing. In these cases the type of intersensory integration involved is tactile-auditory (and this obviously is the method blind children use).

Our field is, unfortunately, beset by much evangelical fervor. One method or another is praised beyond all others. However, remediation must be centered in the child, not in method. It is only by painstaking analysis that one can set up a sensible remedial program for each individual case.

On the basis of a warm and secure therapeutic relation that entails respect for the child's individual rhythm of growth, the finding of effective remedial methods can be a joint adventure. Only if the pupil is himself heavily involved in the active exploration of what works best for him, only if he is a participant rather than an object of manipulation, will he learn to compensate for his particular deficit.

In the best of cases the experience of years of failure leaves deep scars. As our youngsters proceed from junior high school to high school, and mostly very much earlier, they become either profoundly discouraged or so angry that all learning becomes distasteful to them. As these children get older it becomes more and more difficult to distinguish between a primary learning disability related to psychiatric factors and emotional difficulties arising from defeat.

Let me therefore make a plea. Twenty-five years of experience with bright but educationally disabled children has taught us that a good number of them need not have required extensive remedial help had their difficulties been diagnosed earlier. A timely boost and relatively little assistance would have obviated the need for later remediation. We can predict which children are likely to fail even *before* they enter first grade. Postponing formal reading and setting up flexible groups that allow for filling in perceptuomotor and oral language gaps will lessen the remedial load with which we are no longer able to cope; it will also reduce the number of educational and emotional casualties in our schools.

Language Deficits in Children
with Developmental Lags

As remedial therapists working with children who present difficulties with spoken, printed, and written language we are in an ambiguous position. We are not in the usual sense educators. We certainly are not psychotherapists. The children referred for language and learning difficulties frequently come with a file of reports from specialists which lend themselves to very different interpretations.

Consider the reports from the teacher, the neurologist, and the psychiatrist on a fifth-grade boy referred to us for remediation. The teacher states that the boy reads two and a half years below the class average, that his spelling is bizarre, and that he absolutely refuses to write a composition. His marks in math are not impressive either. She describes the boy as an underachiever in terms of his high intellectual potential. His performance is curiously uneven. By now he is so discouraged that he can hardly bear to try. Perhaps he is just lazy.

The neurologist writes that this boy's prenatal, natal, and postnatal history is ambiguous. He was a little late passing developmental milestones. He did not use phrases until the age of thirty-three months. He has always been moderately hyperactive. The electroencephalogram (EEG) is negative, as is the classical neurological examination, except for mild cerebellar signs which might or might not be significant. At any rate, his coordination is poor, not so much for large muscle activities as for graphomotor skills, to wit, his atrocious handwriting. He appears to suffer from a learning disability (which is the reason he was referred in the first place) probably on the basis of minimal brain injury.

The psychiatrist believes that as a result of neurotic conflict the boy presents an arrest in ego development and has insufficient psychic energy available for academic requirements. Punitive handling has complicated the situation. The parents are confused, angry, and guilty. The child's failure is experienced by them as a severe narcissistic blow.

Reprinted with permission from Yale University Press, from *The Psychoanalytic Study of the Child* 30:95–123. 1970.

All of these diagnostic labels—underachievement, learning disability, minimal brain injury, arrested ego development—have some essential validity. None of them, however, takes into account the complex interactions between physiological and psychological aspects of functioning, interactions which in turn are crucially affected by the emotional climate of the child's home.

I shall attempt in the following pages to discuss some of the characteristics of a number of children referred to clinics and offices with a variety of dysfunctions that escape precise classification. Many of these youngsters present atypical developmental patterns that are reflected not only in perceptuomotor deficits but above all in failure to master receptive and expressive aspects of language that require a high level of central integration. Among such children I have singled out two groups whose maturational delays and imbalances are fairly striking.

In view of the reciprocal relationship between language and developing ego functions, the question is raised what linguistic deficts mean in terms of children's psychic structure.

The problem of labeling and its implication for referral and therapy is taken up. Two cases are briefly discussed because in spite of similar physiological deficits, they did well with different kinds of management.

Language Development and Deficits

The children whom I shall describe, rather than discuss in terms of labels, range from two to eighteen years. The severity of their dysfunction extends from mild to severe. Some are in need of assistance at the preschool level. The difficulties of others do not become evident until they are faced with academic demands. Their difficulties are recognized relatively late because the children did not appear to be atypical, at least at first glance.

Nevertheless, these children are different. They present varying degrees of perceptuomotor deficits, uneven development, inconsistency of response, lability of affect, and little resistance to the normal stress and strain of growing up. They are vulnerable children. They exhibit symptoms singly or in a variety of combinations: irritability, poorly established early sleep and feeding rhythm, the disorganized and global motility typical for younger subjects, occasionally severe disorders of body schema and praxis, motor clumsiness, primitive perceptual and visuomotor experiences, fluctuations in attention, and a lowered threshold for anxiety. They have trouble with organizing and integrating experiences into cohesive wholes. The management and patterning of all kinds of information, perceptual, linguistic, and conceptual, present difficulties.

These children show no evidence of a circumscribed cerebral insult of the kind found in individuals who have suffered the loss of a previously established function. They do not present positive signs on the classical neurological examinations and the EEG. Nor do they suffer from significant sensory deficits or marked intellectual impairment.[1] Their difficulties are less gross. Ajurriaguerra (1966) points out that the effects of even subtle interference with central integrative processes are less drastic but far more global in younger than in older individuals. The less differentiated and the more plastic the organism, the more diffuse and more generalized are the symptoms (and at the same time the greater is the potential for compensatory adjustments). Whatever may have happened to the central nervous system of these children (and I specifically exclude children with verifiable brain injury, for example, epileptic children, etc.) happened to a system in the process of formation and can be assumed to have interfered with maturation and integration in many areas and on many levels of physiological and psychological functioning.

The more complex a function the more vulnerable it is. Language is a highly differentiated function; it is thus not surprising that we find linguistic deficits frequently in conjunction with other disturbances. Early linguistic difficulties are red flags in terms of subsequent academic failure. Even more significantly, they interfere from the very earliest age with developing ego functions that are essential for learning and for the child's total adaptation to his world.

Language comprehension requires ability to process intricately patterned inputs. Our children have difficulty breaking up the totality of a pattern and synthesizing parts into wholes. Their perceptual organization is diffuse. How do these babies, who have trouble analyzing and structuring patterns, make sense out of the buzzing confusion in which they are embedded? How do they detect the inherent regularities in the swiftly flowing stream of speech?[2]

Normal babies begin very early to respond selectively to many linguistic events (Friedlander 1970). Seemingly passive infants apparently do an enormous amount of discriminative listening.

Lewis (1963) describes how children learn to understand language. They first respond to the intonational features which carry the emotional load of communication and are an integral part of the

---

[1] These children are often called "organic." The concept, according to Clements (1973), has been broadened of late to include a wide spectrum of dysfunctions, sometimes based on genetic variations.

[2] The discussion of the crucially important communicative, interpersonal aspect of language is beyond the scope of this paper.

mother's affectively-colored caretaking activities. Very slowly, phonemic patterns become intertwined with situational and intonational
features until, gradually, as further differentiation takes place, phonemic patterns become dominant relatively independent of the
situation.

The mother's ongoing vocal and verbal exchange with her baby
differs from her communication with older children and with adults in
rate, rhythm, and dynamic accent. It provides the matrix from which
spring early communicative attitudes as well as the enjoyment in
verbal give-and-take, which is essential for language acquisition and
later learning. The mother caresses the baby with her voice; she tailors
her own utterances to his specific developmental needs; she endlessly
repeats sounds, words, and phrases, thus providing him with the data
that allow him to detect and to organize the recurring intonational and
phonemic signals into more or less stable categories. Wyatt (1969)
describes this interaction as a mutual feedback based on unconscious
identification. Piaget (1923) calls it "contagion verbale."

Language develops in the matrix of a close mother-child bond.
There are mothers who do not tune in, who either fail to provide
carefully dosed stimulation and feedback or who swamp the baby with
their verbalizations, thus failing to make him aware of the crucial
features of input.

The children I am discussing may fail to take advantage of the cues
provided by the mother. They may not stimulate her to engage in vocal
and verbal play. As a result, those children who need stimulation most
usually get least. Some of them may not even separate out speech from
the background of noise. They may experience speech as a diffuse
undifferentiated flow. At eighteen months when normal children
begin to discover phoneme and word boundaries, these children are
bathed in a sea of sounds and do not grasp the underlying schemata.

By the age of three or four, normal chidren are quite familiar with
the small connective words, the number, space, and time markers that
provide a set of relations and are the framework for the organization of
experience. The child who lacks understanding of such words lives in a
confusing universe, and this confusion may in turn interfere with the
organization of his inner and outer cosmos. He is limited to the here
and now. His world has few shades and few signposts.

The child who is unable to deduce from the incoming messages
the phonemic and syntactical rules underlying the surface structure of
language tends to tune out. He has learned *not* to listen. Difficulties
with processing input and withdrawal into fantasies interact. Missing
the more subtle aspects of communication, the child finds the pull of
fantasies more compelling, and invests less and less in listening except
when the message is highly cathected and verbalizations are relatively
short.

Kagan et al. (1960) point out that certain children fail to acquire the set of symbols that would allow them to conceptualize important aspects of their experience. The acquisition of these symbols, however, depends on adequate interpretation, and in order to conceptualize experience the child must understand the grammatical structures that provide him with linguistic options.

Both receptive and expressive language represent intricate structures. It is precisely with the structuring of perceptuomotor, affective, linguistic, and conceptual configurations that our children have the greatest difficulty. Such difficulty with structuring is typical for delayed or disordered development. Development, according to Werner (1957), proceeds from relative globality and lack of differentiation in the direction of increasing articulation and hierarchic organization. Successive stages of development are characterized by the emergence of new forms of organization and novel structures of increasing complexity. The performance of the children we work with could therefore be expected to be more primitive, more global, and less differentiated than that of children whose developmental course runs more smoothly.

Among the numerous children who present maturational delays I have picked out two subgroups—prematurely born and educationally unready children—because their maturational lags and imbalances in all areas of functioning appeared to be striking.

Prematurely Born Children

In the course of a reading prediction study (de Hirsch et al. 1966a, 1966b) we had an opportunity to investigate 53 children born before term with birthweights ranging from 2,240 grams to 980 grams. By comparing these children with a control group, we hoped to learn something about maturational deficits. Children born before term are by definition immature at birth, and there is some evidence that some of this immaturity may persist for varying periods of time.

We excluded those children who had been diagnosed as brain-injured, whose IQs fell a standard deviation below or above the norm, who showed sensory deficits, and who, on psychiatric evaluation, presented symptoms of psychopathology.

We saw the children two or three times between the ages of five and a half and eight. While there were considerable differences among them, I could, without prior information, distinguish most of the prematurely born from those born at term, which suggests that the prematures had certain characteristics in common. I would say that I recognized them because they somehow looked "unfinished" and "immersed."

With regard to those features that were treated statistically, one aspect measured was motility patterning. The prematurely born children hopped across the room, if indeed they were able to hop, like four-year-olds. The entire body was involved. Differences in motility patterning between prematures and controls were statistically significant in the direction of greater globality in the case of the prematures. Some of them were hypoactive and tended to slump. Most others were entirely at the mercy of a thousand environmental stimuli.

Their visuomotor gestalts were both primitive and fluid and only rough approximations of the designs to be copied. They flowed into each other and were rotated in space. In the visuomotor area differences between prematures and controls also reached statistical significance. The children's ability to imitate tapped-out patterns, to respond to auditory gestalts, and to reproduce them was inferior.

As a group the prematurely born brought to mind Bender's observations on "primitive plasticity" (1966).[3] One could say that their maturational status resembled that of younger children. At kindergarten age those born at term surpassed the prematures in 36 out of 37 tasks. On 15 tasks the differences were significant statistically. Among the 15, eleven were verbal tasks. Recognition of words, heard, language comprehension, word-finding, story organization, and ability to categorize were all significantly poorer in the prematures than in controls. It is of interest that in no single oral language dimension were the prematures superior. Differences in favor of controls were overwhelming on the so-called prereading tasks.

Twenty-eight months later, the performance of the prematurely born children in reading, writing, and spelling—all of which require a high level of neurological integration—was poorer than that of controls.[4] Statistically treated aspects of this study thus demonstrated that,

---

[3] Bender uses the term "plasticity" the way embryologists use it: "as yet unformed but capable of being formed;" and she uses it primarily for schizophrenic children. See also de Hirsch (1965).

[4] In a study of the interplay of prematurity, intrafamily dynamics, and "idiogenic" cognitive organization, Caplan et al. (1963) found a preponderance of cognitive disorders in the prematures as compared to controls. In their sample of 16 subjects the differences between the two groups were even greater at ages eleven to twelve than they had been between the ages of six and seven.

The discussion of the relationship between cognitive and linguistic dimensions has gone on for generations and cannot possibly be reviewed here. It is well known that language stabilizes perception and also serves as a mediator for nonverbal performances (Luria 1961). Verbal children talk themselves through a puzzle (this is how subjects with good linguistic endowment compensate for perceptual deficits). Language makes possible operations such as categorization and serializing. It allows the individual to determine the common property of things and to group them into larger entities, thereby facilitating the shift from associative to cognitive levels of operations. Thus, what Caplan calls "cognitive disorders" in his premature population may be closely related to linguistic deficits especially at higher age levels when the two tend to fuse (Vygotsky 1962). See also Scholnick and Adams (1973).

at least at kindergarten age, many of the prematurely born children represented a high risk group in terms of subsequent academic achievement.

Notes added to the children's protocols and an inspection of their individual profiles conveyed a clinical impression of each child's style as a learner. They showed that certain features were common to virtually all the prematurely born children. Clinically, they struck us as disoriented in time and space and as if they did not know how they fitted into the scheme of things. It is of interest that the 16 prematurely born children in Caplan's study (1963) showed identical problems with spatial and temporal categories.

The human figure drawings of our group were bizarre only in a few instances. However, they were crude, stick figures mostly, and they did not look as if they were anchored down. Many were slanted on the page and others seemed to float in space. The premature likewise had trouble remembering the dates of their birthdays, identifying the times of day, recalling past events.

Disorientation in space and time is characteristically found in children presenting disorders of spoken and printed language. Difficulty with sequencing and serial-order manipulations are frequently seen in dyslexic youngsters.

Disorientation in time has, however, other important implications. The pleasure principle operates now. The reality principle demands submission to time. Children have difficulty relinquishing immediate gratification until they have acquired some comprehension of the linguistic structures that denote temporal relationships. In dysphasic children, one observes that their capacity to wait grows with their increasing understanding of linguistic forms that represent the future. Their anxiety decreases. Pain does not last forever, mother will return *soon.* Time concepts and academic performance are closely related. Work requires postponing of gratification in the service of a distant goal.[5]

The prematures' approach to the examiner and the testing situation differed from that of the children born at term. Separation was much harder for the prematures. "Infantile" was the most frequently mentioned term in their protocols. Some had to be taken on the examiner's lap to enable them to get through the testing. They needed massive support and demonstrated little autonomy. Their need for oral gratification was enormous; they devoured masses of candy during testing sessions.

---

[5] Leshan (1952) found time orientation to vary with social class, perhaps because so many deprived individuals have no future, literally or figuratively. There is little incentive to work for uncertain rewards. Goal orientation and a stake in achievement are closely linked to the ordering of life in terms of sequencing. Some groups do not experience life in these terms.

The ego organization of premature children appeared to be loose and fragmented. We were impressed with the ebb and flow of their attention. More than full-term children, they moved in and out of focus. The level of their performance fluctuated. This variability may have resulted from the children's difficulties sustaining psychic energy for longer periods of time, but one also felt that smooth managing of inputs presented difficulties, that some of the children's basic perceptual experiences were unstable, and that their frame of reference tended to shift from one moment to the next.

Their anxiety—Greenacre (1953) described its organic stamp—appeared to be diffuse and amorphous. One cannot but feel that their poorly patterned, primitive, perceptual experiences were contributory factors (see also Kurlander and Colodny 1965).

Many of the prematures impressed one as dependent, passive, and shadowy. They appeared to be immersed in fantasies to a point where they were unable to invest in age-appropriate tasks. I do not want to give the impression that all of our prematures were handicapped; there were some vigorous and lively children among them who had considerable ego strength,[6] but they stood out in the group. And they did not necessarily do well on testing. They were still wedded to the pleasure principle and unable to mobilize their plentiful energy in the service of tasks that were unrelated to their drives. And among the 53 prematures there were, of course, a few who managed very adequately and did not present a significant developmental delay.

It would be a gross simplification to ascribe the relatively poor performance of the prematurely born children solely to the factors just described—to their deficits in the primary ego apparatus, their trouble with early homeostasis, and their lack of power over their bodies and the environment. Surely, the profound anxiety and sometimes despair aroused in mothers by premature birth, the prohibition against the handling and fondling of these babies, the worry over their slow early development (Kaplan and Mason 1960), the guilt feelings because such children are often unwanted, must of necessity have interfered with the mothers' handling of their infants. Psychiatric help enabled some mothers to respond both to the children's legitimate needs for protracted infantilization and to their emerging readiness for autonomy. The prematures' difficulties were inextricably bound up with their mothers' anxiety, which flowed over to these children, thus constituting a configuration in which it was difficult to tease apart crucial environmental, physiological, and psychological determinants.

---

[6] Ratings of ego strength were based on the independent judgment of three observers. We found statistically significant differences between the prematurely born children and controls in favor of the latter.

It is therefore of interest to look at a second subgroup of children whose history is not burdened by their mothers' intense anxiety but who nevertheless show a similar clinical picture.

Educationally Unready Children

Large numbers of five-and-a-half to seven-year-old children are referred to us because of questionable readiness for first grade entrance. This is, of course, a preselected group. However, in the course of a second predictive investigation (Jansky and de Hirsch 1972) we found among 400 randomly selected kindergarten pupils a fairly well circumscribed group whose test performance reflected a high risk of failure in the elementary grades. These children came from a variety of socioeconomic backgrounds; their IQs ranged from high to low.

The early development of educationally unready children does not necessarily present marked deviations. The majority are boys, and many of them are small in size. Bentzen (1963) believes that learning problems in boys may be the response of the immature organism to the demands of a society that fails to make appropriate provision for the biological age difference between boys and girls. Tanner (1961) found that around the age of six, males lag twelve months behind females in skeletal age. Some are very bright; Ilg and Ames (1965) call them the "superior immatures." They retain some of the global responses previously described as characteristic of prematurely born children. They frequently turn the whole head, for instance, when asked to flex the tongue. They have an inordinate need for motor outlets. They are distractible and cannot stick to a task for longer than 10 minutes at a time. Their frustration threshold is low.

Laterality is often ambiguous.[7] Auditory perceptions are not sharply defined.[8] They are poor listeners.[9] They do not follow the line of a

---

[7] In neither of the two predictive studies (1966 and 1972) was ill-defined laterality at this early age predictive for subsequent reading disorders. Identical symptoms mean different things at different ages. A ten-year-old who switches hands during writing would be suspected of central nervous system irregularity because by this age certain functions should be locked into place. McFie's research (1952) suggests that in children with reading disabilities, the neurological organization corresponding to dominance is not normally established in either hemisphere. Subirana (1961b) has found that the EEGs of strongly lateralized children are more mature than those of others. This does not exclude the significance of genetic factors.

[8] In speaking of auditory and visual perceptions in this context, I mean *verbal* auditory and visual perceptions. Many of the children described here have no trouble distinguishing between shades of sounds in the environment and do very well with discrimination among shapes and forms.

[9] During the course of development children become sensitive to successively different aspects of their environment. At age four and five the "critical" time for learning to listen may have passed.

simple story; they do not suggest alternate solutions. Some appear to be so preoccupied with the psychosexual conflicts typical of this particular age that they cannot listen to directions. Others simply have trouble interpreting all but the most primitive grammatical constructions. They cannot sort out, for instance, the difference between "the dog chases the boy" and "the boy chases the dog," or the difference between "mother's cats" and "mother cat." Their kindergarten teacher may complain about their trouble following directions. Visual verbal forms also are unstable. Letters such as p and q appear to pivot. Directionality continues to be an arbitrary matter. *Tap* and *pat* look more or less alike. Indeed, in some cases, ground and figure are not sharply differentiated. When presented with the word-matching section of the Gates Reading Readiness Test, one six-year-old told me angrily: "It's just a jumble, it looks like ants crawling around the page." While this was, of course, a phobic response, it also reflected the child's inability to structure and organize the printed configurations on the page into some kind of pattern.

Some of these children learn to compensate for their earlier plasticity. With the help of conceptual and contextual clues they become good readers. (Ability to compensate depends largely on cognitive endowment, ego strength, and environmental support.) The overwhelming majority, however, are stuck with often severe spelling disorders. They do not remember the overall gestalt of the word, or its internal design. They have little "physiognomic" ability. Words never become familiar or stable enough for recall. The children may do relatively well on a spelling list, but fail to reproduce correctly the identical words when they are embedded in a sentence. They are unable to maintain a linguistic gestalt (French 1953) even when ego functions are relatively unimpaired.

Dysnomia (word-finding difficulty) is frequently seen among educationally unready children. They can match colors, but cannot name them. They forget the names of favorite characters on their TV programs. These are the same youngsters who a few years later have trouble retrieving the names or the sounds of the alphabet. Picture naming was a powerful predictor of reading failure in Jansky's kindergarten screening battery (1972).

Despite high intelligence in many cases (as evidenced by their problem-solving ability and their often superior performance on psychometric tests) one finds a delay in physiological maturation and a lag in ego development which appear to go hand in hand. These children continue to move their bodies globally; their reflex behavior, tonus, and posture belong to a chronologically younger age. Their outstanding trait is impulsivity. They cannot wait; they cannot postpone gratification; and, as Anna Freud (1965) puts it, they cannot "carry out preconceived plans with a minimum regard for the lack of immediate pleasure yield, intervening frustration, and the maximum regard for the pleasure of the ultimate outcome."

Drive control constitutes a central problem.[10] Aggression is primitive and expressed through action rather than verbally. The amorphous nature of the stimuli on the Rorschach plates tends to arouse disorganized and chaotic responses and makes it difficult for such youngsters to reject aggressive and fairly primitive fantasies. The stories they tell in response to pictures are filled with references to food and longings for early instinctual gratification. The material clearly shows that the children have not begun to move out from a fairly egocentric universe and are preoccupied with conflicts belonging to an earlier psychosexual phase. Wish-fulfilling and magic solutions are ready at hand. Anna Freud's statement (1965) that a measure of advance in ego development and drive control is a necessary forerunner of the ability to work is strikingly demonstrated in the case of these children. They are not ready for formal education. At older ages some of them develop compulsive-obsessivelike mechanisms. At age eight a youngster's Bender copies may be scattered all over the page, while at age thirteen the same youngster might encase each single copy to anchor it down on the page, as it were. These defenses appear to be directed not so much against forbidden impulses as against fears of disintegration (Kurlander and Colodny 1965). Whatever their origin, these mechanisms constitute one more barrier to learning. An important avenue for research would be the choice and the structure of defenses used by these particular children.

Language and Psychic Organization

If one looks at both prematurely born and educationally unready children, the question arises whether lags in ego development and delay in patterning perceptuomotor and linguistic stimuli should be regarded as two separate phenomena or rather as manifestations of a pervasive organismic immaturity[11] that invades all sectors of the personality and interferes with the orderly organization of experience.

---

[10] Lack of control over drives is, of course, not related solely to linguistic deficits. In some cases it appears to be one aspect of the child's biological dysfunction, the "organic drivenness" syndrome. The forces that propel the children appear to be related to their difficulty in organizing their inner and outer cosmos. Secondary conflicts are, of course, the rule rather than the exception.

[11] The concept of maturation as put forward by Bender (1958) is based on the theory of functional areas in the brain and the personality which develop longitudinally according to a recognizable pattern. A maturational lag, then, could be defined as a retention of primitive experiences in perceptuomotor gestalts, body imagery, and conceptualization of time and space.

In the prematurely born children, maturational deficits are in all probability related to the original physiological lag and one might ask, as Weil (1961) does, whether the organism's inherent tendency to structuralization and the capacity for integration are weaker in these children than in others.

In the educationally unready children, one might hypothesize a physiological variant. Orton (1930) and his pupils, most Scandinavian researchers (Herman 1959; Hallgren 1950), and Owen et al. (1971), who tested the parents and siblings of dyslexic children, maintain that reading and spelling difficulties are found in given families. This is borne out by the large number of family files piling up in our clinics and offices. That severe immaturity may be genetically determined was postulated by Zangwill (1962). It is possible (though I have no way to prove it) that it is not the reading and spelling disorder per se which is genetically determined, but rather the underlying maturational defect that is reflected both in deficits of spoken and printed language and perhaps also in delays in the structuralization of the ego.

It may be worth while to trace in greater detail the specific and intricate meshings of lags in both the linguistic and the psychic organization, what Edelheit (1968) calls the deeply rooted reciprocity between language and ego development.

Linguists are primarily concerned with the formal properties of language. The main interest of academic psychologists centers around the role of language in cognition. Both disciplines have largely neglected to probe the part language plays in the child's growing ability to define himself, to gain control over drives, and to cope with reality demands. It is to the psychoanalytic literature that one must turn for more penetrating insights into the relationship between linguistic and psychic structure (Atkin 1969; Edelheit 1968a, 1969; Rosen 1967; Peller 1966; Katan 1961; Waelder 1960; Balkanyi 1964; Kolansky 1967; Frank 1969).

Rappaport (1961) speaks about the repercussion of the organic dysfunction on the epigenesis of the ego. This implies, however, a cause-and-effect relationship, and does not take into account the interactions between the two. While a severe lisp, for instance, may interfere with the child's social relationships, it should not be overlooked that a need for oral gratification may enter into lisping and in turn reflect attitudes which might be unacceptable to the group in the first place.[12]

---

[12] To assume, as does Rousey (1969), that other specific sound substitutions, such as f for th, reflect highly specific emotional constellations—in this case, a disturbance in the early and significant relationship with the father—seems to be a gross simplification. Among other things, it neglects to take into account the inherent laws of phonemic development.

Rappaport ignores the fundamental fact that the development of language is a major determinant in the differentiation and growth of the ego itself. Indeed, Edelheit (1969) considers the ego as a language-determining and language-determined structure.

Verbal signs heavily reinforced by intonations reassure the child that the mother will return even if she is gone for a while, and they thus contribute to object constancy. In the children discussed here, the very perceptual experience of the mother is probably more fragmented and more diffuse than that of others. Being unable to stabilize their experience by means of language, they are doubly handicapped. It would be of interest to explore the possibility of a delay in development of object constancy in organic children and to investigate what such delay, if any, means in terms of the children's adaptation to and trust in the world.

The appearance of the ego as a psychic structure and the emergence of verbalizations occur more or less simultaneously during the last two phases of the separation-individuation process (Mahler 1971). Rosen (1967) states that the symbolic use of words is the most crucial step in the process of individuation. Since individuation itself seems to be a prerequisite for the development of language, it is clear that these processes are reciprocal and that disturbance in one will be reflected in the other.

Children probably have some sensorimotor schemata that give rise to a vague and fleeting sense of self before they use words. It is quite true that without a fairly well developed sense of self, of being separate, verbal dialogue cannot take place. On the other hand, the distinction between the *me* and the *not me* is enormously strengthened when the child understands and uses concepts such as *mine* and *I* (Peller 1966). One sees this clearly in schizophrenic children. Their unstable ego boundaries are mirrored in their severe communicative deficits. Their idiosyncratic use of language reveals the dominance of archaic and primitive affects and drives. Words for these children are not necessarily tools for adaptation to reality or for communication.[13] As in dreams, words are played with, condensed, truncated (Werner and Kaplan 1963); they tend to express instinctual needs.

In young children one can observe the many ways language fluctuates depending on its use for the primary or the secondary process. Baby talk is an example of the use of language in the service of regression. Syntactical constructions change into more primitive ones,

---

[13] This becomes very clear when one compares the language deficits of dysphasic and schizophrenic children. The language of the latter may reflect the displacements and condensations of the primary process, while in the former, verbalizations, no matter how primitive, serve mainly the secondary process (de Hirsch 1967).

word-order rules no longer hold, phonemic profiles flatten out, iterations of sounds and words become more frequent, sentence melody
changes in the direction of nursery rhymes, and singsongs often
accompany rhythmic movements. Pitch rises, and the oral gratification
function of language moves into the foreground. A little later, the
child's language changes back into more age-adequate linguistic forms
and the cognitive and communicative functions of language reassert
themselves.

Listening to a four-year-old talk to himself while he plays with his
train, one may notice initially that his verbalizations are in the service
of mastery. As the play changes and the train comes to stand for power
and potency, syntax dissolves, novel words are invented, meanings
are used idiosyncratically, pitch fluctuates. In other words, as the child
slips back and forth between the different levels of organization, the
formal features of language reflect these changes.[14]

Katan (1961) describes how the externalization of magical and
omnipotent fantasies by means of words renders these fantasies less
dangerous and contributes heavily to reality testing, one of the crucial
functions of the ego. Dysphasic children take much longer than others
to emerge from their magic universe. Lacking verbal concepts, they
have far fewer opportunities to test their fantasies against reality,
which is one of the reasons why the differential diagnosis between
autistic and dysphasic children is often difficult to arrive at.

Inner processes enter consciousness by being associated with
their verbal representation (Frank 1969). Verbalizations help establish
control and reduce acting out. Many years ago we worked with a
four-year-old who had been referred by an analyst because of a
moderately severe receptive-expressive aphasia and who could not be
retained in his nursery school because of severe hyperkinesis and
uncontrolled aggressiveness. Thomas did not strike us as a particularly
hostile youngster. His aggression was somehow different from that of
neurotic children; it had a quality which has been described as "organic
drivenness." Since the boy was unable to reconcile his behavior with
the demands of the environment, there were many secondary conflicts. Moreover, he suffered from feelings of guilt about being bad, as
do many such children. Some two years later, when he had acquired
reasonably effective, if primitive, verbal tools, I heard him say upon
entering the room, "This is one of my days, take the junk [toys]

---

[14] Vygotsky (1962) distinguished between the "meaning" of a word and its
"sense." Sense, he says, contains all the private and perceptual associations of the
word. He talks, of course, about inner speech which, he maintains, is saturated
with "sense." It seems to me that in the egocentric speech of young children (Piaget
1923), which accompanies their fantasies during play, we find the same saturation
with the "sense" of words—verbalizations drenched with affect rather than related
to thought processes.

away—it sets me off." The fact that this youngster had learned to label his behavior and the underlying feeling states meant that he was no longer entirely delivered to the forces that drove him.

Anna Freud (1936) wrote:

> The association of affects and instinctual processes with word representations is stated to be the first and the most important step in the direction of the mastery of instinct which has to be taken as the individual develops. Thinking is described in these writings as an "experimental kind of acting, accompanied by displacement of relatively small quantities of cathexis together with less expenditure (discharge) of them" (Freud 1911, p. 221). This intellectualization of instinctual life, the attempt to lay hold on the instinctual processes by connecting them with ideas which can be dealt with in consciousness, is one of the most general, earliest, and most necessary acquirements of the human ego. We regard it not as an activity of the ego but as one of its indispensable components.

The ontogenesis of language cannot be separated from consciousness, which, according to Edelheit (1968a), confers meaning and structure on the world and which includes an awareness of self, an awareness that is an essential condition of superego development. Waelder (1960) felt that a prerequisite of superego formation is the capacity for introspection and the ability to stand back and regard the self from an imaginary vantage point.[15] It implies the capacity to abstract, which in turn is intimately bound up with language.

It was fascinating to watch the parallel emergence of superego precursors and linguistic forms in another dysphasic boy who was started on a language-stimulation program at the age of thirty months. As his speech improved, he was able to talk about his difficulties with self-control, and after a particularly stormy session, he stood himself in front of the mirror and said: "Brian, you are a horrid little boy."

Piaget (1932) says that cognitive development must have reached a certain stage to enable the child to internalize moral values. While this is undoubtedly true, one might raise the question whether the internalization of moral demands does not also require the ability to use certain linguistic options. Conscience implies a choice. "I would like to swipe the candy, but *if* I did, I would feel bad." The nonverbal child might or might not swipe the candy. If he did, he might anticipate punishment, but in the absence of linguistic options his chances to internalize moral values would be limited.

---

[15] It should be added that this also includes an awareness of the tool of language itself as revealed in the linguistic jokes most seven- and eight-year-olds delight in: "Did you ever see a butter fly?" (Gleitman 1973).

If linguistic development were in some ways related to superego formation, one would expect deaf individuals to be delayed in this respect. There is a great deal of new research directed toward the relationship between cognitive and linguistic dimensions in deaf children (Furth 1974), but very little work has been done on the ego and superego development in youngsters who have profound hearing losses. Lesser and Easser (1972) say that the deaf show a relative lack of the self-observing ego, a conscience formation different from that to be expected, and they add that deaf children regress easily to primary process thinking. The few deaf individuals I have observed closely appeared to follow very rigid rules of behavior (which does not necessarily mean that they had internalized a value system). It was evident that they dealt in absolute categories. Things or people were either black or white; there were few shades because these children did not have at their disposal sophisticated and differentiated linguistic tools.

It is, of course, essential to stress that in innumerable cases, physiological lags and neurotic conflicts resulting in arrested ego development or regression to an earlier psychosexual phase may have independent roots, but nevertheless interact. The seven-year-old who has failed to solve conflicts belonging to the oedipal situation, and who does not catch on to reading in the first and second grade because of a constitutional weakness in the language area, will look on his failure as a conclusive confirmation of the grave doubts he has about himself. His failure intensifies feelings of helplessness and impotence, which in turn prevent him from using his compensatory resources. We encounter this kind of interaction day in and day out in the children referred for language and learning disabilities. Specific weaknesses provide a convenient focal point for phobic responses.

The Implications of Labeling for the Choice of Therapy

Calling our children "brain-injured," no matter whether or not we add the word "minimal," is unjustified in the absence of positive signs on the classical neurological examination and a conclusive history of cerebral insult (Birch 1964). This label, furthermore, does not account for genetic variations. It is an inferential diagnosis, conveying to the parents and to the environment, including the children themselves, that they are physically and mentally crippled. Saying that they suffer from minimal cerebral dysfunction also constitutes an inferential diagnosis, but it has at least the advantage that the term refers to processes rather than to structure.

If one were to describe these children rather than label them, one might say that their experiences in a number of areas are less stable, more fragmented, cruder, and above all far less under the control of the ego than those of other children. To say that their experiences resemble those of younger subjects is valid, but the fact that they are actually older, and thus encounter a different environment and expectations, results in significant developmental imbalances[16] as well as in a different structuring of their defenses.

Bender (1955) feels that a maturational lag reflected clinically in primitive patterning is precisely what constitutes nonfocal brain injury.

Conrad (1948) in his work on adult aphasia speaks of the phenomenon of "dedifferentiation." We observe in our children simplified organizational schemata and what is probably a defect in differentiation of more complex gestalts.

Starting with early sensorimotor experiences and continuing all the way up to higher psychic functions, our children appear to have difficulties responding to and integrating gestalts, a difficulty which may be reflected in delayed development of the integrative function of the ego. Evidence of problems with gestalts is seen clearly in the lack of flow in the children's handwriting, in the absence of sentence melody when they read aloud. Pick (1931) called it "Sprachgefühl," feel for language.[17] One also sees it when after months of painstaking work, the dyslexic youngster suddenly integrates subskills, takes off, and reads. Watching the process, one feels that it does not consist of adding one skill to another, but rather that the gestalt suddenly jumps out (de Hirsch 1954).

It would be fascinating to inquire whether the tendency to fragmentation, the difficulty in grasping wholes, and the instability of the gestalt experience influence the formation of the very easiest object relationships. Perhaps these children are slower than others in linking need gratification with the percept of the person who provides it.

Unfortunately, the problem of labeling is not an academic one, since in a large number of cases the label determines the choice of therapy. The child who is said to present minimal brain dysfunction may receive appropriate medication. However, he may miss out on the psychological support from the psychotherapist who lends him his own ego attributes—interest in mastery, pride in achievement, and willingness to push through. He has nobody to turn to if he needs help with the secondary conflicts arising from his situation. On the other hand, the youngster who has been correctly diagnosed as suffering from lag in ego development may be exposed to years of interpretative

---

[16] The problem of "critical" periods comes up in this context: the time (and it clearly varies for different functions) in which basic organizations and structures are laid down (Connelly 1972).

[17] Many years ago Pick (1931) said that the process of language do not consist of a collection of elements, rather they are from the very beginning patterned structures ("gestaltete Strukturen").

therapy to the neglect of his educational needs which tend to snowball and result in additional problems and conflicts (A. Freud 1974).

In my experience, the preschoolers who have significant linguistic deficits and lags in readiness skills do best with an intensive relationship therapy. This can be done either by a psychotherapist who can simultaneously carry out a careful language-stimulation program in the framework of his own approach and who can work with the mother; or by a language therapist who has some idea of the psychological implications of the child's behavior, who has learned to listen to what the child is trying to say even on a nonverbal level.

Weil (1973) suggests educational therapy for such children before latency, in preparation for analysis. The educator, on the other hand, must be alert to signs which point to the necessity for psychiatric intervention.

In many cases, the contribution of specific handicaps is slight and the child's educational difficulties are directly related to neurosis. While the decision in such cases is relatively clear-cut, it is not always easy to convince the parents. They often come to us precisely because we are *not* psychiatrists. Consulting an educator seems to be less threatening. Furthermore, the parents may previously have been told that the child's problem is "developmental," "organic," or "familial," and it may be difficult for them to understand that such conditions do not exempt the child from conflict but are, rather, precipitating factors.

There are other children whose significant neurophysiological lags are closely intertwined with their psychological problems. Some of them are so preoccupied with intruding fantasies that they are unavailable for remediation and have no psychic energy available for academic requirements.

Tonia is an example. She was a small, dainty, little girl with a tiny face and masses of very dark hair. The child looked anxious and somewhat distraught. There was a frantic, worried air about her. She had been rejected for the second time by every private girl's school in town, a blow to her parents. She was currently in the third grade of one of the more acceptable public schools in the silk-stocking district in Manhattan. She managed in math, but she was nevertheless at the bottom of her class in reading, writing, and spelling, although she scored an IQ of 125 on the verbal and one of 112 on the performance section of the WISC. She hated school, she had no friends, and her mother said she was totally unable to concentrate.

There were no doubts as to Tonia's specific deficits. At this late date she reversed the letters in her own name and signed her drawing: "Msi Tonai" (for Miss Tonia). She transposed sounds in words and scrambled words in sentences even in speaking. Her verbalizations were rushed, indistinct, and poorly organized. She told endless stories in which people went to and fro, but it never became clear what they were doing and why they were there.

Tonia's responses to the CAT pictures raised more questions than they answered, but they pointed to sexual preoccupations. The bathroom picture, above all, elicited a good deal of excitement.

Tonia's mother told me that the child's early development had been uneventful, except for speech which had been late to emerge. Tonia had nightmares during which she twitched all over. She did not easily talk about her feelings, the mother added. Apart from her failure at school, the main complaint was "stubbornness." It was only when I specifically asked about toilet training that I got the full story. Tonia had stopped wetting early. Bowel training, on the other hand, had been a traumatic affair. The child was afraid of the toilet, she refused to perform, and suffered from extreme constipation. The nurse became terribly upset, as did the mother, with the result that the child held on to her stools for as long as 10 days. Suppositories and enemas were not particularly helpful and produced endless scenes. The power struggle lasted for nearly two years, but things straightened out when the nurse left.

I suggested that the parents discuss Tonia's problems with an analyst. Nothing came of it, however, because they could not bring themselves to go any further.

In the meantime the child had settled down in the office,[18] and although she would much rather have played and often looked longingly at the dollhouse, she did try to apply herself to the educational task. The returns were woefully limited. Tonia's many spatial and linguistic difficulties continued to plague her. Above all, she was unable to stay with any one activity. "Things run around my head like squirrels," she said. She asked innumerable questions, not taking the time to listen for the answers. She became more and more restless swaying in her chair and complaining about her peers: "They think I'm crazy and dumb, but I'm not, am I?"

Over the next few months it became increasingly evident that Tonia was intensely preoccupied with sexual fantasies in which beatings played a predominant role. None of these fantasies was elicited; they would spill over against her wish; she appeared to have no way of defending herself against them. Not only did they make Tonia feel terribly guilty, but they played havoc with learning. No wonder she was drawn to the dollhouse; play would have given her some outlet for her fantasies.

Since nothing solid was being accomplished, I made another

---

[18] Dr. Jeannette Jansky was the therapist who worked with both of the children described here. She also did the psychological work-ups.

urgent appeal to the parents, who finally agreed to send the child into analysis while continuing with remedial work. The analyst was a man, which initially eliminated some of the transference problems that might otherwise have been troublesome. The remedial therapist was quite capable of dealing with the vicissitudes of the analytic process as it intruded into the educational situation. Tonia soon understood which kinds of material belonged to the remedial setting and which to the analyst's office. Above all, the analyst and the therapist were in close contact.

There were no very sudden changes; but when one looked at the child two years later, she was a different girl. What had apparently happened was a developmental spurt that was reflected in both the physiological and the psychological segments of the personality. One might ask whether such a spurt would by itself have worked the changes we observed. I do not think so. I believe that the analytic process, by relieving the child of preoccupations belonging to an earlier psychosexual phase, enabled her to respond to teaching and to compensate for her specific deficits.

The stubbornness that had so upset the mother was now in the service of autonomy and adaptation. Her academic work improved considerably because Tonia could bend her energies to the task at hand. She was accepted in a private school. Her spelling still was quite poor; her compositions were vivid but not exactly elegantly form-ulated, and she still had trouble with punctuation. She read with pleasure and she now had a few friends.

In Tonia's case remedial work and analysis were carried out simultaneously. She would have fallen too far behind if remedial help had been postponed. Without analysis, on the other hand, she would not have been accessible to remediation.

Nick's case is different. His specific difficulties were, if anything, more massive than Tonia's. To begin with, the family history of language difficulties was heavily positive. In the past we had worked with two other members of the father's family, and we had seen three others in consultation because of delayed speech development and various disorders of printed and written language.

Nick immediately impressed us as strikingly immature physiolog-ically. Although he is in the fourth grade, his second teeth are just coming in. He was a slight, blond boy with a charming face, but when we first saw him more than three years ago he looked as if he had not quite jelled. Nick was incredibly hyperactive, as a result of which his family found it difficult to cope with him. His kindergarten teacher had called him a "buzz-bomb." Sitting still was a major problem. For the past two years he had been on Ritalin which helped in the learning situation. His drawing of a human figure was quite primitive, his Bender copies those of a much younger child. He had a terrible time managing the pencil and his hand tended to shake because he had to press so hard to control it. Nick's oral language was quite immature. He had not incorporated basic syntactical rules and would cheerfully say: "I dag clams" because he had the vague feeling that the past tense of *dig* is irregular. He would tell one excitedly that they had a *firebrush* close to the house when he meant a *brushfire*. Nick was (and up to a point still is) a clutterer and appears to lack anticipatory schemata—his verbal formulations are quite poor. Nick had a dysnomia of gigantic proportions—he could not recall color names until he was seven years old.

It is easy to see the implications of these deficits for learning the letters of the alphabet or, for that matter, their sound equivalents—Nick had to tie the shape of the letter and its name to some concrete clue in order to remember it. His retention of whole words was terribly poor as well. It took him forever to learn to recognize the printed word *kitten:* he was apt to lose it when he saw it in different contexts. He simply could not hold on to the verbal visual gestalt. If only he had had a feel for the flow of a sentence, it would have been easier for him to compensate for his perceptual instability by guessing from the surrounding syntactical and contextual configurations what the options were. Unfortunately, he had no feel for it. It was the combination of perceptual instability and linguistic deficits that accounted for his massive reading disability.

Psychologically, Nick was a solid boy. He had the age-appropriate conflicts which he handled rather well. He had his difficulties; his boiling point was low, and he was very easily frustrated (in his case there were good reasons for it). Yet, he never gave up, even when he was occasionally close to tears. He was fiercely jealous of his younger brother, but nowadays he is occasionally amused by him. He treats him the way he treats his animals—Nick lives surrounded by lizards, two dogs, three cats, and a much beloved snake—roughly but good naturedly.

Nick is bright. He does well in math, and he is a collector of facts. He is a vivid, entertaining boy with a delicious sense of humor, and he has many friends. He more or less owns the office. He has been coming for over three years, which means that his unusually devoted mother had to drive him four times a week from one of the Connecticut suburbs to Manhattan.

For the first time this year Nick is beginning to look like a latency boy. He is much less hyperactive, but during lessons he wriggles in his chair. In spite of intensive efforts his handwriting still is atrocious and his spelling remains quite poor, though it is less bizarre than it had been. However, he is developing a feel for the flow of a sentence. It makes all the difference because it helps him guessing from context and to compensate up to a point for his continuing perceptual instability. To everyone's amazement he is now reading at the mid-third-grade level, and the other day he wrote a composition half a page long. For Nick this is a tremendous achievement. The next year will probably show further physiological changes and we expect considerable gains.

Nick illustrates the gross physiological immaturity described earlier in this paper. In his case one would be entitled to speak of a maturational defect rather than a lag. While his deficits will become less obvious with ongoing development, I believe that one will find residuals in later years. I feel sure, nevertheless, that Nick will in the last instance do well. He is determined to be an explorer, an excellent illustration of his ability to sublimate his hyperkinesis and to use his passion for animals.

What enabled this grossly immature youngster to cope? In contrast to many other physiologically immature children, he has a great deal of ego strength. His capacity to relate is impressive. He uses his therapist constructively. It is this relationship that enabled the boy to mobilize the more than normal quantities of energy he needed in order to benefit from remedial measures. I feel (though it would be difficult to prove) that in some of these children a very close identification with the remedial worker is a powerful factor in neurophysiological maturation.[19] Another asset in his ability to work. In contrast to many other immature children, he has made the shift from the pleasure to the reality principle. Finally, he had the full support of his family.

Remedial therapists confronted with sometimes conflicting reports from a variety of specialists need some awareness of the complexity of the presenting symptoms. They must realize that an identical configuration of deficits may or may not result in failure, depending on the child's inherent strength and the kind of support he can draw upon to compensate for his deficits. Without such awareness, they will not be in a position to make appropriate referrals, nor will they be able to map out adequate remedial strategies. No matter which specific techniques are employed, the therapist will have to work with the child's affects in order to mobilize the energy he needs to compensate for early adaptive failure.

Summary

This paper attempts to describe a group of atypical children whose sometimes severe physiological deficits represent one aspect of a

---

[19] This statement is of course debatable since maturation has been defined as the organism's inherent tendency to evolve new structures relatively independent of environmental influences. Koffka (1935) stated that any perceived gestalt is the product of inner organization *and* training. Schilder (1964) felt that training and stimulation play a significant part even in those functions in which maturation of the central nervous system is of primary importance. This is true, above all, during transitional states.

pervasive organismic immaturity that is reflected in difficulties with integration on all levels—perceptuomotor, linguistic, cognitive, and in terms of the ego's organization. The specific constellation varies from child to child. The impact on the child's functioning depends on his ability to mobilize his adaptational resources. The child's genetic endowment, including his greater or lesser vulnerability to stress; his prenatal, natal, and postnatal history; the emotional climate in which he is raised; the social scene of which he is part—all interact in complex ways.

The crucial role of the home and, more specifically, of the nature of the mother-child bond has not even been touched upon and is beyond the scope of this paper. Suffice it to say that at the very earliest ages the characteristics of the children discussed here tend to alter the normal response patterns of the mother (Thomas et al. 1963; Weil 1970a), which in turn modify the child's perception of self and contribute to his pathology. I refer here to what Weil (1970a) calls the "multifaceted complimentary series of interactions."

The premium our society places on success is another factor that enters the situation in the case of learning-disabled children. It is against the background of the mother-child communication, non-verbal and verbal, and the demands of the larger society that the difficulties of these children have to be assessed.

Patterning and Organizational Deficits in Children with Language and Learning Disabilities

with Jeannette Jefferson Jansky

Introduction

Among children referred with the label learning disability, there is an identifiable and distinct group that presents specific difficulties with the organization of complex patterns. Such children exhibit one or several dysfunctions in behavior, motility, memory, attention, perceptual and perceptuomotor functioning, and the processing and generating of language. Depending on the examiner's bias, they may be classified as brain injured, as presenting deviational development, or as having maturational lags. Occasionally some are diagnosed as borderline schizophrenic or as suffering from atypical ego development. Whatever the label, problems with the organization of both internal and external events are at the very core of their difficulties.

Gestalt theory, which is concerned with the organization of experience and its arrangement within the observer into a cohesive view of the world, offers a useful framework for conceptualizing the behavior and performance of these particular children, a framework that transcends several diagnostic categories.

Gestalt theory claims that there exists in the organism an inherent tendency to apprehend and respond to organized configurations and that this tendency to impose structure[1] is a basic principle of psychophysiological functioning. Piaget (1971) says that a predisposition towards organization exists even before the organism has experienced the external environment. Experiences are not recorded on a blank field, but are integrated into constantly changing structures. Form,

---

[1]The authors use the term "structure" not as it is used in psychoanalysis, but in the much broader sense, that is, structure as enduring form impressed upon the flow of energy.

Reprinted with permission from The Orton Dyslexia Society, from *Bulletin of The Orton Society* 30:227–239. 1980.

according to Wertheimer (1944), depends on the relationship between the whole and its parts, which mutually determine each other. Gestalt theory deals with the dimensional and organizational aspects of experience and refers not only to part-whole relationships, but also to figure-ground contrasts.

While classical gestalt theory was limited to visual phenomena, the theory, as explained by Werner and Strauss (1941), is applicable also to higher processes. Instability of figure-ground relationships can exist on the conceptual as well as on the visual level. In the group of children discussed here, marked difficulty with organization of patterns implies a reduction in complexity, a "primitivisation" of gestalten (*Strukturvereinfachung*) perceptually, conceptually, and perhaps also, in the realm of psychic organization.

Description and Symptomatology of Organizational Deficits

The descriptions and formulation that follow are drawn from clinical observation.

Organizational Difficulties

Organizational deficits permeate the children's personal style. Their hold on their daily life is precarious. They often look disheveled and their rooms are chaotic. They may be pulled about by their fantasies (and their defenses against them may not always be effective), but in a more fundamental sense, their tendency to drift appears to be related to their inability to organize their experiences adequately.

Their difficulty with managing time is an example. Awareness of time is, of course, an ego function and related to the ability to postpone gratification. But time is also an inherent dimension of language, and for children with language deficits, the *now* is what counts. Clinically, they appear to lack an inner clock, a lack which may be related to a basic dysfunction in organization and planning.

Many of the children are flooded with anxiety, an anxiety that differs from that of normal children for whom it serves as a signal and leads to defensive mechanisms and symptom formation. Disorganized children are overwhelmed by poorly sorted out impulses and impressions and thus they are not always sure how they hang together and how they fit into the scheme of things.

The ability to manage schemata, that is, organized configurations, changes as a function of age. This ability clearly does not depend solely on organismic factors. Individual life experiences contribute to the children's competence in structuring the perceptual, linguistic, social, and affective field. To be embedded in a nurturing environment enhances the baby's chances of making sense of his world. Chaotic surroundings, forever shifting caretakers, and exposure to an over-whelming array of stimuli in the absence of a consistently available and caring adult are bound to contribute to disorganization.

But, taking into account the indisputable effects of age and life experience, one must nevertheless acknowledge that ability to manage complex patterns varies from one individual to the next. Among youngsters of the same age and intelligence, there are those whose difficulties with the analysis and construction of complex patterns are far more pervasive than are those of others.

These phenomena are readily observable in infancy. Those babies with a diffuse and unstable perception of the mother, and those able to recognize her voice only much later, may be delayed in achieving object constancy. Precursors of a deficit in pattern management are evident also in babies who, on the vegetative level, fail to establish adequate feeding and sleeping rhythms.

At a later stage, these children may have trouble patterning their motor behavior. According to Birch (1964), and this is important, the children are not hyperactive in the sense that their movements are excessive quantitatively, but their movements differ qualitatively in that they are random, imprecise, and poorly directed.

Most children with organizational difficulties are distractible and easily pulled from one activity to the next, probably because they are unable to defend themselves against the onslaught of a host of stimuli and cannot respond selectively to the field. Figure-ground separation is one of the basic mechanisms by which the individual organizes the environment. Difficulty with pulling out from a chaotic universe the figure, i.e., what Gibson (1963) calls the "focal point" in stimulus arrays, may be one reason for their distractibility. These children's troubles with figure-ground organization were vividly illustrated in a mother's story about her ten-year-old whom she could take to Saks department store, but not to Bloomingdale's. Bloomingdale's, she said, "unhinges" him.

Ambiguous Laterality

Ambiguous lateralization, a normal occurrence in young children, continues to be a feature in the older subjects in this group. It is usually ascribed to uncertain hemispheric differentiation. This, in turn, raises the question of whether such lack of differentiation reflects a diffuse internal organization.

The children find it hard to organize proprioceptive, tactile, per-ceptual, social, and affective experiences into a cohesive body image. This is reflected in their poor drawings of the human figure. These drawings are poorly articulated and very primitive. Often they are slanted on the page, testifying to the youngsters' weak spatial organization.

One can observe similar difficulties in their reproductions of the Bender gestalten. Some children in the group fail to respond to and reproduce the essence of the gestalten, violating the integrity of the individual figure by cheerfully superimposing one design upon another. Others have trouble organizing visual space and scatter the designs on the page so that they look windblown.

Organizational Problems with Language Processing

The organizational deficits mentioned so far involve relatively simple asymbolic functions. The management of complex symbolic activities, such as language, requires far more sophisticated pattern-processing strategies.

Far earlier than has previously been known, infants are actively engaged in seeking out the recurring patterns in the swiftly flowing stream of speech. For children with pattern processing difficulties this is a formidable task. They are bathed in a sea of sounds, there are few boundaries, and little stands out from an amorphous background. Such children find it hard to break up the sequence of only vaguely perceived impressions into meaningful and clearly defined units.

At a somewhat later age, there are other difficulties, holding in mind specific linguistic configurations, scanning incoming ones, and comparing them with those previously stored. Their diffuse reception, furthermore, makes it hard for the children to pull out from the input the underlying linguistic rules that govern both the comprehension and the generation of correctly constructed sentences. As a result, the children's acquisition of language is often delayed and on close examination their language development shows significant receptive gaps.

Output, i.e., expressive language, mirrors the children's diffuse reception. Their characteristic expressive oral language dysfunctions will be taken up in the section on cluttering, a symptom that is typically found in children with organizational problems.

Perceptual Instability

Reading disabilities are purported to be related to perceptual disorders, but "perceptual instability" would be a far better term. Configurational problems may show first at lower levels: children may fail in spite of frequent exposure to identify the characteristic gestalt of single letters. Both letters and word gestalten evidently look different to them from one context to the next and are recognized one moment only to be missed minutes later. For these youngsters, left-to-right progression is an arbitrary matter. Indeed, some may read as well upside down as right side up. To certain youngsters who fail to learn to read, the printed page may look like a bewildering meaningless design. One seven-year-old said disgustedly, "These scribbles look like ants running around the page." Although this is, as mentioned earlier, a phobic response it describes the child's experience vividly.

The salient point in all of this is the children's enormous difficulties maintaining linguistic gestalten. The verbal configuration apparently shifts from one context to the next.

Their spelling clearly reflects this phenomenon. Many youngsters compensate for their reading difficulties very early by means of intelligent use of contextual and linguistic options. But it is far more difficult to compensate for perceptual instability in spelling than it is in reading. The children may manage spelling lists, but they lose the overall gestalt of the word as well as its internal design when the word is embedded in context. Because the physiognomic quality of certain words is weak, children mix up "faceless" words such as *wear, where,* and *were,* in spite of the fact that the semantic and syntactical functions of these words differ (de Hirsch 1954). In the final analysis, poor recall of the way words look distinguishes the poor speller from the good one because spelling depends mainly on the retrieval visual-verbal configurations. For the weak speller, gestalt of the word is never stable enough to become familiar.

Cluttering

The cluttering syndrome,[2] which should not be confused with stuttering, is a paradigm for a pervasive organizational language deficit. As such, it includes nearly all of the features characteristic for language impaired youngsters.

Cluttering youngsters tend to be distractible and their motor patterning is usually inferior. Their auditory memory is quite short and they present auditory discrimination difficulties. As for articulation,[3] the children telescope words, disregard phonemic detail (Masland and Case 1965), and simplify sound clusters. In other words, their verbal gestalten are primitive. Some children's articulation of single phonemes may be correct in isolated words, but disintegrates when sounds are embedded in phrases and sentences. Their articulatory difficulties are related to their inability to program and organize sounds into longer and phonemically stable configurations. When the affect load, or the burden of having to express complex thoughts, becomes too heavy, all linguistic systems—phonemic, semantic, and syntactic—break down.

---

[2]The cluttering syndrome was not recognized in this country until eighteen or twenty years ago. It was first described in Europe by Lieberman (1900) and, above all, by Freud (1934) and Weiss (1935). See also subsequent publications by Weiss (1950; 1964), as well as by de Hirsch and Langford (1950); Arnold (1965); and Luchsinger (1959).

[3]There are children who cling to infantile speech patterns as a way of hanging on to more childish ways of functioning. There are also those who regress, who at five or six years of age use the speech that was normal for them at the age of two or three—pitch, modified forms, etc. These are not the children we are discussing here. Nor do we mean those who, as a result of brain lesion show dysarthric features, nor those who have problems with the peripheral speech apparatus.

Nearly all clutterers have severe word-finding difficulties, dys-
nomias, which should not be confused with meager vocabularies.
They seem to lack clear-cut word images. Many of them report that
they have the word "on the tip of their tongue" but that it will not
emerge. Unable to plan ahead, they fail to form anticipatory schemata
of what the sentence is going to say. They cannot as it were, "cast a
syntactical shadow" (Grewel 1970). They make false starts; they use
innumerable fillers; their sentences hang in midair; and their output is
loose and disjointed. Sequences invariably present difficulties.

The following is a word-by-word transcript of a recording made of
a clutterer, a highly intelligent eleven-year-old girl who reported on a
movie she had seen the night before. While she had done very well
with the WISC Similarities subtest, which requires only short verbalizations, she fell down when it came to extended discourse.

> It was The Silent Movie. It, it just wrote wrote our things . . . you
> know . . . It was, like, it was it was like Blazing Saddles. It was
> just about three men who were trying to get . . . a movie . . .
> called The Silent Movie. They were trying to make a movie and it's
> just about how they finally did get the movie and where they went
> and stuff, and it's really good . . . and it tells, like, it's just . . . it's
> called, I'm not exactly sure what they're called, but they're trying
> to stop these three men. It's hard to describe . . . (sighs) . . .
> Yeah, and, let's see, what part . . . it's to just how they're chasing
> them and they're trying to . . . um . . . Wait. There's another
> part that . . . it's important . . . Oh, and then their manager was
> in the hospital, and they were going to tell him about the movie.
> Started playing TV tennis with this brain thing . . . with the
> equipment that was attached to his head . . . stuff that was stick-
> ing out of his head . . . and it was attached to, like the like the
> radio thing. You know what it's called, like it, it tells whether he's
> alive, or, you know, that screen, and it shows balls going along, or
> it shows, it's going like this (gestures) . . . and then at the end
> they make the movie and it was a great hit, I left out a few parts,
> but they were not that big you know . . .

What the transcript does not show is the fast rate and the monotonous quality of the girl's speech. Inflection and intonation, like punctuation and paragraphs in writing, are carriers of meaning and serve to
structure output. Nor does the transcript reflect the clutterer's characteristic dysrhythmia, so striking to the listener.

Note the dysnomia, the overuse of pronouns, the lapses in grammar, the fragmented, simply constructed sentences, and the enormous difficulty bringing the story to a conclusion.

The same girl's compositions (her written utterances) are as diffuse as is her spoken discourse. There is a lack of hierarchical structure. The linkage between ideas is loose. Cause and effect are not developed logically. In spite of it, some of the thinking is original with unexpected connections and sometimes surprising insights. It is not the substance that is at fault, but the organization.

Clutterers write the way they sound. Their dysrhythmic disorganized handwriting, with its frequent omissions of sounds and words, reflects their dysrhythmic and disorganized speech. Words run into each other, testifying to trouble with word boundaries on this level as well. The graphologist Roman-Goldzieher (1962) was able to pick out from a large sample of handwriting specimens the written work of clutterers. In thirty-five years of experience, the authors have hardly ever encountered a clutterer who was a good speller.

The fact that the clutterer's organization of spoken language (which uses auditory channels) and of printed language (which makes use of visual pathways) are equally poor speaks against the frequently advanced theory that every learning disorder can be classified according to specific modality weaknesses. That this is not the case has been confirmed by the findings of Jansky (1970). Such weaknesses do exist; there are some who do much better visually than auditorily. But the organizational deficits of poorly patterned children are neither primarily auditory nor primarily visual-spatial; they represent a more basic weakness in dealing with complex structures and patterns in both modalities.

Differential Diagnosis

The symptomatology just described does not hold, of course, for all learning-disabled children. How does one distinguish among them? It is easy enough to separate out those learning-disabled children who are mentally retarded, who are sensorily impaired, or who are grossly brain-injured. This, however, leaves a heterogeneous group of youngsters that have been given various labels such as maturational lags or minimally brain-injured. It is among this heterogeneous group that further differential descriptions are needed so that we can have a clearer picture of the subgroup with organizational deficits. We are dealing with description, with phenomenology here; Gestalt theory serves merely as a theoretical framework for what is observed.

Bender's Group

In separating children with organizational deficits from other learning-disabled youngsters, their superficial resemblance to schizophrenic children must be noted. The term *plasticity*, coined by Bender

(1966b) for schizophrenic youngsters and those with maturational lags, implies a pervasive organismic lability which is somewhat reminiscent of that seen in children with organizational or gestalt deficits. Bender describes as typical for her group disturbances in visceral and autonomic functions, difficulties with perception, motor patterning, mentation and language, and severe deviations in the social and affective realm. She stresses the children's tendency to regression, their isolation, their precarious hold on reality, their thought disorders, as well as their autistic responses and their symbiotic relationships.

Unlike the children in Bender's group, children with organizational deficits present no autonomic or visceral disturbances. They are not bizarre, regressed, or withdrawn. They do not suffer from thinking disorders. Their affect is not flat. In contrast to schizophrenic youngsters, they demonstrate communicative intent. Above all, both their disorientation and the resulting anxiety have a different flavor from that of psychotic children.

There is, as might be expected, some limited degree of overlap between the Bender group and the one described here. One thinks especially of similarities in the Bender Gestalt protocols. The human figure drawings of poorly patterned children also remind one occasionally of the group described by Bender, but with one major difference: the total absence of bizarre features. In both we find evidence of primitivization.

The fundamental difference between children with organizational deficits and borderline schizophrenic youngsters is their capacity for relationships. They are available; they form affect bonds. Although their social techniques are sometimes crude (a few suffer from a degree of social dyspraxia) they have friends. And their response to remedial therapy is much more positive than that of schizophrenic or borderline youngsters.

Severe Language Disorders Without Organizational Deficits

Clearly, not all language-impaired children suffer from pervasive organizational deficits. There are many whose well-circumscribed dysfunctions are limited to the verbal realm. These children are not distractible. They do not present disorders of attention, and their perceptuomotor and visuomotor competence is often above average. They do tend to be literal and, at times, compulsive and their verbal conceptualizations are poor. Verbal mediation of both internal and external events is deficient and, as a result, the children appear to be relatively primitive; their view of the world lacks shades. On the WISC-R their Verbal IQ is usually significantly lower than their Performance score.

Such a child is typically referred with a family history of language disorders. He may be a well-organized youngster, one who does very well with activities involving spatial conceptualization, but with severe formulation difficulties. The ability to tell a story is woefully inadequate, and word-finding difficulties are enormous. In order to retrieve the word *dwarf*, for example, one such child had to visualize the cover of the book *Snow White*. Beyond it, having lacked verbal representation of feelings at an early age, such a child may have missed out on some very fundamental experiences so that verbal inadequacy blocks expression of feelings even at later ages.

The Target Group: Language Disorders Associated with Organizational Deficits

This target group is comprised of youngsters in whom disorganization is pervasive and affects both verbal and nonverbal functioning. To give a rough idea about the relative size of this group: of 42 youngsters, ranging from two and a half to eighteen years in age whom we are presently seeing for a variety of language and learning disorders, admittedly a selective group, approximately 23 belong to this subgroup.

Their dysfunction in school is striking and looks, of course, different at different ages. But as a group they show a responsive intelligence as manifested in average or better IQ. Of course they function very unevenly on tests. Their weak performance on Object Assembly and Block Designs, for instance, is probably related to difficulty with order of patterns laid out in space. On the other hand, the clinician often finds highly elevated scores on Similarities and Vocabulary, scores which are counterbalanced by depressed Information and Arithmetic ratings. Low Information is probably related to word finding difficulties, and poor Arithmetic to an inability to hold the set in mind. Good Vocabulary and Similarities scores, on the other hand, reflect a feeling for word connotations as well as considerable ability to form verbal generalizations. In any case, their reading and spelling levels fall way below that suggested by their overall IQ.

They show no evidence of significant neurological impairment, although there seems to be some neurophysiologic difference (cf. Denckla 1978), mostly on a familial basis.

The emotional resources of youngsters in this group are often excellent. Genuinely responsive to others and aware of their reactions, they often attract adults and children by their warmth and spontaneity. At the same time their boundless energy may be diffuse and unfocused. They appear to be readily propelled by their drives and feel guilty about them. Impulsivity is common, leading to some antisocial acts, such as snitching small objects or engaging in mild sexual acting out. One can observe what Anna Freud describes as "lack of harmonious synchronization of the various developmental strands."

In such children, inability to reject stimuli from the unconscious may interfere with the transition from the primary to the secondary process. It is suggested that the ego's thrust toward organization, as well as the capacity to develop age-appropriate defenses may be less predictable in these children than in those whose experiences of their world is tighter and better defined.

Neglect of the concept of organization has led to occasional misinterpretation of behavior. The rigid and even obsessive-like defenses that some very impulsive children develop cannot be attributed exclusively to intrapsychic conflict. It may, in some instances, be a direct response to fear of disintegration, in Goldstein's sense (1939)[4] of, literally, falling apart. The particular mixture of impulsiveness and compulsivity frequently encountered in clinical practice has been insufficiently explored in children with learning disabilities.

It would be absurd to say that these children are conflict-free. It is, in fact, likely that conflict intensifies their tendency to fly apart. But at least some of their conflicts, by no means all of them, may be secondary ones. An impulsive adolescent's acting out may be primarily related to physiological factors, while his attempt to reconcile his misbehavior with an internalized moral code results in secondary conflicts.

Some Therapeutic Remarks

It is now the fashion to proceed during therapy by the so called skill building approach, that is to say, the end result is conceived as a stone edifice in which every single stone is essential. This atomistic approach is, in our opinion, essentially wrong. An example from speech will illustrate what we mean.

A four- or five-year-old, for instance, whose speech is unintelligible because his output is rushed, disorganized, and defective, will benefit from a modelling approach. During play the therapist repeats the child's own utterances in short slowed-up form; she clears up his speech, as it were, and provides him with a model that is intelligible and well organized. As a consequence there is often no need to work on single sounds. They fall into place, and if they do not, there is time to institute work on specific substitutions or omissions later on.

Reaching out for the whole gestalt also applies to work in content areas. The child must be oriented first to the framework, to meaning. Then he can fit specific information into the slots which have been provided for him.

---

[4]Tolpin (1978) maintains that fear of disintegration, lack of cohesiveness of the self, is not based on neurotic conflict, but rather on a developmental deficit related to very early parental neglect and consequent failure to evolve adequate integration of the self. Fears of disintegration as discussed here are related, rather, to the catastrophic reaction described by Goldstein (1939).

These children are not difficult to work with. They are very ready to form a treatment alliance. In the process, the therapist must sometimes lend the child her own ego, since the relationship to her serves as a prime organizer of experience. This helps the youngster not only to structure content (and we conceive of structuring not as external manipulation such as shutting out extraneous stimuli or working with heavily programmed materials and mechanistic drills), but means orientation and clarification of the child's world on a deeper level. The bond between child and therapist creates an atmosphere in which learning is infused with meaning and becomes stabilized. In this "love" relationship a figure is constructed that is memorable for the pupil. With this kind of approach the performance of poorly organized children often improves dramatically. Although vestiges of disorganized speech, oral reading, and spelling may be observed in cluttering adults, the fact that there is considerable improvement nevertheless means that one deals with a potentially intact ego.

Summary

It is postulated that organizational deficits are basic to and characteristic of the subgroup of learning-disabled children discussed here and that these deficits set them apart from youngsters in other diagnostic categories. Such gestalt deficits are, we believe, related to central nervous system differences, including differences in genetic programming, although it is obvious that an inadequate infant-mother bond and a chaotic social milieu are major contributory factors.

The dysfunctions of the group described here range from mild to severe. They are more striking in younger individuals, but it would be a mistake to attribute the deficiency to transient immaturity. Underlying difficulties with the organization of highly patterned configurations are masked or compensated for at older ages, but they still exist and can be observed in the cluttered speech and continuing writing and spelling problems of some adults. In younger individuals they are reflected primarily in difficulties with spoken, printed, and written language, but they are observed in other areas as well. Because of the looseness of their associations and because the children are diffuse and disoriented, they may be labeled as borderline schizophrenic. However, the ability to cope socially, their relatedness, and their positive response to remediation points to the absence of severe psychopathology.

Gestalt theory has served as a theoretical framework for the phenomena observed. Smooth language functioning is conceived as a correlate to adequately perceiving and to responding in terms of organized configurations. The disorganization of children described is severe enough to compromise the imposition of order on the endless stream of internal and external stimuli. Disorganized children can be helped, but not necessarily by attacking a multitude of specific weaknesses by way of the now fashionable skill building approach. While working with specific skills is useful up to a point, difficulties with managing complex schemata is a more basic deficit and must be addressed primarily globally. Therapeutic strategies for disorganized youngsters are developed in the context of a close identification with the tutor who clarifies the child's world and helps him to structure himself and his environment.

Part IV

THE CHILD WITH LANGUAGE DISORDERS

Clinical Note on Stuttering and Cluttering in Young Children

with William S. Langford

Stuttering has been the subject of speculation for two thousand years. Therapy followed in the wake of theory. In the middle of the 19th century, surgery was considered the best way to treat the disorder (Burdin 1940). Later on the German school of Kussmaul (1910) and Gutzmann (1898, 1910) advised the training of speech muscles for better coordination. At the present time there are two fairly sharply divided schools of thought as to causation and treatment. One regards stuttering as an anxiety neurosis with obsessive-compulsive features (Kugelman 1946) and recommends dynamic psychiatry as the pre-ferred treatment. The other, represented by Orton (1937) and Bluemel (1930, 1935), considers stuttering as essentially a neurologic disorder.

In recent years numerous studies have been made of the constitu-tion of stutterers. Pulse rates, respiratory patterns, the type and rate of voluntary motor movements, electroencephalographic patterns have been investigated as well as the chemical constituents of the blood and metabolic rates. As yet there has been demonstrated no distinctive pattern for the stutterer. It would seem that there is a common fallacy in both the basic theories and in these investigations. Most workers, even those who distinguish between primary and secondary stutter-ing, deal with the disorder as if it were a single clinical entity.

Close observation of the stuttering of young children has led the present authors to believe that stuttering cannot really be regarded as a specific clinical entity.

In the consideration of stuttering the following questions would seem important:

    1. Are all disruptions in the rhythmic flow of speech to be considered as stuttering?

Reprinted with permission from American Academy of Pediatrics, from *Pedi-atrics* 5:934–939 copyright American Academy of Pediatrics, 1950.

2. Are some disturbances in the rhythmic flow of speech related to other dysfunctions in the language area?

3. Do such disturbances signify something fundamentally different at different age levels?

4. Is it possible to judge from the symptom alone whether we are confronted primarily with a manifestation of anxiety or predominantly with a specific language disorder?

5. Should therapy differ according to what we believe to be the outstanding etiologic factor in a specific case and should it differ with the age of the patient?

In answering these questions we must bear in mind that the speech of infants is characterized by a basic pattern of repetition. The very young child does not say *ma*, but *ma-ma*. This occurs in all early speech; *da-da, bow-wow, choo-choo, ta-ta, wa-wa* are typical. There is a repetitive character in what we call vocal play of the young child, the activity in which he first experiments with sounds and gains valuable auditory and kinesthetic experience as well as essential oral gratification from playing with sounds. The speech of the two- or three-year-old child has a similar tendency. Repetition of sounds, syllables, words or phrases belongs to the normal speech pattern of this age group. Davis (1939) and Fischer (1932) have found that one in every four words of the entire speech output of the child between the ages of two and four is repeated in one form or another. These repetitions consist of easy effortless clonic iterations executed at a normal speed, at an age when the young child's intellectual and emotional drives far outstrip his technical ability to handle speech as a tool. Such iterations tend to decrease with age and disappear in the large majority of children. Labeling these iterations as stuttering is in no way justified.

The following is a sample of speech of an intelligent thirty-one-month-old girl playing with her older brother:

> Tommy, Tommy, push the wheelbarrow, push the wheelbarrow. It's m-mine. I want the blocks, blocks. I want it. G-give it me. I build a tower, look I build a high tower, yes, I b-build build the tower, it's high, look, high.

The pediatrician can do much to ease the concerns of parents who, noticing these normal iterations, mistake them for stuttering. He can help to lessen their preoccupation with the act of speaking and to withdraw attention from it. He can discourage perfectionistic attitudes in general and particularly as they pertain to speech.

Although most children fall into this category there is another, smaller group that has similar symptoms but at a later age. Many of these children start talking late, i.e., at thirty-six to forty months or even later though their development is otherwise normal and their intelligence as measured by formal tests is average or above average. These young children have considerable difficulty in enunciating sounds. They have a limited vocabulary and show immature sentence construction but with it a marked drive to express themselves. They often talk with extreme rapidity. Frequently their motor speech patterns are so poor that their speech is practically unintelligible. Most of these children show clonic iteration of sounds but at a later age than is normal. Their trouble with word finding is more obvious.

Investigation of the family background of these children frequently reveals a history of language difficulty: a father who started speaking late and who is a poor speller; a paternal uncle who stuttered when a child; an older sibling who has trouble in learning to read. Mixed laterality patterns are often found in the family background; a certain percentage of these children themselves show confusion in motor leads or a delay in the establishment of a functional superiority of one side over the other. Some of them exhibit a degree of dyspraxia (Orton 1937).

Billy is four years three months of age. His father, who stuttered when a child, is a poor speller and had originally been left-handed but had later been switched to the right hand. The paternal uncle has a slight lisp. Billy's first cousins on the father's side also have difficulties in the language area. One of them has a fairly severe reading disability; the other, aged three years two months is not yet using more than a few isolated words. Billy himself was late as far as onset of speech is concerned. His first words did not come through till he was thirty-two months old; he began using sentences at thirty-seven months.

The boy rated an IQ of 91 on the Stanford-Binet test, but came out with an IQ of 118 on the Merrill-Palmer. His auditory memory span is short. Coordination is good for the long muscle groups but only fair for the small muscle groups. So far Billy has not established a functional superiority of one hand over the other: there are about 60 percent right-handed responses as against 40 percent left-handed ones. The boy is friendly and at ease with both children and adults. He presents no outstanding nervous symptoms though he will once in a while use his poor speech in order to gratify infantile needs.

Curious George, the story of a monkey, is being read to him. "B-b-but wy doeth de man want to catth im?" (But why does the man want to catch him?) When Billy gets bored with a lengthy explanation he says, "Do on, do on." Sometimes he says, "Go on, mee want to do on." By this time he is getting excited. A picture will evoke a train of thought and he will talk about a monkey he has seen at the zoo. "Ee wath a bery big monkey, bery big and wee bed mm im . . . pea peanuts peanuts." (He was a very big monkey and we fed him peanuts.) On seeing George break out of jail, Billy will become more and more excited: "Dorth ith a bery thmat monkey, bery thmat ee ith." (George is a very smart monkey, very smart he is.) Then he says with conviction, "Mee mee wont wike to be a monkey a monkey a monkey ith too wittle, too wittle mee would be a tiger tiger." (I wouldn't like to be a monkey; a monkey is too little; I would be a tiger.) During all this output, repetitions of syllables, words, and phrases are loose and easy.

It is important for the pediatrician to watch closely the clonic iterations of these children. Are they characterized by normal speed? Is there a tonic component? As long as there is no evidence of tonus there is no reason to label this type of verbal expression as stuttering. Should the boy—and it is well-known that more boys than girls are subject to this difficulty—have trouble with the production of specific sounds, it might be wise to provide him with technical help in the handling of speech as a tool. Smoother production of sounds, a larger vocabulary and better sentence construction might well result in a decrease of the original iterations as the child becomes better able to express himself in terms of words.

The speech of these children closely resembles a type of disturbance seen at all ages and known as cluttering (Froeschels 1946, 1948; Weiss 1935; Florensky 1933; Freund 1934). Cluttering is basically a dissociation between thinking and speaking. All of us are familiar with the child or adult who has an enormous drive to talk but who seems to get lost in the middle of his sentences. It appears as if he could not plan a phrase ahead. A clutterer will sometimes omit the verb or some other vital part of the sentence, thereby impairing the logical presentation of his ideas. Tempo of speech is speeded up by quickly racing thoughts, but the speaker seems undecided as to the choice of a specific expression. He lacks clearcut word images and he does not easily put his thoughts into words. Speech is disorganized and again we find a tendency to repeat words, phrases and, at times, whole sentences in the same way as we have observed it in the group of youngsters previously discussed. It is of interest to note that neither adults nor children show much awareness of this type of difficulty; fear and tensions are not noticeable during speaking. In spite of the tendency to disorganization in the language area not every cluttering child is bound to become a stutterer. The familial factor in the cluttering symptom is impressive, a fact which has led a great many workers to believe that stuttering is hereditary (West, Nelson, and Berry 1935). This, however, is not substantiated by experience. A predisposition to disturbance in the language area—if by language we understand the use of symbols for expression—may well be constitutionally determined. Orton (1937), in his important contribution to this field, has stressed the familial factor in reading, spelling, and speech disabilities. Case histories of cluttering children frequently show a familial background (Weiss 1935).

Stuttering and cluttering both represent nonfluent speech. Tension and anxiety, which are essential features of the stuttering symptom, are not constitutionally determined. They are, rather, the outgrowth of pressures, emotions, and feelings which have been superimposed on and fixed to an underlying unstable mechanism. Cluttering children need not necessarily become stutterers, but they often do (Pichon 1948).

In the development of stuttering, what happens to the original iteration of words and syllables? Froeschels (1942–43) has described the development of the symptom: the first easy repetitions are slowed down; *ta-ta* is no longer produced in normal tempo, the tongue presses a little too long against the alveolar ridge in the production of the *t*; delay results. Froeschels calls this phase, which already contains a tonic element, tono-clonus. It is only later that the child will use an exaggerated amount of pressure during articulation in an effort to overcome the first speaking blocks. This will result in pure tonus. Its pattern engenders fear of the speaking situation and this, in turn, sets up spasms at various levels of the peripheral speech mechanism—at the level of the larynx, the tongue and the lips. Breathing disturbances, with accompanying muscular movements, follow and hypertonicity involving the whole body may ensue. A vicious circle is completed; fear of the speaking situation results in additional spasms and severe spasms lead to increased fear.

Since the majority of youngsters easily get over their early clonic repetitions and since a large percentage of what we term cluttering children do not become stutterers, the question needs to be asked: why do some children develop this particular pattern? Increased emotional tensions at a more or less crucial time in language development might make for stuttering in a child whose speech mechanism is not too rugged to begin with. Normally, speech development takes place at an emotionally critical period of the child's life. This is the time when infantile gratifications, particularly oral satisfactions, are being withdrawn, when toilet training is being instituted and enforced, when destructive and aggressive tendencies are being discouraged, when the young child is being subjected to various social pressures and is expected to begin to pattern his responses so that he becomes a responsible member of the family group. Often enough in the midst of these pressures he is presented with a younger brother or sister. Many children are permitted no outlets of any sort for their hostile impulses. During this period of early childhood they find it difficult to maintain a steady emotional equilibrium in satisfying their own needs and at the same time meeting the demands made on them by their environment.

A child with a none too stable neuromuscular speech equipment may well show his emotional disequilibrium in stuttering rather than in another symptom such as enuresis or vomiting. In fact it is rare to see stuttering as the only symptom of emotional maladjustment in a given child.

Parental tension and anxiety are important factors. Anxiety in parents or in the adult closely associated with the child, no matter how it is expressed, is communicated to the youngster and leads to emotional disturbance. In some families, especially where some member has or has had trouble with speech, the child's sounds are apt to be watched with anticipatory misgiving often long before he utters a sentence. In other families without such more or less specific sensitization to speech, undue attention to the child's speech productions may be the result of parental tension and anxiety expressed in perfectionistic, oversolicitous, or other equally deleterious attitudes. Where such anxiety and overwatchfulness are fixed on the child's verbal expression, the resulting emotional disturbance is most apt to be reflected in his speech. (Where the parental concern involves other aspects of the child's functioning, he usually obliges by developing a symptom in the area of the parental concern). Wendell Johnson (1938, 1942) has demonstrated that labeling a young child as a stutterer almost inevitably leads to more speech trouble. Nagging and constant admonition tend to change easy clonic repetitions into something much less benign. To sum up: parental anxiety, undue attention directed to speech, perfectionistic attitudes, reinforced by the child's own secondary gains will tend to make a stutterer out of a youngster whose speech apparatus is still immature and who has a low threshold of stability in the language area. In such children careful attention must be paid to general emotional adjustment. They use their language disability as a psychologic mechanism in the parent-child relationship and at times to oppose a hostile environment. An awareness of this and close observation of the type of speech difficulty will assist the pediatrician in guiding parents. He often has the oportunity to help them to a more relaxed and happier acceptance of their child. Such help at the right time may well make the difference between severe stuttering and a mild cluttering.

There is yet another group of children in which no family history of language difficulty is present nor is there any confusion in motor leads. Many children in this group talk early and fluently. They begin stuttering, seemingly out of the blue, at any age, as early as three and as late as fourteen years of age. The stuttering sometimes follows an emotionally traumatic incident which seems to serve as a precipitating factor. These children most often give a long story of emotional disturbance prior to the onset of the stuttering, symptoms of personality disorder such as recurrent vomiting, fears, sleep disturbances, feeding problems, enuresis, or persistent thumb-sucking. In these cases pronounced tonic elements and accompanying muscular movements, generally a feature of the individual who has been stuttering for some time, appear very early. In this group stuttering definitely seems but a symptom of an emotional disturbance involving the total personality, the expression of severe underlying anxiety which appears to disrupt cortical integrative functions with the result that speech reverts to an earlier and disorganized pattern.

Mark B. is five years seven months old. He is the younger of two children; his older brother, Simon, is eight and a half years of age. Family history is free of language disturbance. The mother, who herself is a tense and anxious person with high blood pressure, describes her husband as "very nervous." As an infant Mark suffered from severe colic and cried continuously. From the time he was seventeen months old he vomited after most meals, especially on occasions when his mother forced him to eat things he did not like. He was a difficult child, Mrs. B. says, "and I used to hit him a lot." Mark produced his first words at sixteen months and his first short sentence came through when he was not quite two years old. By the time he was three years, the boy talked fluently and easily, showing only a few sound substitutions normal for his age. At the time Mark was four and a half years old, his brother was kept home from school for several months recovering from rheumatic fever. The children fought a great deal and it seems that one night Simon had pretended to choke the younger boy. Shortly afterwards Mark started to stutter and continued stuttering even after his brother went back to school. On examination the stuttering pattern was seen to consist of severe tonic blocks, many of them at the level of the larynx so that at times the child could not get a word out. Blocking was accompanied by various muscular movements, above all by jerking up of the head.
"My — — — brother won't let me — — — play. If — — — I go downstairs in the m—orning he could k — kill me cause cause he is jealous. If — — I go with Daddy he makes a picnic — no, — — I m — — m—mean a racket." At times Mark is practically free from blocks: "I can't sleep at night times." At other times blocking is so severe that he flushes with the effort to bring a word out. "Mummy has too — — m—much trouble, must — — force — — — — Simon to eat — — — — I eat too much. I f — f — fight too much." In this example, note should be taken that blocking is most severe on emotionally laden terms.

The fact that in some stuttering one can recognize crude movements of sucking, chewing, and swallowing has contributed to the psychoanalytic theory that stuttering is a neurosis associated with the persistence into later life of early pregenital components (Coriat 1942–43). This theory has not been adequately corroborated.

Occasional cases are seen in which the stuttering exists as an hysteric conversion symptom. We have observed several cases of hysteric stuttering involving predominantly respiratory and laryngeal structures in children who had experienced emotionally traumatic tonsillectomies. Children with hysteric stuttering or those in whom it appears after psychic trauma need the early help of the competent, well-trained child psychiatrist.

A good deal has been written to prove that emotional difficulties are not only the cause but frequently the result of stuttering. Obviously the child who is constantly frustrated in his attempts to express himself, the child who cannot communicate effectively with others, the child who is being teased by his playmates because of his speech disability will develop secondary emotional disturbances. The pediatrician meets with this problem in the child at an early stage; if he is alert to recognize it and to deal with it, he will be of inestimable value to both child and parent.

Summary

The early clonic iterations of the child between twenty and forty months are a part of the normal speech patterns of growing children. As a rule reassurance of the parents and withdrawal of attention and concern from speech are all that is necessary.

There is a group of children who start speaking late and whose familial background shows evidence of difficulty in the language area and delay in establishing a functional superiority of one side over the other. Many of these children have trouble with the enunciation of specific sounds, with vocabulary, and with sentence construction. In spite of at least average intelligence these children handle speech poorly. They often show a great number of clonic iterations at an age when most children have already discarded them. Their handling of speech closely resembles the cluttering of older children and adults. Such children frequently need technical help with sounds, vocabulary, and grammatical construction. Smoother production of speech and slowing up of speed will often bring about a reduction in the original iterations. The pediatrician should be aware of the fact that emotional tensions and conflicts tend to become fixed to a speech mechanism that is none too stable in these children. The cluttering child may easily turn into a stutterer.

There is a larger group of children who show no familial difficulty in the language area, who talk early and quite well, and who abruptly develop stuttering at some time during childhood. Some of these children display other symptoms of emotional disorder; others seem to function effectively in most areas but express their emotional conflicts principally in stuttering. These children should be referred for psychiatric help early.

In older children who stutter, a careful differential diagnosis is necessary to determine the relative importance of specific language and emotional factors in pathogenesis. If existing emotional difficulties seem to be the result rather than the cause of the stuttering, a more specifically technical therapy is favored; in cases where emotional factors are outstanding a psychiatric approach is to be preferred.

Speech is a means of expression of the personality as well as a means of communication; severe dysfunctions in speech then may reflect a personality disorder or a disorder of interpersonal relationships or both. In the child, however, speech is also a tool which he masters as it develops. A speech difficulty in the growing child must be evaluated from both points of view.

Developmental Word Deafness
and Speech Therapy

The speech therapist leaves to others the ultimate decision as to whether a child's inability to understand the symbolic meaning of words and sentences is related to focal agenesis, to actual cerebral pathology, or whether it constitutes, as Dr. Orton suggested, a physiological variant. The speech therapist leaves to others the ultimate decision as to terms: word deafness, idiopathic language retardation, receptive audio-mutism, or congenital auditory imperception.

The speech therapist is immediately concerned with the child and his mother who comes to the clinic and says: "My youngster is three and a half and he uses hardly any words. He pays no attention to anything one says." Or with the father who worries about six-year-old Peter who has trouble expressing himself. Peter will do things but he won't talk about them; besides, if he does talk one can't always understand what he is trying to say. He seems to have some sort of jargon of his own and he runs his words together in a monotonous kind of voice. The family is sure that Peter is alert; he certainly is the first to hear an airplane overhead or a car approaching the house, but somehow one can't get him to listen and he isn't a bit interested if one reads him a story. He isn't easy to handle, either; he is awfully active and never sits still for a moment.

Saying that the speech therapist is not primarily interested in terminology does not mean that he can do without a sound working hypothesis. Obviously, the therapeutic approach will differ essentially according to the clinical picture. A widespread organic defect, developmental delay all around, regional auditory loss, deep seated psychopathology, or a primary selective language deficiency, each of these calls for different treatment. Having determined in a given case that we do actually deal with specific linguistic retardation, it remains to be further established whether the child is only unable to cope with the instrumentalities of language or whether his failure with symbolization is related to a receptive disturbance. Since all processes involving

---

Speech given at The Orton Society, October 1952.

perceiving, conceptualizing, and expressing meaning through language are closely interrelated, this is not always easy. As a matter of fact, there is nothing more challenging in our field than the differential diagnosis in the case of a three- or four-year-old youngster who has no verbal tools, who shows no interest in verbal communication, and who is moreover so difficult to reach that we need all our empathy, all our skill, our intuition, and knowledge to decide upon even a tentative hypothesis. In the rare case, such a child is sent to us after extensive clinical evaluation; such evaluation includes, of course, careful prenatal, natal, and postnatal clinical history and all available medical, neurological, psychiatric, psychometric, and audiometric data. Since the diagnosis of both acquired and developmental word-deafness is arrived at by a process of elimination and not directly, it may be permitted to comment briefly on the process of elimination.

To begin with auditory factors: audiometric testing procedures have improved so much during the last few years that the difficulties in assessing regional, in particular high frequency, losses have been greatly reduced. Speech thresholds are now being determined in addition to pure tone ones. The child, however, suspected of a degree of word-deafness shows so much auditory inattention, his auditory memory span as tested by repetition of nonsense syllables is so short, he is so little interested in acoustic phenomena that he is difficult to test, and, as a matter of fact, such youngsters come to us frequently with contradictory audiometric findings. In the youngster under three or four the task of testing becomes, of course, still more formidable because of lack of motivation. The Psycho-Galvanic Skin Resistance Test techniques are being perfected, and this, which dispenses with the conscious participation of the patient, may eventually prove to be the answer. There is, however, at least in the case of the very young child, no substitute for clinical observation; the speech therapist will have to take careful notes over a period of weeks on the youngster's responses to all types of auditory stimuli. Even where there is no peripheral hearing loss, responses will tend to be inconsistent and reaction time frequently delayed. We must not forget that in the normal youngster also interpretation of material heard is acquired through a process of learning. Active integration and acceptance on the part of the child are required. In our youngsters responses are sluggish because, for a variety of reasons, they are unable, some of them perhaps deep down unwilling, to make the effort involved in the interpretation of certain types of acoustic stimuli. Direct tone introduction by means of the Urbanschitsch whistles which Froeschels recommends (these whistles contain both fundamental and harmonic overtones), sometimes elicit reliable clues.

Frequently a child is referred to us with a psychological report saying that his IQ is anywhere from 80 to 150 on a standard intelligence test. Needless to say, such a report is by no means satisfactory. Since language is intimately related to other psychic functions of a non-language character and since linguistic disturbances must be evaluated in terms of agnosias and apraxias, we need a careful qualitative analysis of the youngster's performance in all areas, perceptual, conceptual, visuomotor, and social. We should know whether the test results show a significant discrepancy between tests involving language responses and other types. Our children sometimes have trouble with form concepts or with orientation in space; occasionally they show tactile defects. All information which throws light on performance in these areas is important. Oseretsky's tests, for instance, which measure children's motor age, confirm Dr. Orton's findings that dyspraxic features are relatively frequent among children suffering from severe language disabilities. The Bender Gestalt will tend to reveal lags in visuomotor function, a Goodenough will often enough show not only defective manual skills but also immaturity of body image. Our children should be submitted to several kinds of projective techniques. I, personally, would like to see the Marble Board and the Goldstein-Scherer sorting tests included since they furnish important data about possible brain damage and deficiencies both in the perceptual and conceptual realm. Extensive psychological testing is, of course, not always possible at low age levels. Nance tests standardized from ages two to seven, which can be administered by pantomime and require performance responses only, may be helpful in some cases. In many instances, however, our children are so difficult to reach that we are lucky if we get any formal testing done at all. The Vineland Social Maturity Scale is, in many instances, the only measurement we do get. Here again it is only painstaking clinical observation which enables us to differentiate between delayed general development, pseudoretardation resulting from language deprivation, and specific linguistic deficiency.

Once in a while the speech therapist is furnished with the information: no neurological findings. However, the classical neurological examination and even the electroencephalogram do not always reveal minimal signs of central nervous system lesions. These might appear later at the time the child tries to master a function as complex as is language, even where there is no evidence of other cerebral pathology. For the differential diagnosis between acquired and developmental word deafness such minimal neurological signs are of great importance, and symptoms such as perseveration, stimulus-bound behavior, forced responsiveness to unessential details, instability of figure-background relationships, which have been observed in the brain injured child, should therefore be noted carefully. Studies as they are being done in Dr. Bender's department at Bellevue Hospital by Dr. Silver and Dr. Teicher, who have investigated tonus, posture, and motility of severely strephosymbolic youngsers, might be significant for our group as well.

The differential diagnosis between psychotic states and word-deafness constitutes a most difficult problem, primarily because some of the outstanding symptoms, to wit: profound auditory inattention, a tendency to echolalia and sometimes, though by no means always, restricted verbal output, are found in both. Data on the past history of the child are, of course, valuable. However, here again it is only prolonged clinical observation, the qualitative evaluation of the child's total behavior, the study of his psychosocial attitudes that will enable us to decide whether we are confronted with a total or partial inability to communicate at any level, verbal or nonverbal, or whether we deal with a limited response only as far as spoken symbols are concerned. Anyone who has spent time with a twelve- to eighteen-months-old baby knows that there is a constant stream of give and take between child and adult. The baby smiles, he plays peek-a-boo, he teases, he reacts to the adult's facial expression, to the tone of his voice; in other words he relates in a thousand different ways. If our patient does not communicate, if he plays well but always by himself, if our smile and our frown mean little or nothing, if he does not relate, be it only by aggressive gestures, he is in all probability not a word-deaf child.

It took a four-year-old boy who had, with adequate warrant, a profound distrust of adults fifteen weeks to establish a relationship to the therapist. When he finally did relate, he began to respond to words. His resistance to verbal communication was his defense protecting him against a hostile environment. We are now observing another bright four-year-old, referred because he does not respond to and does not use language. Mark's hearing is excellent, he plays beautifully, but always by himself. He has many bizarre fears and a number of obsessive traits. He has never permitted anyone to fondle him. Now, after three months, he occasionally smiles and he uses single words, but he does not really use them for purposes of communication. He plays around with these words or he repeats them mechanically. While a severe language deficit of this kind would, of course, affect such a child's total behavior, I feel sure in this case that Mark's emotional disturbance is not secondary to language deprivation. I am persuaded that he is an autistic youngster and he will be referred to the psychiatrist.

Once peripheral auditory factors, mental retardation, and psychopathologies have been ruled out in the etiology, the speech therapist will proceed with further testing. Careful investigation of the child's laterality and a family history of handedness and language are of importance. In cases where a functional superiority of one hand over the other has not been established, an attempt will be made to determine a preference. The therapist then goes on with the task of assessing the youngster's ability to interpret spoken words, to associate sequences of verbal symbols, sound patterns, with meaning. Auditory impressions in the form of words and sentences obviously do not occupy the center of our child's psychic field. The figure, in Goldstein's sense, the gestalt, the sound sequence, is insufficiently differentiated from the background. In very severe cases, words are being treated as if they were noises. To the very young child we show a series of pictures and objects and ask him to point to the appropriate one when we call out its name. Some youngsters are able to focus their attention on single words only, but fail when it comes to sentences. We therefore give them simple directions to carry out, carefully eliminating all visual and situational clues. We play with the doll house and make suggestions: "Pick up the baby, push the chair, find the stove," and so test the child's ability to interpret words strung into sentences. Ability to repeat single words has little significance. The child might respond to the auditory stimulus only and not to the concept behind it. His memory for sound patterns might not be good enough to allow him to establish a stable relationship between object and word. As Dr. Orton pointed out, immediate recall does not prove anything for retention. From the older child we expect response to more elaborate verbal material. While playing a game of picture lotto we might discover gaps in his understanding of relatively simple word concepts. Words like *swing, vacuum cleaner, frigidaire,* are sometimes missed by an alert six-year-old. Questions have to be graded in terms of difficulty since comprehension of language varies, of course, with the complexity of the material. I refer to the boy mentioned by Dr. Orton who understood a question only when it was broken up for him into two different parts.

Many observers have failed to comment on the fact that our type of child often shows delayed responses. His threshold of excitability for verbal material is apparently high and interpretation therefore takes longer than in the normal youngster. This would explain why so often the mere repetition of exactly the same stimulus is effective. For testing purposes we give the older child soldiers and Indians to play with, a little fortress and ask him to act out the story as well as we tell him. The soldiers march and catch the Indian chief who is taken prisoner. The Indians attack to free him and so forth. Our type of child will tend to miss out on the gist of some of the story. The process is then reversed and the youngster gives the directions, thus providing an opportunity for the therapist to judge the fluency and accuracy of his verbal output. As the child directs the action, large gaps in vocabulary, poor motor speech patterns, defective inner language as manifested by paragrammatism, a disturbance of syntactical relationships, and inadequate organization of spoken material will soon become evident. We are interested also in the child's capacity to function on an abstract level.

To this purpose we ask him to sort out from the doll house all articles belonging to furniture. If he includes eating utensils, and if at a later stage he has trouble grasping the meaning of metaphors and proverbs, then he very probably has difficulty with categorical performance which, according to Goldstein, is essential for the highly symbolic level requisite for language function.

I would like to illustrate some suggestions as to therapy with two necessarily abbreviated case histories: one of a very young child, another of a nearly seven-year-old youngster. In discussing these cases I am not primarily concerned with fairly intricate diagnostic aspect but want to limit myself as much as possible to the discussion of therapeutic techniques which are essentially the same whether we deal with a case of acquired or developmental word deafness.

Maureen

Maureen was hospitalized in May 1946, at the age of three and a half, with the complaint not only that she had lost what speech she had had previously (and there had apparently been very little of it), but that beginning in December 1945 she had paid less and less attention when spoken to and that she now seemed unable to understand the language of others. The medical history was negative except for an episode of unexplained fever and a fairly severe fall down a flight of stairs with, however, no loss of consciousness or vomiting. Maureen was then the middle of three children. Her mother had not paid much attention to her; she said she had been afraid to make her older girl jealous and not too long afterwards another baby had been on the way.

Maureen is a highly intelligent youngster: on the Merrill-Palmer done at some later date she scored over 130. At first a profound hearing loss seemed likely; however, repeated tests over a period of time have proved that a peripheral auditory difficulty is in no way a significant factor. The progressively more and more favorable results of these tests are themselves of interest. In 1950 the audiogram showed a 25 dbs. loss in the right and 30 dbs. loss in the left ear for frequencies of 2000 and over. In 1951 a 20 dbs. loss in the right ear only for frequencies of 4000 and higher was established. When Maureen was first seen, she responded to all types of noises but looked confused when one talked to her. At that time she used her left hand fairly consistently.

The child presented a complicated picture because she seemed so very withdrawn and showed on occasions some waxy flexibility. Both a schizophrenic episode as well as word deafness were considered in diagnosis by Dr. William S. Langford, the head of Pediatric Psychiatry at Columbia-Presbyterian Medical Center. In the fall of 1946 he started working with Maureen once weekly and her mother was seen regularly by the psychiatric social worker, Mrs. Katherine Wickman. The child responded to treatment and began to communicate by way of smiles, gestures, and inarticulate vocalizations, though she did not respond to the spoken word. An electroencephalogram was ruled out so as not to traumatize her any further. In April 1948, she was referred to the Language Disorder Clinic. I remember her as a most attractive but highly suspicious little girl who played beautifully but scowled when spoken to. We spent several weeks playing with her and had her listen to musical records, something she enjoyed. All pressure in the language area was carefully avoided. Maureen's first need was the assurance that she was very important to the therapist; at the beginning she could not tolerate any other person in the room.

Finally, when she seemed ready, she was shown three large pictures pasted on cardboard, representing a house, a doll, and a chair. She was then asked to point to the correct picture when its name was called out. It took her about six weeks to associate each picture with its verbal symbol and still longer to carry the association over to the actual object. Associations were dramatized through play and repeated endlessly till they "stuck." After three more weeks she had mastered six more concepts. We were then employing smaller pictures that she could take home after every session in a little red pocketbook of which she was very proud. Shortly afterwards she pointed to her hat when I remarked how pretty it was; this was the first time she had interpreted a word from conversation.

Maureen was never asked to repeat or produce a word. The word was provided for her, played around with, incorporated in motor activities and highlighted. However, after another month she was willing to repeat words after the therapist, and a little later she used her first words spontaneously although the world of spoken symbols still meant very little to her and although auditory attention still was very defective. By November, seven months after therapy was started, she produced her first two-word sentence and from then on progress was fairly consistent. That year we sent Maureen to a small nursery group headed by an intelligent and understanding teacher who helped her in her relationships to other children and gave her opportunities to use words in communicative situations.

During therapeutic sessions, normal verbal stiumli were repeated, prolonged, accentuated. All sensory avenues, visual, auditory, kinesthetic were used so as to reinforce associations. Units of speech were reduced to very small ones, tempo was slowed up and words were dramatized as integral parts of actual situations. They were never presented out of their meaningful context. All teaching was done through play. The order of acquisition of words followed developmental lines—first nouns, then verbs. Grammatical unity like *under*, *inside*, had to be acted out. I remember spending the better part of a morning rolling a ball between Maureen's feet so as to get the concept of *between* across. Pronouns and abstract concepts like *people* or *family* and, later on, concepts like *pride* presented great difficulties. It was hard also for Maureen to accept the fact that an orangey-red color and bluish-red both came under the heading of *red*. She showed something of the abnormal concreteness which Goldstein discusses in brain-injured individuals; categorical behavior, that which involves abstract and generic functioning, was inadequate.

For a long time Maureen's motor speech patterns were extremely poor, and since she resisted correction, little was at first accomplished in this area. We simply could not afford to sacrifice her drive towards expression and communication for better enunciation. Auditory training, however, designed to bring auditory impressions into fuller consciousness, was added to the program. I have found such training helpful both in cases of peripheral and central disturbances. For one thing, central conductive pathways might suffer if not sufficiently stimulated. Then again we are able to increase auditory memory span by appropriate therapy. Auditory training is still more important in some of the mixed conditions we occasionally encounter, the cases where a slight peripheral loss complicates and aggravates a central difficulty.

In 1950 an electroencephalogram was done on Maureen. The report says: "Abnormal record, with predominance of abnormality over the entire right side of the brain. There is some suggestion of greater irregularity over the parietal cortex. The character of the disturbance is more suggestive of organic than of functional change. This pattern is not the type generally observed in the primary behavior disorders." It is of importance to add that by this time Maureen had become entirely right-handed; she had shifted spontaneously, so that we might assume that the originally nondominant hemisphere had taken over the language function. Obviously it is the ability to comprehend and to use language symbols that is most strikingly affected in cases of this sort; however, we should not overlook the fact that practically all of them show dysfunctions in other areas as well. We happened to give Maureen a Bender Gestalt a few days ago and she showed a striking tendency to verticalization; she rotated the horizontally directed figures to the vertical position. This tendency, which in most children disappears around the age of seven or eight, reveals a lag in visuomotor maturation not infrequently found in children suffering from severe language difficulties.

Maureen is now ten years old and has just entered fifth grade in public school. She is doing well and is now an adjusted if somewhat bossy little girl. Being able to read is helping her with her motor speech patterns on which she now works conscientiously. She still requires assistance with grammatical forms, retention of new verbal material still is inferior, but she has on the whole done remarkably well and prognosis is excellent.

Steven

Steven was admitted to the Language Disorder Clinic in October 1950 when he was six years and ten months old. He was referred because of unintelligible speech and behavior problems dating from the time he first went to school. The psychologist described him as a boy of high average intelligence. His Rorschach did not reveal any severe psychopathology though it did show a number of conflicts. At the Clinic he presented no behavioral problems of any kind but was restless to a point where it was impossible for him to sit still. He either walked around or stood next to his chair. He played constructively and imaginatively and was interested in a variety of subjects from boats to birds and all kinds of sports. His motor coordination in both large and small muscle groups was poor. Medical history was negative except for resuscitation at birth.

His mother had been sick a good deal and showed some depressive features. She worried over Steven and said he never paid attention when one talked to him. There was a history of language disturbance in the familial background. Steven's sister also had been very late in starting to talk and she had a fairly severe stutter. One paternal uncle had used baby talk long after he had entered school. Several members of the family had trouble with spelling and were reported to be left-handed. Steven himself had established a right-handed dominance only recently.

The boy's motor speech patterns were extremely poor, his grammar very defective, and his vocabulary severely limited. During the first interview the therapist was impressed with the fact that Steven showed large gaps in understanding of spoken material. He also seemed to watch the speaker's mouth a good deal of the time although he was able to hear whispered sounds spoken behind his back. He was therefore referred to the audiometric department. His first three audiograms were very inconsistent. Steven's auditory attention fluctuated to such a degree that results were contradictory. It was finally established, however, that the boy's hearing deviated only 15 dbs. on the whole frequency range and that a peripheral auditory difficulty was not a significant factor in his condition. Neurological examination was negative.

We worked with Steven over a period of four months concentrating entirely on the receptive aspect of language. In a relatively short time the mother reported that the boy was more prepared to listen at home and that he had become interested in some simple stories read to him. His vocabulary grew but was still deficient. Motor speech patterns left much to be desired and grammatical construction was extremely slow in improving. Inner language undoubtedly was still defective. Steven's restlessness had decreased somewhat but since we felt that his public school could not cope with the problem, we referred him to a school for the deaf which had a special section for children with aphasic-like difficulties. We have not seen Steven since, but the point I want to make is that in a case like his it would be a waste of time to work on articulatory patterns primarily. Only after the disturbance is recognized to lie in the receptive aspect of language function are we able to institute effective therapeutic procedures.

Summary

1.   Orton and a number of other authors as well have shown that disturbance in the receptive aspect of language is a clinical entity of a primary nature and can be differentiated from conditions like genuine or pseudomental retardation, regional auditory deficiency, and psychopathologies.

2.   Word-deafness is a disturbance in the mechanism of association. In a severe form it is probably met with but rarely except in cases of cerebral trauma, which incidentally might go unrecognized till the language phase is reached. However, a relatively large number of youngsters referred for retarded linguistic development or for severe dyslalia show a similar condition although nothing in their history or neurological status points to cerebral pathology. Orton says that these youngsters suffer from developmental word-deafness. Their trouble with the instrumentalities of language is not a primary kind, but secondary to a receptive disturbance. These children do hear sequences of sounds, but they fail, at least up to a point, to associate these sequences with meaning. Both their recognition and their recall of sound patterns are poor. Failure to appreciate that the resulting paucity of language, the paragrammatism, and the poor motor speech patterns are related to a receptive difficulty will result in wasteful and ineffective therapeutic efforts.

3.   Orton pointed out that children suffering from severe language difficulties have basically trouble with sequences, with temporal sequences in the case of the word-deaf and dyslalic youngster, with spatial ones in the case of the strephosymbolic child, and with sequences of motion in the case of the dyspraxic youngster. It would be of interest to follow these leads and investigate whether these phenomena resemble the configurational difficulties reflecting disturbance in figure-background relationships as they have been observed in the brain-injured child.

4.   Our children undoubtedly have difficulties with patterning not only of perceptual but also of behavioral responses. Obviously some of their emotional difficulties are of a derivative nature, the direct result of frustration and deprivation. A neurotic superstructure is the rule rather than the exception. I feel, however, that some of the motor restlessness and distractibility of these children is of a primary nature, a direct outcome of their inability to integrate and organize relational and emotional patterns, one more indication of their physiological-psychological immaturity.

5.   Treatment proceeds along holistic lines and always takes in the whole child; it is never confined to his language difficulty only. Without initially satisfying the youngster's emotional needs, effective therapy is impossible. An excellent transference from patient to therapist is *sine qua non*. Since these children have been exposed to pressure where speech is concerned, many of them resist, consciously or unconsciously, remedial teaching. This attitude has to be reversed. We have first to create a functional readiness for speech. Communicative situations have to be meaningful and satisfying. All of the youngster's abilities, interests, and skills have to be used. The multiple approach serves to reinforce associations. As in other aphasic conditions, the imagery type of the patient, preponderantly visual, auditory, or kinesthetic plays an important role in the choosing of preferred pathways. Since auditory imagery is frequently weak in this type of child, kinesthetic and visual associations have to be used to a large degree. On the other hand, therapy is directed towards fortifying auditory attention. The relationship between the object and its representative symbol needs to be stabilized. To this purpose intensive and repeated stimulation is required. Words are repeated over and over again, tempo is slowed down, verbal material is reduced to small units. Words are dramatized for the child till they become an integral part of a highly motivated situation. Abstract concepts are made concrete in a variety of ways.

6.   Prognosis is favorable, particularly if the condition and its receptive character are recognized early and if therapy is directed accordingly.

Word Deafness

with Jeannette Jefferson Jansky

The term *word deafness* has been used in the literature with refer-ence to both children and adults; the present discussion is confined to word deafness in children.

The word-deaf child is entirely or partially unable to comprehend spoken language. In some of the milder cases all that can be observed is a time lag between reception and interpretation of the verbal stimulus. There may or may not be difficulty in attaching meaning to sounds other than language, such as the ring of the telephone or the bark of a dog. Occasionally there is trouble with localization of sounds. How-ever, the disturbance is essentially on the verbal symbolic level, and these children are often good at interpreting the inflection of the speaker's voice or his facial and bodily expression. The degree of expressive language impairment varies. Language may be non-existent, limited in quantity, or poor in quality; jargon may be sub-stituted for meaningful speech.

The diagnosis of word-deafness is appropriate only when sig-nificant peripheral auditory loss, mental retardation, and psycho-pathology are ruled out as major contributory factors. Differential diagnosis is by no means always easy (particularly in the case of young children) and can be arrived at only by a process of elimination.

It was Kussmaul in 1877 who first coined the term word deafness when referring to patients who had difficulty with comprehension of speech. Allen (1951) divided the historical development of the concept into four phases. During the first phase from 1828 to 1868 the tendency was (with only a few exceptions) to regard word-deaf children as idiots. During phase two (from about 1868 to 1900) the expressive aspects of the disorder were emphasised, and Hale-White, Golding-Bird, Bastian, and others described children who had a language all their own. During phase three, lasting through World War I, there was

Reprinted with permission from South African Speech and Hearing Association, from *Journal of the South African Logopedic Society* :13–14. 1957.

a shift back to the receptive field. During the fourth phase the study of traumatic aphasias resulting from the first world war gave new impetus to these investigations. Wallin (1927) first suggested that the disorder might be more widespread than was generally recognized.

Worster-Drought's (1943) description of the syndrome is basic to present understanding of the disorder. He said that the speech of these children, once it develops, is monotonous, indistinct, and often complicated by what he calls verbal aphasia. He feels that the disturbance is probably the result of a biological variation in the nature of an agenesis. Froeschels (1949) focuses interest mainly on the auditory inattention of word-deaf children and recommends therapy directed towards this aspect of the syndrome. In 1937 Orton drew attention to the hyperactivity of word-deaf children and to their delay in developing a master hand. He was particularly interested in what he calls "developmental" word deafness—cases which did not show a reliable history of brain injury but in whose family background there was ample evidence of various forms of language disability. Ewing's study (1940) showed that of ten children who had been diagnosed as word-deaf, six had high frequency losses, thus pointing up the necessity for careful hearing evaluation. Nance (1946) described intelligence evaluation of word-deaf children by means of tests not requiring comprehension and use of language. Goldenberg (1950) stimulated by Bangs' study done in 1948) did an exploratory investigation on fourteen children said to be word-deaf, by comparing their performance with that of ten normal youngsters and found that intellectual retardation, brain injury, and regional hearing loss accounted for numerous cases diagnosed as being word-deaf. Carrell and Bangs (1951) asserted that trouble with language comprehension was but one aspect of a more widespread syndrome and suggested that disturbed visuomotor function, poor abstract performance, inferior figure background discrimination are worth while investigating. de Hirsch (1952) took up some problems in differential diagnosis and drew attention to the fact that profound auditory inattention, tendency to echolalia, and paucity of language are features found both in word-deaf and in autistic children and that only prolonged clinical observation of the child's total behaviour enables the clinician to discriminate between the two. She emphasized the fact that while not all word-deaf children show a positive electroencephalogram or gross neurological signs, observation of their performance reveals perseveration, stimulus-bound behaviour, severe hyperkinesis, and difficulty with control. In a later publication (1953) she stresses these children's basic gestalt difficulties. Myklebust (1954) throws light on behavioral symptoms of word-deaf children. He feels that their disturbance on the cortical level makes for difficulty with integration in most areas of functioning. Strauss (1954) in his very important contribution to the problem views word-deaf children as brain-damaged. Brain injury, he says, results in poor development of basic sensory-motor schemata and thus leads to difficulty with language reception and expression.

The latest study in the field by Jansky (1955), who with de Hirsch investigated in detail twelve word-deaf children, points in the same direction. Diagnosis of word deafness in this investigation was arrived at after other possible etiology had been ruled out. The audiograms of some of the children studied showed some inconsistency. However, careful testing (including the psychogalvanic skin resistance test) proved absence of a significant peripheral hearing loss in every single case, though some patients manifested marked delay in response to verbal stimuli. All twelve children were carefully evaluated as to intellectual potential. In addition to a quantitative analysis (the children's IQs ranged from dull normal to superior), they were analysed qualitatively so as to assess functioning in areas other than language. All twelve cases were studied by signs of withdrawal or other psychopathology and only if it was possible really to reach the child was the diagnosis of autism ruled out. Jansky closely investigated the receptive aspect of language by testing the children's interpretation of both words and sentences. Inability to attend to verbal material, need for frequent repetition of linguistic stimuli, excessively short auditory memory span were all found to be of interest. The categories of articulation, intelligibility, quantity of verbal output, pitch, and rate were evaluated so as to assess the children's competence in terms of the expressive aspect of language. The children's body image, their perceptual, their motor, and their visuomotor performance were studied, as well as figure-ground discrimination. In addition, other soft neurological signs—evidence of disorganization, impulsiveness, distractibility, rigidity, and perseveration—were noted. Laterality was evaluated in the framework of the child's ability to deal with spatial relationships. The results of Jansky's study showed that in word-deaf children language deviations are accompanied by disturbances in other areas of functioning and suggest that their performance is similar to that found in youngsters with verifiable brain injury.

Severe word deafness is not a frequent syndrome. When it occurs there is often a history of anoxia, birth injury, hemorrhage, convulsions, or erhyroblastosis fetalis due to the RH factor. In cases where neurological and encephalographic tests are negative it has been usually inferred that one deals with what is generally called developmental word deafness. However, Strauss' findings indicate that diffuse organicity can be inferred from severe motor area as well as from behavioral and language symptoms in the absence of a positive electroencephalogram and gross (as opposed to soft) deviations in the perceptuomotor and visuoneurological signs. One therefore feels inclined to assume that many of the cases diagnosed as developmental actually do present diffuse, nonfocal, and probably mild organic signs on a central level.

The writers agree with Strauss that word-deaf children have trouble with fundamental sensory-motor schemata. They feel that the inability of these youngsters to respond to the highly complex patterns as they are presented in spoken speech is but one aspect of their difficulty with perceptuomotor and visuomotor configurations. They have trouble structuring the perceptual field and experience speech in a diffuse, undifferentiated manner. The figure, be it the spoken word or the sentence, does not stand out from the vast number of un-organised stimuli constantly impinging on the organism. Thus, words fail to have meaning. The word-deaf child's attempts at speech, mo-notonous, indistinct, formless, and slurred reflect equal difficulty in organization and differentiation.

From these theoretical assumptions certain conclusions can be drawn for therapy:

1. While word deafness in severe form is a rare occurrence, it is probably insufficiently recognized that a relatively large number of children referred for dyslalia suffer from mild receptive language disturbances, even where there is no significant peripheral hearing loss. Failure to recognize that the resulting paucity of language, the paragrammatism, and the poor motor speech patterns have a receptive basis results in wasteful and ineffective therapeutic efforts.
2. Inconsistent audiograms are fairly typical for word-deaf children.
3. A time lag in response to auditory stimuli is not always due to a hearing deficit, nor is it necessarily an indication of mental retarda-tion. It might occur as part of the word-deaf syndrome and repre-sent difficulty with differentiation and integration of the essential feature of an auditory experience.
4. Since the latest studies have shown that hyperkinesis and distracti-bility are important features of the syndrome (many of these chil-dren are explosive and disorganized) it would follow that they need help with structuring their environment. The number of stimuli has to be reduced, and a relatively simple frame of reference has to be set up before language training can be undertaken.
5. Since it is assumed that the difficulty of these children is primarily one of organization of complex auditory configurations, the cutting down of the configurations into shorter units is thus a prerequisite of treatment. Speech must also be slowed up, dramatized in actual life situations. Constant repetition of verbal stimuli is needed to facilitate the integration of the material of experience with the linguistic symbols representing them.

Language Investigation of Children Suffering from Familial Dysautonomia

with Jeannette Jefferson Jansky

The purpose of this paper is to describe the language and related performance of twelve children diagnosed as having familial dysautonomia. This syndrome was recognized as a clinical entity and described by Riley et al. (1949) and more fully defined in two papers in 1952 (Riley) and 1954 (Riley, Freedman, and Langford). A team, consisting of the pediatrician, a neurologist, psychiatrist, psychologist, psychiatric social worker, statistician, and the writers investigated in detail twelve of these children.

According to Riley (1952), familial dysautonomia "is characterized by evidences of vegetative dysfunction, such as excessive perspiration, drooling, erythematous blotching of the skin, intermittent hypertension, and defective lacrimation; hyporeflexia and emotional instability are also present."

Riley (1954) also says:

The most striking identifying feature is the failure of the patients to produce normal quantities of tears when crying . . . Other frequent manifestations suggest diffuse involvement of the central nervous system, such as difficulty in motor coordination with retarded motor development, absent or diminished deep tendon reflexes, and relative indifference to pain. Particularly distressing symptoms occur in many of the patients. Some take the form of frequent episodes of bronchopneumonia in infancy, others of distressing cyclic vomiting associated with severe personality change. The death rate due to secondary disease, such as intercurrent infection, has been high.

Reprinted with permission from American Speech-Language-Hearing Association, from *Journal of Speech and Hearing Disorders* 21:450–459. 1956.

In relationship to the syndrome, the following factors are also of interest: genetic factors, blood pressure lability, and inadequate control of body temperature.

Procedure

At the Pediatric Language Disorder Clinic, Columbia Presbyterian Medical Center, twelve patients suffering from familial dysautonomia were studied. The age range was from three years six months to twelve years ten months. There were seven boys and five girls (see Table 1). The intelligence of these patients was not assessed quantitatively since it was felt that in children with organic involvement an intelligence quotient is not representative of actual intellectual potential. All but one child were evaluated more than once. The interval between the first and final sessions was from eight to twenty-one months. The second series of observations was used to test some performances refused by the younger children the first time. It also provided an opportunity to observe certain aspects of maturation. Recordings were made of each child's speech. A parent (in most cases the mother) provided the history. A series of tests was presented to each child and the results evaluated on the basis of some of the available norms and clinical experience.

In certain categories tested, norms could not be defined since specific criteria have not as yet been established. Moreover, some

Table 1
Sex and Age Distribution and Intervals Between First and Last Tests

Child	Sex	Age when First Seen	Age when Last Seen	Interval in Months
1. D.B.	F	4.7	5.8	13
2. K.E.	M	10.6	12.1	19
3. A.G.*	M	3.6	4.8	14
4. J.G.*	F	6.11	7.11	12
5. J.H.	F	12.10	14.4	18
6. P.K.	M	5.3	5.11	8
7. G.L.†	M	6.0		
8. R.N.	M	4.3	6.0	21
9. E.S.	F	5.6	6.10	16
10. J.S.	F	3.7	4.9	14
11. H.R.	M	9.10	11.5	19
12. M.W.	M	6.2	7.4	14

*Brother and sister.
†Child seen only once.

performances were only judged grossly since the task set for the team was to get an overall picture of the functioning of these children.

Language disturbances were defined as disturbances of speech, reading, and writing. Ability to read printed and written language was not tested due to the fact that eight out of the twelve children were under seven years of age at the initial testing and two of the remaining four had such severe visual defects as to render them virtually unable to cope with printed symbols.

Language was regarded as patterned behavior. Underlying those language disturbances which are not primarily emotionally determined, there are significant deviations in motor, perceptual, visuomotor, and conceptual performances that become apparent only after careful investigation. Therefore, tests were included which might give information as to the child's integrative and organizational capacities.

Testing of the emotional aspects of communication was not included since the team's psychiatrist and psychologist carefully investigated these areas.

The following criteria were used in the areas investigated:

History

Sitting and Walking

Using the Gesell (1940) developmental norms, a child was said to be late in sitting alone if he had not done so by nine months. Walking without support was judged to be late if the child was not able to manage by eighteen months (Gesell et al. 1940).

Words and Phrases

If the first words had not been spoken by twenty-four months, the child was felt to be late in this respect (Gesell et al. 1940) The child was judged to be delayed in combining words only if he had not done so by thirty months. (Gesell points out that by twenty-one months combinations of words are encountered in nearly all normal children.)

Present Status

Motor Coordination

Gross motor skills like gait, running, and balance were observed; also activities demonstrating finer motor control.

Gross Coordination.

a. Gait. Ataxia, awkwardness, unsteadiness, and tumbling were considered to be deviations.

b. Running. Running, according to Gesell (1940), begins at two years. If the child could not run at all or if he stumbled or had difficulty in running twenty feet at the age of three and one-half years, he was judged to be inept.

c. Balance. According to Myklebust (1954), using standards taken from Bayley, a child of approximately forty-nine months should be able to hop on his right foot two or three times. In his Tests of Motor Proficiency, Oseretsky (Doll 1940) provides criteria for judging balance in children from four to sixteen years of age. Adhering grossly to his standards, balance was felt to be poor if, at the appropriate age, the child was unable to perform the skill required.

Fine Coordination. The child was observed in manipulation of small objects, in insertion of pegs into a board, and in graphic activities. If tremor, severe awkwardness, frequent dropping of objects, or fumbling occurred, or if the child of six or over handled a pencil particularly clumsily, his finer motor performance was considered to be deviating. It should be added that only ten out of twelve children were tested in this area since the severe visual difficulties of the remaining two obviously interfered with finer motor control.

Visuomotor Ability

The Bender Gestalt test (Bender 1938) was used to evaluate visuomotor functioning. This test has been found useful in the diagnosis of cases showing some central involvement. According to Silver (1950), the Bender Gestalt test measures the following complex series of functions:

(a) the visual function, that is the reception of visual stimuli;
(b) the integrative function, in which the visual stimuli are sifted through the experiences and the organic matrix of the individual, and thus interpreted;
(c) the motor function, in which the visual percept is translated into the motor activity of drawing.

Since the Bender Gestalt test has been standardized as to age, deviations from the standard were judged to be manifestations of inferior visuomotor ability. Only ten out of twelve children were tested for reasons already cited.

Patterning and Organizational Capacities

According to Strauss and Kephart (1955), it is in the area of organization of relationships that children with central disturbances have trouble. Out of the mass of incoming stimuli the individual has to construct certain patterns and schemata. From the multitude of such schemata were chosen some which are involved in spatial, temporal, and figure-background relationships as being particularly pertinent to language.

Temporal Organization. In the auditory area the ability to grasp and reproduce sequences was tested by giving the children a series of tapped out patterns to imitate. This seemed to be a significant test, since for spoken language organization in time is an important factor. If the child was unable to imitate tapped-out patterns the length and complexity of which were increased with various age levels, he was felt to be inferior in temporal ogranization.

Spatial Organization. Adequacy in this area was judged by performance on the Bender Gestalt test (1938) and the Goodenough Draw-a-Man test (1926). The latter was chosen because spatial concepts are originally derived from a person's image of parts of his own body and their relationship to each other. Vernon (1952) emphasizes the close parallels between development of spatial concepts and body schema. Gross difficulties with spacing of the configurations, overlapping of figures, poor use of the framework of the page, or rotational tendencies on the Bender Gestalt, as well as severe deviations in proportions and relationships of body parts on the Goodenough, were noted as evidences of difficulty with spatial organization. Parallel investigations were done by Galefret-Granjon (1951), who uses these tests among others for evaluation of spatial relationships in cases of dyslexia. Only ten of the twelve children were tested for spatial organizational ability.

Figure-Background Organization. According to Goldstein (1939), inability to distinguish between the foreground and the background of a given motor, sensory, or ideational configuration has been found to be a significant phenomenon in brain-injured individuals.

Figure-background organization was judged by performance on the writers' adaptation of the Strauss-Lehtinen cards (1947), which were flashed by hand for just less than a second. Exposure time was increased for the younger children. When a child missed three or more figures after two or more exposures of each card, his performance was felt to be deviating in this area. Eleven children out of twelve gave responses to this test; the severity of the visual defect in one of them made it impossible for him to respond to the stimulus.

Biological Functions Related to Language

Those biological functions were tested which are made use of in the process of speaking; namely, breathing, swallowing, chewing, and sucking.

Breathing. In his evaluation of breathing in cerebral palsied children, Palmer (1949) considered breathing unsatisfactory if it was arrhythmic or explosive. If either were observed in children with familial dysautonomia, or if, in addition, severe hypotonicity and excessively fast rate were noted, breathing was felt to be deviating. Fairbanks (1940) does not necessarily consider shallow breathing a departure from the normal pattern.

Swallowing. Swallowing was judged to be atypical when initiation was difficult or delayed, when gagging occurred, or when part of the bolus of food was expelled in the process.

Chewing. Chewing was felt to be deviant if the process seemed inordinately time consuming, if the child usually used his incisors, if jaw movement was limited, or if, instead of using his teeth, the child's chief means of breaking down food was by pushing it with his tongue against the palate.

Sucking. Sucking was said to be poor if the child of three and one half or older was unable to suck or did so only with great difficulty.

Movement and Control of Peripheral Speech Organs

The control of lips, tongue, and velum was observed, as well as diadochokinesis and drooling.

Lip Movement. Movement of lips was felt to be deviant if the child was unable to purse and spread the lips, if excessive movements or overflow were noted, if there was pull to either side, if lip movement was stiff, and if closure was poor.

Tongue Movement. Tongue movement was said to be unsatisfactory if extension was limited, if after the age of four the child was unable to flex the tongue to both sides, or if, after the age of five, voluntary elevation was absent or poor.

Velar Movement. Velar movement was judged to be inadequate if very sluggish, if elevation was absent, or if movement was asynergic.

Diadochokinesis. Using West's (1937) definition, diadochokinesis was accepted as being "the act . . . of repeating at maximum speed some simple, cyclical, reciprocating movement." The child was given four consonant combinations to repeat. If movement was arrhythmic or slow, or if the child under the age of five was unable to continue two combinations for five seconds, diadochokinesis was said to be inferior.

Drooling. Drooling was placed in this category arbitrarily since in the case of children suffering from familial dysautonomia it is difficult to determine whether drooling occurs on the basis of hypersalivation, of poor control of articulatory movements, or because of difficulty with swallowing. If drooling was observed it was noted.

Voice

Deviations noted in vocal functioning were those in quality, pitch, loudness, and tonus; also fading.

Quality. Using Fairbanks' (1940) designations, nasality, breathiness, hoarseness, and harshness were marked as deviant.

Pitch. Pitch was judged to be atypical by three of Fairbanks'

(1940) criteria: too high, too low, or inflexible. The criterion of poor control as manifested by sudden fluctuations between too high and too low a pitch was added.

Loudness. Deviations were assumed to be present if, according to Fairbanks' (1940) criteria, voice was too soft or too loud; or if, in addition, there was poor control of loudness.

Vocal Tonus. Vocal tonus was observed and extreme hyper- or hypotonicity were noted as deviant.

Fading. Fading was observed in a separate subcategory, although in some cases fading was felt to be a function of hypotonicity or possibly of poor control of loudness. Fading was assumed to be present when there was marked decrease in loudness as the child progressed from syllable to syllable in a word or phrase. Since it is difficult to measure fading by objective means, clinical judgment was used to gauge deviations.

Language

Receptive Aspects.

a.   Hearing. Crude hearing tests required the child to choose from a toy box specific objects the names of which were whispered from a distance of approximately four feet behind his back. If the child failed the same stimulus twice, gross hearing capacity was considered uncertain enough to warrant further investigation.

b.   Understanding. In judging understanding of verbal material, interpretation both of single words and of a connected story was tested. In the former, the child was asked to point to pictures named by the examiner.

In evaluating understanding of connected verbal material, the three- to four-year-old child was asked to tell the point of a story which involved a single incident; the four-to-five-year-old one involving some concept of time; and the six-year and older child a joke involving a verbal absurdity. If the child failed at the appropriate level, understanding of verbal material was judged to be poor.

c.   Auditory Memory Span. In testing auditory memory span, the child was presented with syllables containing different consonants and vowels such as *bah-moo*. Since consonants and vowels were combined as Beebe (1944) did in her study, her norms were used. Beebe required the child of five to seven years to repeat four nonsense syllables, the child of seven and above to repeat five nonsense syllables. In this study, the four-year-old was expected to repeat three nonsense syllables instead of four. Auditory memory span was considered to be short if the child's performance fell below these expectations.

Expressive Aspects.

a.   Articulation. Using Templin's (1953) findings, articulation was considered deviant if, by the age of eight for boys and seven for girls, errors in vowel and consonant pronunciation were observed. For the younger child, intelligibility was considered a crude indicator of articulatory ability. If it was not possible to understand the essence of what a child of four, five, or six said, it was concluded that one of the factors involved was poor articulation.

b.   Intelligibility. Intelligibility was rated separately. The criterion for judging intelligibility was the ability of the trained listener to understand the child's verbal output at least on second repetition.

c.   Rate. Rate of speech was considered deviating if too fast, too slow, or fluctuating between the two.

d.   Rhythm. Rhythm was judged to be poor if staccato, jerky, or if there were clonic iterations or tonic manifestations interrupting the flow of speech.

Organizational Aspects.

a.   Grammar. Grammatical construction was observed in the child's spontaneous conversation. Grammar was considered poor if a child used immature forms for his age. Criteria were taken from the material presented by McCarthy (1954) on this subject. Taking age level into consideration, deviations included excessive use of incomplete sentences, a disproportionate use in a sentence of any part of speech, and difficulty in using any but the present tense.

b.   Story Telling. The smaller children were asked to tell the story of The Three Little Pigs or The Three Bears. The older ones were required to retell one they had seen on television or at the movies. The performance was considered inadequate if the child beyond the age of four and one-half was unable to produce a very crude outline of the content. If the older child's story was poorly organized, if he failed to get the point across, or if he omitted essential items, he was considered to have done poorly in this area.

Categorical Aspects.

a.   Naming. Goldstein (1948) makes a distinction between naming and the use of words in ordinary conversation. Some children have what appears to be a good use of the idiom on a purely auditory-perceptual basis, while they have great difficulty evoking the word concept when presented with a specific demand. The younger children were shown a series of simple pictures representing common objects. The older ones were given pictures representing words of a higher order of abstraction; they were required to be more specific in their responses. If the children at appropriate age levels had considerable trouble in evoking names, they were considered to have difficulty.

b.   Definitions. Since children over five years are expected to define objects in terms of function, inability to do so at this age or older was judged to be a sign of weakness in categorical development. Older children's responses were judged qualitatively. If the definitions of the children were found to be more than usually concrete for their age level, they were assumed to have difficulty with categorical performance. Only ten children out of twelve were tested since the remaining two were still under five years of age by the time of the second testing.

Findings and Discussions

Data on each child's performance in every category were based on clinical observations. A child's performance was classified as deviant if a deviation was clearly present and consistent and there was little or no doubt that abnormality existed. All marginal performances were considered to fall within the normal range. Table 2 shows the number of patients tested who were rated as deviant in each category.

The results should not be considered final because of the subjective nature of much of the examination, because of the absence of a control group, and because the broadness of scope involved in the testing of a multiplicity of items allowed the outlining of only general trends. Since certain developmental processes were involved, the wide age range also presented problems. Two separate, though interacting, factors had to be considered: maturation and degree of pathological involvement. However, allowing for these reservations, reference to the table shows that there emerges a fairly well defined picture.

Table 2
Frequency of Occurrence of Specific Deviations

Areas Tested	Total Number Children Examined	Number of Children with Deviations
I. History		
A. Sitting	12	3
B. Walking	12	9
C. Speech		
1. words	12	7
2. phrases	12	8
II. Present Status		
A. Motor Coordination		
1. gross coordination		
a. gait	12	10
b. running	12	11
c. balance	12	10
2. fine coordination	12	12

(continued)

Table 2 (continued)
Frequency of Occurrence of Specific Deviations

Areas Tested	Total Number Children Examined	Number of Children with Deviations
B. Visuomotor Ability	10	8
C. Patterning and Organizational Capacities		
1. temporal organization	12	6
2. spatial organization	10	7
3. figure-ground organization	11	6
D. Biological Functions Related to Language		
1. breathing	12	8
2. swallowing	12	9
3. chewing	12	9
4. sucking	12	7
E. Movement and Control of Peripheral Speech Organs		
1. lip movement	12	12
2. tongue movement	12	8
3. diadochokinesis	12	10
4. velar movement	12	6
5. drooling	12	11
F. Voice		
1. quality	12	10
2. pitch	12	10
3. vocal tonus	12	9
4. fading	12	8
5. loudness	12	7
G. Language		
1. receptive aspects		
a. hearing	12	0
b. understanding	12	2
c. auditory memory span	12	7
2. expressive aspects		
a. articulation	12	6
b. intelligibility	12	6
c. rate	12	10
d. rhythm	12	5
3. organizational aspects		
a. grammar	12	5
b. story telling	7	5
4. categorical aspects		
a. naming	12	8
b. definition	10	6

The findings in visuomotor ability agree with the observations of Goldstein (1939), Bender (1938), and Strauss (1947) who maintain that visuomotor difficulties are frequent in individuals who show a degree of central involvement.

All but one subcategory in the area of movement and control of peripheral speech organs were found to show deviations. This is not surprising since three of them (movements of lips and tongue and diadochokinesis) are probably closely related to difficulties with finer motor control (see Table 2). The only subcategory in which deviations were less frequent is that of velar movement, which half of the children found difficult. It should be stated, however, that precise measurements of velar movements are hard to obtain by means of clinical observations.

Of the ten children out of twelve judged to have poor voice quality, nine were observed to have nasal voices. This fact is of interest, considering that only six children had difficulties with velar movement. Several possible explanations present themselves: (1) The difficulty of measuring velar movement by clinical observations; (2) The question as to whether velar movement as produced under strong stimulation (in response to the command to repeat specified units) is the same as that found during habitual conversation; (3) The relation of action and position of the tongue to nasality (McCarthy 1954); (4) The relationship of the hypotonicity of the children in the dysautonomic group to the relatively severe nasality observed.

Eight of the ten children showing difficulty with pitch had monotonous voices. Attention is drawn to the fact that in some cerebellar conditions voice is strikingly monotonous (Worster-Drought 1953).

The finding of fading in eight out of twelve children might be related to overall hypotonicity, though not unlike monotony, fading is also frequently a feature in neurological conditions. Six of the seven children with deviations in loudness showed poor control. In other words, their voices fluctuated between being too loud and too soft. These fluctuations might possibly be related to fading, since five of the children manifested both fading and poor control. It is likely that tonus, loudness, and fading are all interrelated.

Similar Speech Syndromes

Speech patterns similar to those observed in children who have familial dysautonomia have been reported with other neurological disorders. Worster-Drought (1953) reports speech manifestations in cases of congenital suprabulbar agenesis in which there are:

. . . varying degrees of weakness and spasticity of the lips, tongue, soft palate, pharyngeal and laryngeal muscles, either separately or combined. Speech may be extremely dysarthric, being slurred and indistinct with deficient lingual and labial sounds. In severe cases, the lips, tongue and soft palate may be immobile. Sometimes the child is able to protrude his tongue to a certain extent but is unable to curl it upwards and lateral movements are impossible. In milder cases, the paresis of the muscles of articulation is of lesser degree and isolated weakness of either the lips, tongue or soft palate may occur. Not infrequently, owing to the weakness of the lips and impairment of swallowing, the accumulation of saliva is uncontrolled and consequently the child dribbles continually.

Peacher (1950) points out that in bilateral pyramidal lesions in pseudo-bulbar palsy there is dysphagia and dysarthria. In speech, "respiration and rhythm are largely implicated" if the pontine pathway is involved. In articulation bilabials and lingua—dental consonants and lingua—rugal sounds are most often distorted. Peacher mentions that bulbar speech is usually described as flaccid. Peacher also says that "certain aspects of the dysarthrias are more prominent due to lesions in certain areas, *e.g.*, rhythm in cerebellar implication, articulation in pyramidal involvement, respiration and phonation in the basal ganglia disturbances . . ."

Rutherford (1944) found that in children with extra-pyramidal lesions speech may be louder, lower pitched, irregular, monotonous, and aspirate, which was felt to be due to interference with the respiratory apparatus.

Zentay (1937) describes corticostriopallidorubrobulbar tract lesions as affecting maintenance of "the required tone, rate and depth of respiration, pitch of voice, tempo of speech." He refers to both "hypotonic-hyperkinetic" and "hypertonic-hypokinetic" manifestations. In the former there is hyperkinesis of the vocal cords, involuntary diaphragmatic movements, and in coordination of various movements, all of which results in a weak voice and deviating pitch. In the latter, speech is hesitant, halting, and delayed; it is also lacking in modulation and sometimes blurred.

Robbins (1940) discusses patients with "bulbar speech" as having marked elision of syllables with slurring and high pitched, hoarse, monotonous, and nasal voices.

Comparing the speech picture in the various conditions described in the literature with that of the dysautonomic group one finds hypotonic manifestations in the speech musculature are far more frequent than hypertonic ones. In any case, the speech examination seems to indicate that the whole of the nervous system is implicated. Only further investigation will show whether bulbar speech manifestations, in addition to basal ganglia ones, are of particular significance.

Summary

A study was done of twelve children suffering from familial dysautonomia. Findings revealed that the patients studied had severe difficulties with gross and finer motor control and associated difficulties with movement and control of articulators. They had trouble also with biological activities underlying speech, such as breathing, swallowing, chewing, and sucking. The voices of these children were deviating: quality was nasalized and pitch was monotonous; there was poor control of loudness and a tendency to fading. Auditory memory span was short, though hearing and understanding presented no problems. In the area of expressive language, these children showed fluctuations in rate. Articulation and intelligibility were inferior to what one would expect in the general population. These children's rhythmic abilities did not seem to be particularly good. Difficulty with story telling was relatively frequent. Categorical behavior seemed to be poor. The implications of these findings were discussed in relation to observations of similar speech conditions reported in the literature.

A Case of Motor Aphasia

Mark S., the boy who is described here, represents, we feel, a case of motor aphasia, a syndrome which is found infrequently in children in the absence of a verifiable history of cerebral trauma, significant neuromotor involvement, and the usual classical neurological signs.

A description of the findings might be of interest in the light of Strauss's contention (1954) that there is justification in diagnosing diffuse organicity mainly on the basis of severe dysfunctions in perceptual, motor, and visuomotor performance even in cases which do not show gross neurological signs or a positive electroencephalogram.

If we call Mark a case of motor aphasia (Strauss prefers the word oligophasia) a term which is, of course, borrowed from a comparable condition in the adult, we are aware of the fact that a child's failure to develop essential sensory-motor and perceptual schemata gives rise to a different syndrome from the adult's disturbance which is caused by disintegration of function and a disruption of patterns which formerly had been well established. Obviously, in children, developmental and maturational factors complicate the picture.

Language is patterned behavior and should be considered only in interaction with other patterned mechanisms. The ability to understand and to use both oral and printed language depends in the last analysis on normal performance in the motor, perceptual, visuomotor, and conceptual areas. Severe cases of language dysfunction mostly show disturbances in related fields of behavior and do on close investigation reveal some deviations in organization of temporal and spatial patterning. Mark shows these features especially clearly.

Case History

Mark was first examined in the Pediatric Language Disorders Clinic in November 1952, when he was four and a half years old,

Reprinted with permission from the author, from *Speech* 51–57. 1957.

because of the mother's complaint that he had failed to develop speech. He is the youngest of three children; his older sisters are five and seven years old, respectively. The pediatrician who first saw him noted that the family history of language and handedness was negative. Mark, it seemed, cooperated poorly during examination. Babinski's sign was absent, abdominal reflexes were active. Pregnancy had been uneventful except for some occasional pain across the lower abdomen. Labor was induced by a substance unknown to the mother. It was a full term delivery, no instruments were used, and the child weighed six pounds at birth. Neonatal history was noncontributory. There is no report of cyanosis, respiratory difficulty, or jaundice. There is no history of convulsions. Mark took food well until he was six months old at which time he had bronchopneumonia.

Early development was deviating. The child did not sit by himself until he was a year old. He did not walk without support until he was twenty months of age. Toilet training was started at nine and a half months but was not established until the boy was two and a half years old. The mother says Mark fell out of his crib at least five times at around sixteen or seventeen months. However, he never lost consciousness, bled from his ears, or vomited. General health was good. Mark had no significant childhood diseases but suffered from a chronic cough. The boy ate little and mostly mushy food. He hardly ever fed himself and by the time he was first seen he made no efforts to dress or undress.

Mrs. N. reported that he communicated entirely by nonverbal means, gestures, grunts, and screams and that in this manner he achieved all he wanted. She firmly declared that Mark did not want to talk, but added a few moments afterwards that he had used the expressions: *ma* and *da* and *e* for *yes* at the age of two and a half and that he then had stopped talking altogether. According to her story he started again with the same words a year later but had made no further progress. On the other hand, she felt sure that he understood language of others and was proud of the fact that at four and a half years he was able to articulate the letters of the alphabet (he used grunt-like vowels only) and that he knew his numbers.

An effort had been made to send the boy to nursery school in the early autumn of 1952. However, he had adjusted so poorly that he had to be withdrawn. In January of 1953 Mark was referred for psychological evaluation. The psychologist took extensive notes on her conversation with the mother. She reported that Mark shared his sister's bedroom and had a tendency to walk around at night, getting into one bed after the other, usually settling in his mother's. He had a habit of removing his clothes even in the day time. It appeared that he fluctuated between periods of quiet solitary play and those of marked hyperactivity.

The psychologist did say that Mark's muscular coordination was poor and that he was unable to fasten buttons. She found his figure drawing crude and immature. He rated an intelligence quotient of 91 on the Merrill Palmer performance test. She concluded that the boy presented significant emotional problems, that he reacted to the Oedipus situation in an obsessive-compulsive manner; she recommended parental counseling.

First Investigation by Language Disorder Clinic

In March 1953 Mark was referred to the Pediatric Language Disorder Clinic. We found him a good-looking and very friendly boy. His nails were bitten to the quick. What struck us first when going over his history was the striking discrepancy between the youngster's substantially delayed early motor development and his apparently normal overall intellectual functioning as borne out by the result of the psychological evaluation.

When we examined the youngster ourselves we found outstanding difficulty in coordination of large and small muscle groups. Mark was unable to ride a tricycle, he constantly knocked things off the table, his hands shook, his movements were jerky, and he held a pencil awkwardly. He did not know how to wash his hands although he was carefully shown what to do. He could not walk on his heels. One had the impression that he not only had trouble with the single movements involved but that, as in ideomotor apraxia, he failed to grasp the concept, or one would better say, the gestalt of the act.

When we first saw Mark he was able to extend, flex, and elevate the tongue without difficulty so that it was evident that we were not primarily dealing with a dysarthria. As other motor aphasics, Mark was able to use the muscles of the tongue, lips, and jaw for activities like chewing, swallowing, kicking, and sucking. It is true that he was somewhat dyspraxic, that diadochoinesis was far from good, and that the child still occasionally drooled. However, these moderate difficulties could not possibly account for his total inability to reproduce words. Thus it seemed that not so much the instrumentalities of language were at fault, but a central condition.

Mark showed deviations not only in the motor area. Although he had no hearing loss and responded to whispered words behind his back he confused units like *bird* and *boat*, testifying to considerable difficulty with auditory discrimination. His auditory memory span was extraordinarily short; he could repeat at best two nonsense syllables and even these two he frequently reversed. Since he was obviously unable to keep a sequence of auditorily perceived units in mind, it was thus not surprising that he was totally unable to cope with polysyllabic words. Mark failed not only where symbols were concerned, but was also unable to repeat the simplest auditory patterns, to imitate quite easy tapped-out sequences, or to hum a tune.

In conjunction with Strauss, Goldenberg (1950) reported findings of a test requiring a number of brain-injured children to repeat simple melodies. The patients failed significantly when compared to a control group, since, as the study put it, they were, "unable to perceive or respond to patterning of the tones."

In the visual field Mark was unable to match colors. Visuomotor performance was inferior in terms of his age. As could be expected, his Bender Gestalt (1938) showed poor manual control, figures were superimposed on each other, and some ran off the page. The boy evidently had trouble not only with temporal but also with spatial organization. Apart from some primitivity and a tendency to vertical-ize horizontally-oriented figures (a sign of immaturity by no means abnormal at his age), he showed features typical for the organic child: disinhibition, slight perseveration, and a tendency to be drawn to irrelevant details rather than to attend to the concept of the gestalt.

Mark's drawing of a human figure was not only crude as the psychologist had said, but it was also deviating. He reproduced (and still does) elongated sticklike figures, one of which had two heads. It seemed that his body image (a concept which refers to an individual's awareness of parts of his own body and their relationship to each other) was disturbed, a characteristic feature of the organic child.

On testing laterality Mark showed considerably more right- than left-handed responses. The right eye seemed dominant.

The boy's speech consisted of a few monosyllabic words which sounded like soft grunts. He did not produce any consonants spon-taneously, and he had the greatest difficulty imitating them. Most of the time, as for instance, when he counted, which he loved to do, he made the vowel do for the word. Voice quality was harsh and monoto-nous. While a lack of inflection as Mark showed it might indicate a lack of communicative intent, it might also represent an inability to struc-turalize the verbal output in a way which makes the figure, the meaning, stand out clearly.

That he did have some trouble with discriminating figure from ground was borne out when we showed him our adaptation of the Strauss-Lehtinen cards (1950). It seemed that he could not withstand the attraction of the extraneous stimuli as they are represented by the strongly patterned background, and as a result he failed to perceive the object, the figure.

Mark was without a doubt an emotionally somewhat deviating boy. He was infantile to a marked degree, he had a variety of tics— shoulder shrugging and eye blinking—and he was so obsessive and occasionally became so lost in some mechanical activity or other that one was at first not quite sure how far he was basically interested in communication. However, he did relate to the therapist and most of the time his gestures and inarticulate vocalizations so strongly indicated a need to communicate that one felt he was not an autistic youngster.

While we did not want to exclude the pressure of significant emotional factors, we nevertheless felt during this first investigation that there were valid reasons for suspecting organicity, and we therefore referred the boy for an electroencephalogram and for neurological evaluation.

These are the findings:

> *Neurological:*   Examination essentially negative. No neurological focal signs. There are, however, some contradictory facts. No real signs of organicity, but there is an element of poor coordination, also hyperextensibility of the figures which makes one wonder whether basal ganglia involvement is present. The speech disorder is bizarre. Perhaps there is some motor aphasia though this is hard to support. One might consider the possibility of areas 39-40 of Brodman involvement in the cupular supramarginal gyri of the left inferior parietal lobule. Even here this might be organic or physiologic. Continue speech treatment.
>
> *EEG:*   No focal or lateral signs. Essentially normal for this age group.

We saw the boy a few more times during the spring of 1953 and found that interpretation of language, was, as a matter of fact, not nearly as good as we had assummed at first. To begin with Mark had trouble understanding concepts like *under* or *on top of.* When one exposed pictures and asked him to find the "thing that cuts," he failed to point to the knife. He performed poorly when tested for verbal absurdities and did not object when asked if a boy could use his sledge in the summer.

There were other aspects of the case which were difficult to overlook. Mark, it seemed, was fighting a running battle with his mother and refused everything she wanted him to do. At home (probably because his mother felt fundamentally very guilty over what one sensed was her basic rejection of him), she let him "get away with murder." Mark's sister was the only one who could manage him. At the same time the pressure on the youngster to produce words was tremendous. We learned that daily bulletins were given out over the phone to the family at large on how many sounds Mark had produced that day. It appeared that his negativism had become fixed in an area where he had enormous difficulties to begin with, and as a result he was at first quite resistant to work on sounds and words at the clinic.

Mrs. N. was therefore asked to withdraw pressure as much as possible and was referred to the social worker for counseling.

A Group Experience

We did not see Mark again for six months. A nursery school was found for the boy where he seemed happy, and since this was his first successful group experience it was felt wiser to wait to see what socialization, combined with counselling for the mother, would do for the child. Mark stayed in this group until the beginning of January 1954 when the school felt they could do nothing further for him.

When he returned to the clinic we found on examination that Mark's muscular coordination still was strikingly inferior; he could not even hook together our simple trains. Spatial orientation was as poor as was temporal organization. There was striking overall hypotonicity, occasional associated movements, and whirling along a longitudinal axis.

The boy's chief improvement was in the area of language interpretation. He still missed finer shades of meaning, but by and large he had little trouble understanding verbal material. He seemed a little happier but his tendency to tics, eyeblinking, and shoulder jerking had become more marked.

Expressive speech still was practically nonexistent. Mark communicated still mostly by gestures, demonstrations, and facial expressions. He used a few consonants, such as the medial *d* in *addy* for *daddy*, and the final *s* or *es* for *yes*, but for the most part he omitted them. His voice had the same harsh quality.

Speech Therapy Begun

Treatment was begun in February 1954. Two weekly sessions were scheduled and Mark's mother brought him in faithfully.

There were many times when the boy had to be weaned away from his endless obsessive play with wooden clowns and trucks. The question arose as to the basis for this over-structured and repetitive behavior. While the traffic jams Mark played out with the trucks obviously symbolized his frustration over his inability to communicate, it seemed also that Mark (as do many adult aphasics) clung to repetitive activities bcause they did not frustrate him as desperately as did other more complex ones. He was obsessed with numbers and up to a point he still is. There are of course psychological interpretations for this, but one would have to say also that numbers for Mark simply were safer and more predictable; they did not frustrate him as much as did these very crude verbal tools. The boy was so rigid that for a while he got upset whenever the therapist took off her glasses. This is understandable if one remembers that the child's very perceptions were unstable and that more than others he had to depend on reliable

configurations. Rigidity, moreover, is a way to cope with basic disorganization and Mark, like practically all diffusely brain-injured children, get disorganized easily.

He tends to go completely haywire if he is handled too permissively, and he functions better when given clear and understandable
rules of conduct. He is not as distractible as are some brain-injured
children who often seem to be at the mercy of environmental stimuli,
but he is nevertheless extremely restless. Patterning of behavior is
frequently difficult for diffusely brain-injured youngsters, as is the
patterning of motor, perceptual, and language units. These children
tend to respond explosively and often, to the observer, inappropriately
to stimuli impinging on the organism. This restlessness, together with
his short frustration threshold, made it seem inadvisable to press him
too hard since this would have simply resulted in an increased number
of tics. There were times when one had to help Mark to express within
limits and through play some of his rage and frustration. His anger was
all the more fierce since he had no way of using words as an outlet.
Only his strong attachment to his therapist enabled him to cope with
what Goldstein (1939) calls "catastrophic reaction," the disorganized
response of the organism faced with a task with which he is unable to
cope.

What made things more difficult for the boy to bear was the fact
that his failures were not confined to speech but were distributed over
a wide area. To begin with, he could not throw a ball, nor could he tie
his shoes. His difficulties with finer motor skills were probably related
to several factors; his spatial abilities were poor and he had trouble
placing small objects; his visual perceptions were probably not precisely enough structured to serve as effective leads for the execution of
complex movements; finally, and this is probably the most important,
his lack of inner speech, which is so essential during the learning of a
new motor skill before it becomes automatic, probably played an
important part in his dyspraxia.

Mark had difficulties in the conceptual realm as well. For example,
he found it hard to understand that specific toys belonged to specific
boxes—doll furniture went into a different box from drawing material.
Categorical performance, which consists in the ability to group discrete
elements according to certain guiding principles, is usually weak in
diffusely brain-injured children.

Mark's social awareness also seemed somewhat limited. When we
first saw him he had a somewhat disconcerting habit of kissing relative
strangers whenever he met them and although he has become more
discriminating, he is unusually demonstrative for a boy of his age.

The first thing Mark learned was a number of B words produced
under strong stimulation. He got the word *bang*, for instance, when
banging on the table. The violent motor act one might say carried the

word and was designed at the same time to help his marked hypotonicity. A story was started about Bobby the B Boy who owned
things like *bat* and *ball*, and this story motivated him at least to try.
However, even when he had mastered the separate units (we had first
tried him with the whole unit configuration and failed), he found it
incredibly hard to blend them into a word. The word, not unlike the
motor act, is not a sum of separate elements. It is an integrated
experience, a gestalt, and where there are difficulties in organization
and integration of schematas, as in Mark's case, the task is hard. Not
only did the blending of single sounds present difficulties (even now
diphthongs, which are intimately blended, are very hard for him), but
the combination of words into phrases also presented a major hurdle.
Long after Mark had acquired the words *bit* and *bat* he was unable to
combine them, and only in May 1954, after several months of work, did
he produce a number of two-word combinations.

Like most adult aphasics Mark had little trouble reciting the
alphabet and counting after a fashion. In such automatic responses
(which resemble deeply ingrained motor acts) there is little necessity
for voluntary initiation of a verbal response, and since one of the boy's
most marked difficulties consisted in the initiation of such responses, it
was entirely logical that he did better with final than he did with initial
sounds.

Mark came back to us in September 1954. It took him some time to
get settled in the kindergarten group of a health class in his community, since his wandering around during sessions required a good
deal of tolerance from his teacher.

His voice and speech had changed little but he did produce more
two-word combinations and slowly began to use words such as *oi* (for
toilet), *ain* (for *rain*), *air* (for *chair*) spontaneously. In November of that
year he said "Oh Gee" relatively clearly. Hand in hand with his
increasing number of one- and two-word responses we found improvement in visuomotor organization, and during the past year many
of the marked perceptual and motor deviations have slowly disappeared. However, as quantity of speech began to increase it became
progressively harder to understand the boy, and if one did not know
the contextual framework one could not even guess what he meant.

His ability to retain auditory patterns remained abysmally poor
and in January 1955 we started him on reading in the hope that visual
reinforcement might prove to be helpful. Since auditory patterning is
required in the blending of phonetic units and was thus bound to be
too frustrating for the boy, we started him on the whole word approach
and, in fact, he did not do too badly when short whole word configurations were exposed. After a relatively short time he was able to
read phrases like: "I am a boy," "daddy is a man." He also wrote these
units down and although his printing was almost illegible, reading,
and writing opened new avenues of approach.

By the spring of 1955 Mark repeated consonants in three-word phrases and begin to finish sentences when one started them for him. Before the clinic closesd for the summer Mark's repetition of spoken material had improved markedly and he used several short phrases spontaneously. However, as soon as verbalizations had reached a certain level he was plagued by new difficulties, one of the worst ones being his tendency to reversals of sounds in words and of words in phrases. Since it was the final syllable he heard last, it was the one which stuck best in his mind and he thus invariably started out with the last sound saying, for example, *top* for *pot*.

The space is too limited to give a month by month report on last year's therapeutic development. Mark came back to us in the autumn. He had gone to camp and had responded well to the more structured set-up. He now eats all foods. He insists on practising playing ball. He repeats five- to six-word phrases without visual clues. He dictates the captions to the cartoons we draw for him. While he still has terrible trouble with integration of sounds, he now has a relatively large functional one-word vocabulary and a limited number of phrases he uses spontaneously, a number which increases week by week. Repetition of sequences of sounds on purely auditory basis still is a big hurdle, and while verbal communication has improved it is not yet a serviceable tool. He words very hard indeed, his frustration tolerance is much higher, and his tics have disappeared.

As time goes on maturation and training will facilitate verbal communication. However prognosis is guarded, far more guarded than in the case of another youngster whom we started at about the same time and who has responded much more dramatically. It seems thus that Mark's difficulties are far more severe.

Summary

Mark represents a case of motor aphasia. His trouble with patterning of basic schemata shows in poor organization of auditory visuomotor and motor configurations. His main difficulty lies in the initiation, integration, and retention of phonetic patterns. Treatment aims at helping Mark with structuralization especially in the auditory and motor realm. The setting of additional visual and kinesthetic links is designed to reinforce weak auditory associations. Like most diffusely brain-injured children Mark requires help also with patterning of behavior. While he needs massive support and a good deal of tolerance he does better with consistent rules which give him a framework in which to function.

Differential Diagnosis between Aphasic and Schizophrenic Language in Children

The differential diagnosis between primary, specific communicative disorders, sometimes called aphasic, and those communicative difficulties which are secondary to psychopathology is rarely, if ever, straightforward.

In clinical practice one encounters a continuum of communicative deficits that range from severe defects in the codification of language at one end to those which reflect a pathological orientation to the self, the love object, and the world at the other. There exist, however, some more or less pure cases at either end of this continuum and it might be appropriate to discuss these first.

The consensus during the past few years has been to reserve the term aphasic for cases whose difficulties with the decoding and encoding of verbal symbols are related to demonstrable central nervous system impairment. However, not all children who, in the absence of significant sensory deficits or important limitations in intellectual potential, fail to interpret and use language have histories of brain damage or show positive signs on the classical neurological examination or the electroencephalogram (EEG), Jansky (1960), who investigated twelve children with severe symbolic disorders, six with histories of brain damage and six without, found clear differences between these groups and normal controls in most of the 14 verbal and 14 nonverbal areas tested. No essential differences, on the other hand, were found between the children with verifiable histories of brain damage and those without such histories.

Children who partially or totally fail to interpret or use verbal symbols will be called aphasoid in this paper since, regardless of their histories, the overwhelming majority present a fairly typical constellation of dysfunctions, many of which have been discussed by such researchers as Worster-Drought (1943), Carrel and Bangs (1957), and others.

Reprinted with permission from American Speech-Language-Hearing Association, from *Journal of Speech and Hearing Disorders* 32:3–9. 1967.

While aphasoid children's audiograms may fluctuate, their erratic auditory deficits do not account for their profound inattention to auditory and, more specifically, to verbal stimuli. These children hear, but they do not necessarily understand. They have difficulties with "auding" (Hardy 1965), with perceiving, storing, and recalling the serial order of information received through auditory channels. Masland (1965) says that the essential feature in verbal behavior is the sequencing of auditory events. Aphasoid children distort the temporal sequence of signals (Paine 1965). Their auditory memory spans are extremely short, and they have difficulties in recalling both nonverbal and verbal configurations. They show limited ability to repeat patterns tapped out for them, and they have trouble reproducing digits, nonsense syllables, and sentences in the correct order (Lowe and Campbell 1965).

In these children, moreover, the perceptual field is poorly structured; words do not seem to stand out from the mass of unorganized stimuli impinging on the organism. In a recent experiment Williams (1965) showed that her aphasic group's ability to separate the auditory figure from the background of noise was inferior. Words for such youngsters seem to be experienced in a diffuse undifferentiated fashion as evidenced by their strikingly poor auditory discrimination. Above all, the configuration of the word, as well as its meaning, appears to be unstable (de Hirsch 1965); the word never acquires a physiognomy, as it were; it never becomes familiar. As French (1953) puts it, such children are unable to maintain a linguistic gestalt; thus they fail to assign consistent symbolic significance to input events.

The expressive language deficits of these children are mostly secondary to their receptive disorders and mirror their poorly structured and diffuse intake and their inadequate feedback. The degree of expressive language impairment varies. Speech may be severely limited in quantity, crude and undifferentiated in quality. Lenneberg (1964b) comments on the primitiveness of the utterances of these children. They simplify blends, telescope words, and their verbalizations are only crude approximations of the correct model. Masland and Case (1965) describe children's difficulties with the patterning of phonemic detail. Conceptual deficits and, in particular, difficulties with time and space concepts are pervasive and intimately related to symbolic deficits.

In these children primitiveness and instability are not confined to verbal experiences; they are evident also in immature postural reflexes, global and undifferentiated motility, awkward fine motor control, fragmented human figure drawings, fluid Bender gestalten. The children have difficulties on all levels of organization, perceptuomotor and linguistic; in fact, they have trouble organizing and extracting meaning both from their external and internal worlds. As a result, they look, and often are, disoriented. This disorientation has an organic flavor; it differs from that of the psychotic youngster and appears to be part of the aphasoid child's specific constellation of dysfunctions.

These dysfunctions (we avoid the term minimal brain injury since it constitutes an inferential diagnosis for which criteria vary from one clinical setting to another) may be related to encephalopathies, though there is as yet no way to correlate behavioral signs with specific neurological disease entities (Birch 1964). These dysfunctions may rest on a familial basis as hypothesized by Orton (1937), who felt that word deafness and a tendency to motor awkwardness are prevalent in certain families. Finally, they may reflect a massive maturational lag which has interfered with the early establishment of basic sensory motor schemata. That such a tendency to maturational lags may be genetically determined was postulated by Zangwill (1960).

Regardless of etiology, however, severe difficulties with expression and communication interfere with developing ego functions of mastery, impulse control, and ability to postpone gratifications. The child who lacks verbal tools, who cannot discharge tension and anxiety by way of words, who cannot verbalize anger and aggression is forced to resort to action and remains tied to more archaic forms of coping. Emotional disturbance may be but one aspect of lack of neurological integrity; it is well known that "organic" children are profoundly anxious (Greenacre 1963). Kurlander and Colodny (1965) speak of "primary" anxiety. Ego development is dependent on intactness of the central nervous system and any organic insult is bound to interfere with the epigenesis of the ego. The degree of disturbance varies not only with the pervasiveness and severity of the underlying condition, but also with the ability of the environment to support and tolerate this kind of child whose difficulties with control are severe and whose infantile and dependency needs are far greater than those of others. If one considers further that the speech-deprived child often fails to call forth communicative responses in the mother, it is not surprising to find that even under relatively favorable conditions a measure of emotional disturbance is the rule rather than the exception.

Some of the features which characterize aphasoid children—perceptuomotor instability, figure-ground difficulties, and profound auditory inattention—are found also in a large number of schizophrenic youngsters. Their plastic motility, their tendency to melt into the background, their fluid perceptions, and the primitiveness of their organizational schemes all reflect immature central nervous system patterning. Silver (1950) felt that plasticity is an attribute of the immature gestalt. Bender (1953) discussed the persistence of primitive neural patterning in schizophrenic children; she conceived of childhood schizophrenia as a maturational lag on the embryonic level of development.

In aphasoid children instability and fluidity are confined to the perceptuomotor and linguistic realm; in schizophrenic children, this fluidity is pervasive and involves ego boundaries and the totality of the personality organization. The resulting radically different orientation to the world entails a fundamentally altered attitude toward the language function. Since in schizophrenic youngsters the boundaries between self and nonself are blurred, since there is little distance between the one who sends the message and the one who receives it, dialogue becomes precarious or impossible.

When one explores the various aspects of receptive and expressive language in the aphasoid and the schizophrenic groups, one finds both similarities and differences. However, even when the symptomatology is similar, underlying dynamics may vary.

Investigating the receptive language of schizophrenics is, of course, no easy task. These children are hard to reach and they are sometimes more responsive to stimuli from within than from outside the organism, to wit, their occasional auditory hallucinations.

Both aphasoid and schizophrenic youngsters present limitations in comprehension of visual and auditory events. The failure of both psychotic and brain-injured children to make appropriate selection among stimuli from the environment has been discussed by Farnham-Diggory (1966). Aphasoid children, as a result of their symbolic deficits, have specific difficulties with the interpretation of spoken and printed language. In schizophrenic children as described by Goldfarb (1961), the avoidance of selected auditory and visual input signals must be interpreted in psychodynamic terms.

Hoberman and Goldfarb (1963) demonstrated that schizophrenic youngsters' auditory thresholds for speech, that is to say, for meaningful material, are higher than for pure tones, probably because their experiences are so fragmented that they cannot integrate meaningful information into an already existing framework. In aphasoid children similar high speech thresholds are due to their difficulties with the decoding machinery.

The auditory memory span of aphasoid youngsters is usually extremely short, in striking contrast to that of schizophrenic children whose memory for meaningless material may be excellent and who, for instance, are able to reproduce long TV commercials. In fact, some schizophrenic children, in contrast to aphasic ones, may unexpectedly and spontaneously produce words and sentences of a highly complex structure, testifying to their good auditory memory span and their ability to incorporate sophisticated linguistic rules.

Feedback is distorted in both groups. Feedback in the very young organism, as shown by Wyatt (1958), is provided by the mother who playfully throws back the child's own sounds to him, elaborates on them, and clarifies them. It is only at a later stage that feedback becomes internalized. The schizophrenic child who is unseparated from the mother, or the one who is unable to "tune in," cannot use the mother as a model. The aphasoid youngster, on the other hand, may get the feeling tone of the message, but cannot use the mother as a model because his reception is diffuse and his ability to process and to organize auditory sequences is inferior.

The bizarre and idiosyncratic character of schizophrenic children's expressive language is usually unmistakable. There are at least three striking features in the communication of psychotic children.

The first is the often total absence of communicative intent. Communication requires a complicity (de Ajurriaguerra 1963), as it were, between partners, and schizophrenic children are not in on this arrangement. Their inability to establish stable object relationships is reflected in the absence of communicative intent. In these children, language is not consensually validated, to use Sullivan's (1959) expression; it is not an instrument of interpersonal behavior. Lack of communicative intent can be observed in their impoverished and sometimes wholly inappropriate gestures which do not, as gestures frequently do in aphasoid children, serve to reinforce communication. Verbal output is often severely limited. However, even when the quantity of verbalization is adequate or abundant, the wish or the ability to relate may be absent. The echolalic speech of schizophrenic children with its mechanical, high-pitched, birdlike quality carries a feeling entirely different from that of the occasional echolalic utterances of children with severe and specific language deficits. The aphasoid children may repeat words or phrases for purposes of clarification; they may try words out for size, as it were. Although their voice quality may be somewhat monotonous and muffled, their pitch and inflection (which carry the emotional as against the conceptual load of communication) are largely normal. Goldfarb (1961) described the deviations in pitch, stress, and inflection of schizophrenic youngsters, their sometimes stilted and manneristic way of speaking, and the flat voice quality which reflects flatness of affect.

The second typical feature was described by Schilder (1942). He has pointed out that in schizophrenic language words are no longer referents, but are treated as if they were the things themselves. Words lose their symbolic status; they become concrete entities and as such acquire magic powers. Werner and Kaplan (1963) refer to the "thing-like" handling of linguistic forms. Since in schizophrenia speech is not an instrument of communication, specific words may be heavily emotionally invested, played with, juggled, telescoped, even truncated. As happens in dreams, words undergo condensation, a single word may represent a whole train of thought, sentences flow into each other, there is interpenetration of connotations, syntactical rules are disregarded. In a brilliant chapter, Werner and Kaplan discuss in detail what happens to morphophonological and lexical rules in the language of schizophrenics. Aphasoid children also show severe syntactical deficits. Masland and Case (1965) postulate that their inability to remember sequences interferes with the internalizing of syntactical rules. On the other hand aphasic speech, unlike schizophrenic language, does not show the looseness of associations and the kind of verbalizations which are only tangentially related to what is going on.

Language, with its potential for conceptualization, is normally, of course, a superb tool of the secondary process. Anna Freud (1965) says "verbalization is...the indispensable prerequisite for secondary process thinking." Freud (1957) has demonstrated that schizophrenic communication, and this is a third characteristic feature, is subject to "primary process distortion." Instead of being at the service of the ego, schizophrenic language is tied to early instinctual processes (Laffal 1965). One schizophrenic youngster who came for help with his reading told me, "There is no point in learning to read the letter *k*, it is not nice, it has too many spikes!" For this boy, letters like words, had no conventional objective significance; they did not serve reality or conscious purposes, but instead were experienced in terms of primary processes. In this case, *k* symbolized the child's archaic fears of aggression and retaliation. The fact that symbols are heavily invested with highly personalized meanings probably accounts for the fact that much of schizophrenic language is poorly conceptualized.

Concluding Remarks

The clinician who attempts to make a differential diagnosis between aphasoid and schizophrenic language finds that the two have many features in common: high auditory thresholds for speech, inferior auditory discrimination, feedback distortions, echolalia, limitations in verbal output, and conceptual deficits. Unlike schizophrenic youngsters, aphasic children have short auditory memory spans and they do not present the deviations in pitch, stress and inflection, the manneristic style, and the idiosyncratic use of words which are characteristic of those communicative disturbances that are clearly related to psychopathology.

Clinically, one finds innumerable admixtures along the communicative continuum discussed earlier. A great many youngsters are damaged on both the physiological and the psychological levels of integration. Classifying all language deficits as related either to organicity or to psychosis does not do justice to the complexity of the clinical phenomena. Many psychotic children present significant neurological dysfunctions, and a number of organic youngsters exhibit signs of withdrawal and are only tenuously related to the world around them.

As Rappaport (1961) pointed out, organic dysfunctions and psychological disturbances may use identical mechanisms. Both involve ego functions and, thus, language.

In every case, therefore, the clinician has to evaluate neurophysiological, linguistic, and affective aspects of communication and the often enormously complex interaction between them. He must try, furthermore, to form an impression of the way the child deals with the original insult, be it psychological or physiological, and the effectiveness of the defenses he uses in order to cope. Defensive mechanisms in the two groups, however, may show certain superficial similarities and are thus not necessarily helpful in differential diagnosis. We find obsessive defenses not only in the primarily disturbed where they serve against the onslaught of internal threats from the unconscious, but we also observe obsession-like defenses in organic children. In the latter, such behavior may be used as a defense against severe difficulties with control and a tendency to primary disorganization.

The way a child copes with his handicap depends, of course, largely on the manner in which significant people in his environment respond to his deficit. At tentative assessment of the contribution of the environment is, therefore, an additional task of the clinician.

In many cases only intensive work with the child will shed light on the nature of his deficit. No single aspect of it can be evaluated in isolation; every language dysfunction has to be viewed in terms of the organism as a whole.

Stuttering and Cluttering:
Developmental Aspects of Dysrhythmic Speech

Stuttering has been a subject of speculation for nearly 2,000 years. A few centuries ago, the cutting of the frenum was considered the best cure for the disorder, and it appears to have helped in many cases. In the early 1900s, the German school of Gutzman (1898) and Kussmaul (1910) advised the training of the muscles of the peripheral speech mechanism, so as to achieve better coordination. These two therapies rested, of course, on different hypotheses as to the etiology of stuttering.

Currently prevailing theories can be classified into three groups.

(1) Genogenic theories maintain that the stutterer is biologically different from the nonstutterer (Wepman 1939).

(2) Psychogenic theories conceive of stuttering as a psycho-neurosis, characterized by obsessive compulsive mechanisms; psychoanalytic concepts which stress oral-aggressive and anal-sadistic features belong here (Coriat 1927).

(3) Semantogenic theories postulate that stuttering is learned behavior—a response to the mislabeling on the part of the environment of the early normal syllable and word repetitions as "stuttering." These theories are represented by Johnson (1942) and his pupils.

It would seem that most workers, even those who distinguish between primary and secondary stuttering, consider the symptom to be a single diagnostic entity. On the other hand, it seems legitimate to ask a number of questions:

(1) Are all disruptions in the rhythmic flow of speech to be viewed as stuttering?

Reprinted with permission from Grune and Stratton, from *The Journal of Special Education* 3:143–152. 1969.

(2) Are some disturbances in the rhythmic flow of speech related to other dysfunctions in the language area?

(3) Do these disturbances signify something fundamentally different at different age levels?

(4) Is it possible to judge from the symptom alone whether one is confronted with an expression of a severe psychoneurosis or with a specific language disorder?

(5) Should therapy differ according to the outstanding etiological factor, and should it differ with the age of the patient?

The conceptual framework I am suggesting is heavily influenced by the theoretical position of Wyatt (1958b), although it differs from it in some respects, above all in its greater emphasis on neurophysiological factors. Wyatt emphasizes for stuttering, as does Lenneberg (1968) for central nervous system disease, that symptoms have different meanings at different ages and that there are critical periods when the organism is particularly vulnerable to developmental disturbances.

The focus of this paper will be on the development of stuttering in the young child, since it is in the early stages of the difficulty, before the picture has been obscured by elaborate defense mechanisms, that the symptom is best investigated.

There are three main elements which seem to be of outstanding significance in what, in other disease entities, is called the "spectrum of causation."

First, there is language itself: its phonological, semantic, and syntactical structure, its developmental course from primitive to increasingly differentiated organizations. There is, in the second place, the child with his constitutional language endowment, his inherent weaknesses and strengths, and his resistance and vulnerability to stress, both neurophysiological and emotional. There is, finally, the climate in which the child acquires language, the learning situation, in the social and psychodynamic sense. All three aspects will have to be considered in the evolution of the stuttering symptom.

Language learning in early childhood passes through a series of interrelated stages. Development, according to Werner and Kaplan (1966), "entailed not merely change or numerical increase in complexity, but the emergence of new forms of organizations, novel structures, and modes of operation of a kind eventuating in increased differentiation, increased subordination of parts to wholes and means to ends, increased stability and flexibility of systematic functioning." This is especially true in language development.

The first hurdle in language learning, and we know remarkably little about exactly what happens at this crucial time, is the transition from nonsymbolic verbalizations to symbolic speech (words).

Around the age of eighteen months, the child meets the second big hurdle in language development, the transition from nonrelational to relational speech, from one- and two-word phrases to hierarchically ordered utterances. This is a formidable task, fraught with hazards. The generating of new linguistic structures, the learning of innumerable transformations, the acquisition of thousands of shades of meaning, all place an enormous burden on the child's as yet immature organism. The shift from a relatively primitive to a highly differentiated mode of expression (largely completed by the age of four or five) often produces a crisis in language development. The changeover from utterances such as "baby, cry, eat" to saying, "The baby cries because he is hungry and wants to eat," represents an enormous conceptual and syntactical achievement.

The vocalizations of infants are characterized by a basic pattern of repetition. Babbling, the baby's vocal play when he first experiments with sounds and gains valuable auditory and kinesthetic experience as well as essential oral gratification, is basically repetitive. Repetition of sounds, syllables, and words when the child begins to use symbolic speech are the rule not the exception, as testified to by Johnson (1942). Fischer (1932) and Davis (1939) found that one out of every four words of the entire verbal output of children between two and four years of age is repeated in one form or another. These repetitions consist of fairly easy, effortless clonic iterations of sounds and words executed at normal speed at an age when the organism is still immature neurophysiologically, and at a time when the child's emotional and intellectual drive to express himself far outstrips his ability to generate complex linguistic structures. These iterations (Johnson called them "primary stuttering") should not be classified as stuttering at all. They should be differentiated from compulsive repetitions, which are by no means effortless and which are characterized by phobic fears and anxiety.

Wyatt and Herzan (1962) stated that phobic, tense repetitions, occasionally found in young children, result primarily from separation anxiety. The threat of losing or the actual loss of the love object during a time when the child is battling with an expanding vocabulary and complex linguistic forms results in a two-fold crisis: an interpersonal crisis because the child is still heavily dependent on maternal support, and a linguistic one inherent in this particular stage of language development. Under this double load, the easy iterations may tend to change. As the child attempts to enunciate a difficult word, struggles with a new syntactical construction, tries to express a complex thought, vies for his mother's attention, or tries to keep up with the rapid speech of an older sibling, he gets into a jam and his original iterations begin to change. *Ba-ba* is no longer produced in normal tempo; the lips are pressed together a little longer in the production of the *b* and delay results. Froeschels (1942–43), who described the

symptomatology of stuttering over fifty years ago, called these manifestations, which already contain a slight component, "clono-toni."
Then follow efforts to overcome the first slight blocks, resulting in
more tonus and finally in pure toni. These engender fears of the
speaking situation and lead to involvement of the breathing apparatus,
avoidance strategies, and the many other symptoms which characterize severe stuttering. The result is a youngster who is involved in a
despairing fight with words, a full-blown stutterer.

It is important to remember that the elaboration of complex syntactical forms occurs at a critical time in the child's life when early
instinctual and oral gratifications are being withdrawn; when toilet
training is being enforced, and the youngster is engaged in the developmental struggles and conflicts of what analysts call the anal phase
of psychosexual development; when his aggressive and negativistic
impulses are frowned upon and he is expected to pattern his responses
in a way which makes him a responsible member of the family group;
and when, often, he is presented with a younger brother or sister
(de Hirsch and Langford 1950).

The mother is, of course, the primary love object and also the
child's language model. Wyatt (1965) said that language is fostered by a
process of reciprocal identification between mother and child. From an
early age, the nurturing figure feeds the baby sounds and words much
as she feeds him food. Thus, a disruption of the mother-child bond
results in a severe trauma, no matter whether the disruption is the
result of physical separation or of psychological withdrawal on the part
of the mother (e.g., if she is depressed or preoccupied with a younger
child). While the disruption of the mother-child bond probably represents the most important single factor in terms of stress, any severe
anxiety or conflict, if it occurs at a period when language is not yet
safely established, will tend to disrupt a function which is, like all
biologically new functions, still highly vulnerable.

Since most children pass through the normal phases of sound and
word iteration and since all of them have to struggle with complex
linguistic forms, and all of them are exposed to the normal strains of
growing up, why do some become stutterers while others do not?

Let me offer some tentative answers: In the first place, children
vary enormously in their ability to withstand stress. Stress situations
are handled more easily by some than by others. In the second place,
stress varies in intensity from one situation to the next. There are
stresses that are so severe that they cannot be integrated, even by a
robust psychological apparatus. In the third place, some children's
linguistic and neurophysiological organizations are more resistant to
assaults than are those of others. There are some youngsters who,
perhaps on a genetic basis, may have a predisposition to vulnerability

in the language area. Their speech tends to break under a relatively light load.

Such children are often very late in starting to talk. Masland and Case (1965), better than anyone else, have described the dysfunctions of these children in both the receptive and expressive aspects of language: They have strikingly short auditory memory spans and severe difficulties with auditory discrimination. Their indistinct speech output mirrors their diffuse intake. It is characterized by a disregard of phonemic detail, telescoping of words, omissions and substitutions, severe word-finding difficulties, rudimentary syntactical constructions, a tendency to reverse the order of sounds in words and of words in sentences, and an inability to generate the linguistic transformations expected at their age.

Masland and Case (1965) also discussed the deviations in stress and inflection which are typical of the speech of these children. Since their overall language development is delayed, they iterate sounds and words at a somewhat later age than is usual, at first no more frequently than do other children; but, as pressure for verbal communication mounts, and as their ability to integrate perceptuomotor and linguistic schemata lags further behind their often complex ideas, their iterations become more numerous and even minor tensions and conflicts transferred from other spheres of life may become fixed to the already-frustrating speaking situation. In these children, the contribution of psychological conflicts need not be great; minor ones will suffice to bring on an increase in clono-toni and even occasional speaking blocks. Not all of these children develop into stutterers; most of them "grow out of it," which means that with increasing neurophysiological maturation and the development of adequate defenses they learn, up to a point, to cope with the linguistic load. A tendency to verbal disorganization may, however, persist into adulthood (de Hirsch and Langford 1950).

The speech of these children closely resembles what is called cluttering and occurs at all ages. First described by Freund (1934) and Weiss (1935), cluttering is basically a disassociation between thinking and speaking. The cluttering child or adult has an enormous drive to talk, but somehow gets lost in the middle of his sentences. He seems unable to plan ahead; he cannot form anticipatory schemata of what the sentence is going to say (de Hirsch 1963). Weiss (1967) described it as a kind of idling in the speech motor, a blanking out. Clutterers use "fillers" because they are undecided as to the appropriate grammatical construction that should follow. Such individuals seem to lack clear-cut word images and they mostly have severe word-finding difficulties. The tempo of their speech is speeded up by quickly racing thoughts; their sequencing is faulty; their speech is marked by transpositions of syllables or words, iterations of sounds and phrases. Articulation is undifferentiated. While individual sounds are usually correct in isolation or in small units, articulation breaks down when the organizational load becomes too heavy. Organizational weakness in all areas is an outstanding feature in these children. Paralinguistic dysfunctions, above all monotony, are frequent; disturbances of attention are very much in the foreground.

Clutterers have short auditory memory spans and diffuse auditory discrimination; many are tone-deaf and lack a sense of rhythm. Feedback mechanisms seem to be faulty. In contrast to stutterers, however, they have little awareness of their difficulty; there are no phobic signs and there is a striking absence of anxiety.

Difficulties are not, however, confined to the verbal area. If one listens to the jerky, dysrhythmic speech of clutterers and then looks at their jerky, dysrhythmic handwriting, one will find that that papers such individuals write look exactly the way they sound (de Hirsch 1961c). The same basic disturbance in patterning seems to be operating on various levels of integration. Both motor and verbal gestalten lack sharp contours; intake and output are diffuse and unstable. One sees it in the fluidity of the children's copies of the Bender gestalten, as well as in their highly erratic spelling. Word configurations seem to shift; the spelling of a word may be remembered on a spelling list, for instance, and lost when it is embedded in context. Clutterers and individuals with spelling disabilities (and they mostly go together) are unable to maintain a linguistic configuration (French 1953).

Bender (1966) says that instability is the characteristic feature of the immature gestalt. In cluttering individuals immaturity is not confined to the verbal realm. One finds primitive motility patterning, poorly differentiated fine motor coordination, and delay in development of body image. Zangwill (1962) believes that immaturity of central nervous system patterning may be genetically determined, and it is true that cluttering, in combination with other language dysfunctions, such as reading and spelling disorders, is frequently seen in members of the same family.

Children with cluttering-like speech do not have to turn into stutterers but they sometimes do. Their disorganized and immature linguistic organization forms the basis on which the phenomenon of stuttering may be superimposed, as a result of emotional stress and conflict.

This kind of hypothesis would answer two questions which have plagued researchers in the field of stuttering for some time: (1) Is stuttering inherited, since in so many cases several members of a family are afflicted? Stuttering is *not* inherited, but a tendency to a labile language organization might be. (2) Why do we find so many more boys than girls who stutter? The answer to this may lie in the greater physiological immaturity of boys, as compared to girls, which has been well documented by Tanner (1961) and Bentzen (1963). The greater immaturity and instability of central nervous system patterning and the resulting tendency to linguistic disorganization would account for the fact that there are many more stutterers and reading disability cases among boys than among girls.

Not all stuttering is based on cluttering. The child who has spoken clearly and smoothly for years, who shows no other signs of disturbance in printed or written language, but who suddenly starts stuttering, belongs in a different category. Stuttering in such cases reflects not a linguistic but a psychiatric disturbance and has to be treated as such.

Case Studies

In the following, two cases will be presented which illustrate some of the theoretical concepts discussed here:

Martin

Martin was first referred to us because of his unintelligible speech. Family history of language and handedness was positive. The mother had stuttered as a child and was a slow reader. Her brother, an architect, had always been an atrocious speller and read little. Her sister had been late in starting to talk. The mother said she herself was more or less ambidextrous; her older daughter was left-handed and this older child was later referred to us because of difficulties with reading. Martin's mother was Rh negative and he had required a transfusion at birth, having been jaundiced. He had always been a robust youngster and early developmental milestones, except for speech, had been passed at a normal rate.

When we saw the boy for the initial interview, he was three years and three months old, a charming, darkhaired fellow with sparkling brown eyes. He had no trouble separating from his mother, which was good for his age. He was anxious to bat, although he was not particularly skillful and proceeded to hit himself in the teeth. Nor was he dextrous stacking our wooden clowns; fine motor skills were poor. He preferred the use of the right hand, but there were also many left leads. Visuomotor organization was inadequate: instead of hammering the nails into their holes, he simply pounded them into the board, hitting his thumb. He could copy a circle, but not a cross, and he drew something which faintly resembled a human figure.

Auditory memory span was three nonsense syllables. Understanding of language was adequate; Martin roared when he was asked if a dog can fly, and he was quick to see a joke. There were many articulatory difficulties: "hoo ah veh" meant his "shoe is all wet." Units were short and he had, even for this age, enormous difficulties with word-finding; when presented with the picture of a stove, he called it "mummy cook." He showed some easy clonic word and syllable iterations, but they were not dramatic. His language tools were undoubtedly very poor, but he was so vital a boy and so bright, that we thought we should give maturation a chance. His mother wrote us during the summer that Martin's iterations had disappeared and that articulation was less and less of a problem. However, ten months after the initial interview she called us again because Martin was stuttering severely.

When we saw him on this second occasion we were again impressed with his vitality. His specific difficulties were, however, much more striking because he was older. Auditory discrimination deficits were far more noticeable; he confused words such as *Fred* and *thread*. Articulation had greatly improved, and his remaining errors no longer interfered with intelligibility. His naming difficulties continued to be striking; he had a terrible time trying to formulate his ideas and relied heavily on gestures. As he began to deal with more abstract material such as *magic* or *God*, his problems increased.

His stuttering was moderately severe. There was, for the first time, tension in the peripheral speech mechanism, some accompanying facial grimacing, and a tendency for the breathing apparatus to become involved. His stories suggested a heavy tie to the mother and the ambivalent relation to the father typical of this age. The stresses and strains of this developmental phase, which is characterized by severe feelings of rivalry with the father, were complicated by the boy's linguistic frustrations. This was a youngster who had many ideas and whose conceptual development was advanced, but who was entirely unable to express himself. As a result, he felt weak, impotent, and unable to cope.

We took the boy on for therapy and worked with him twice weekly for about fourteen months. At first, verbalizations were kept to a minimum. Martin played a great deal with a sword and with a large ball or (his own idea) he sat in a house he had built himself out of cardboard bricks. The therapist fed him candy from a spoon through an opening in the wall. Thus, he was allowed to go back to a more infantile level of functioning, sitting in an enclosed safe place, being fed. No interpretation whatsoever was attempted. Slowly there was some give-and-take in terms of words and phrases. The therapist echoed Martin's verbalizations, slowing down the rate and shortening the units. It all seemed immensely reassuring to the child, and in about eleven weeks the speech blocks were greatly reduced in number at home and were almost absent at the office.

Very slowly we started working on Martin's poor linguistic tools, helping him with his word-finding difficulties above all. Attempts to teach him to formulate his thoughts were postponed until he felt comfortable about his speech; after a few months this became the core of the program. Graphomotor activities were stressed and this proved to be a difficult area for Martin; he was afraid to try. His father was a painter and the association father-powerful-owner of mother-wonderful with the pencil and Martin-small-powerless-unable to wield his magic instrument was hard to overcome.

After fourteen months of treatment, Martin's language tools were by no means impressive and his fine motor coordination still was poor, but there were no more signs of stuttering and he was better able to express his feelings and ideas. We told his mother to watch his reading, and he did at first have some difficulties. He still is, and probably always will be, a poor speller.

Nancy

Nancy was referred to us by her pediatrician because of severe stuttering. She was introduced formally by her mother as "Miss Nancy." She was a dainty, somewhat solemn little thing, quite feminine, and very, very bright. She brought in a china cat, to whom she referred as "Mr Big." She asked her mother to come along to the playroom, but could easily be persuaded to settle for the door to the waiting room being left open. Nancy then sat herself down in front of the doll house, first putting Mr. Big to bed. This served as an excellent pretext for whispering, rather than talking in a normal voice, while she played with the dolls. "One mustn't wake up Mr. Big." Nancy said.

The child seemed quite ritualistic and she spent a lot of time simply putting the dolls in and out of bed. There wasn't much fun in her play, it was so repetitive. When she was persuaded to come to the bathroom and play with water (which she was quite hesitant to do) she simply filled the container and emptied it over and over again. Playing with water clearly made her a little nervous because it was messy. She was distressingly clean. She was offered a baby bottle to play with, but felt uncomfortable with it. Once or twice eye blinking was observed.

Nancy stuttered most of the time, showing moderate to severe tonus, more so when her mother was present, less so when whispering. The symptom itself consisted of frequent toni, prolongations of initial sounds, and some complete blocks. She was highly articulate, using complex grammatical constructions, and she had an enormous vocabulary. There was little spontaneity, however, little room for imagination, and much stylized behavior.

The interview with Nancy's mother confirmed the impression gained from observing the child. Family history of language was negative. Nancy was an only child, born by Caesarean section. Because of her father's job, she had been subjected to an unusual number of environmental changes. For the first two years of life, she had been cared for by a pleasant housekeeper, who accompanied the family. The mother said Nancy had started to "converse," as she put it, at age two. She must have been extremely cautious and perfectionistic at a very early age; she used to practice words in her bed before using them in conversation.

When Nancy was two years old, a temporary nurse took over. Following this, the family had a maid who came in by the day and of whom Nancy became very fond. When she was three, another nurse came to live with the family and, according to the mother, things went along fine.

The summer before Nancy was referred to us, she and her parents had lived in New York City in a furnished apartment for three months, with Nancy's original nurse in charge. It was at that time that the pediatrician discovered that she was underweight and suffering from a celiac condition. He put her on a very strict diet. Shortly afterwards, when the parents and Nancy moved to their own apartment, her beloved nurse left for good. Nancy was told of her leaving three days before it happened, and it was at that time that speech hesitations were first noticed.

A new nurse, who had since been dismissed, had changed all of the child's routines and had become upset when the little girl occasionally touched herself in the genital region; she had slapped Nancy's hand and used words such as "dirty." Stuttering dramatically increased and Nancy became so afraid to speak that she would whisper and cover her mouth while talking.

Lately she had become difficult at night, saying a dozen times in an hour that she had to go to the bathroom and carrying on to such a degree that the mother for the first time spanked her energetically, with the result that Nancy's speech, which had improved a little after the nurse's dismissal, deteriorated again. The mother said that Nancy had always had an imaginary companion, but that Mr. Big was much more in evidence than he had ever been before.

The mother sounded both upset and guilty. She seemed to be a very perfectionistic person, who intellectualized a great deal. Being afraid of primitive and instinctual gratifications herself, she probably did little to support the need for them in her child. Unexpressed pressures for grown-up behavior seemed heavy, but the mother seemed unaware of them.

Nancy appeared to be well on the way to a severe obsessive-compulsive system; she needed help as soon as possible, and it seemed essential that the mother be included in therapy. Consequently, Nancy was referred to a child psychiatrist who did beautifully with both mother and child. When I saw Nancy once more, a little over a year later, there was no trace of stuttering. Nancy was far less well-behaved, less clean, much freer, and more able to reach her basic productive potential. The mother told me that she herself still was a meticulous housekeeper, but that she was now able to get some fun out of Nancy, even if the child functioned at a more instinctual level.

Considerations for therapy

Both Nancy and Martin had done well with entirely different approaches based on different etiologies. The report on Martin's treatment illustrates our therapeutic approach. We feel, as does Wyatt (1965), that stuttering therapy should be initiated as soon as possible after the appearance of the first compulsive repetitions. Early intervention is imperative because the symptom itself arouses so much anxiety in both the parents and the child that it tends to be self-perpetuating. In occasional cases, a series of sessions between the mother and a psychiatric social worker will suffice to resolve an acute conflict, thus preventing the setting in motion of complex psychological feedback mechanisms.

Regression is the goal of therapy with the child himself. The aim is to reintegrate the child on a less complex linguistic level. Wyatt (Wyatt and Herzan, 1962) attempts to return the child to a state before the mother-child disruption took place. Our rationale for the same therapeutic approach is a different one. We feel that by infantilizing the youngster (by giving him added oral gratification and closer body contact, and by temporarily reducing the demands for grown-up behavior), we establish him on a more primitive level of verbal communication, thus lightening both the emotional and the linguistic burden. In the framework of a less intellectually demanding, more infantile relationship, there is room for nursery rhymes, for singing, for play with sounds, for word-matching games. In this verbal back-and-forth between therapist and child, sentences and phrases become shorter, dependent clauses drop out, conceptualizations are reduced; in other words, for a period of time, the child gives up the struggle with complex linguistic organizations for which he is not ready.

At the same time, the permission to behave in a more infantile manner makes it easier for the child to resolve his conflicts centering around demands to give up early instinctual gratifications and, in some cases, eases the competition with a younger sibling, who is granted more infantile pleasures. With adult support, the child weathers the twofold emotional and linguistic crisis and will be able, after a while, to move ahead to a more highly-integrated linguistic phase and to more grown-up gratifications. Conflicts belonging to a later developmental phase will rarely disrupt speech because by that time the child's neurophysiological maturation has reached a level which makes him more resistant to linguistic disorganization.

Those children whose inherent linguistic endowment is vulnerable, however, need help with the instrumentalities of language for a long time, since in their cases, stress and conflict will tend to be expressed in an area which is already shaky. In the absence of conflict, these youngsters' articulatory problems usually clear up, but their difficulties with word-finding, with organization of verbal output, and with formulation persist, and most of them wind up (as will Martin) as poor spellers.

Therapy for older stutterers presents different problems. In the severely phobic older stutterer, the symptom has usually become part of the individual's defensive system and is often inaccessible to non-psychiatric therapy. In those cases which present a large cluttering component, the prognosis for speech training is much better.

Conclusion

To answer the original questions: Not all disruptions in the rhythmic flow of speech should be labeled stuttering. Some dys-rhythmic manifestations belong in the category of cluttering and are related to other language dysfunctions. Careful observation of the individual, as well as of the symptom itself, provides clues for differential diagnosis.

Dysphasia—Autism

We are concerned here with a puzzling group of children who are sent to us between the ages of two and a half and five years because they present massive diagnostic and therapeutic problems with verbal communication. They are referred with a variety of labels: developmentally deviating, schizophrenic, word-deaf, autistic. Most of the parents have made the rounds from one evaluation center to the other and each resulting diagnosis reflects the examiner's experience and personal bias.

A Case Study

In this paper, I will discuss a little girl referred to us because she showed severe lags in language development. I would like to present her, not because we have a satisfactory name for her case but, on the contrary, because children like Claudia present deficits that defy any simple labels.

Claudia, the younger of two daughters, was four years and nine months old when I first saw her mother for an initial interview. Her father is of Argentine descent, rather a demanding individual, but, like most Latin men, deeply fond of his daughters. The mother grew up in this country; her parents had immigrated from Portugal. English only is spoken in the home. Except for Claudia's sister, who has trouble spelling, family history of language difficulties is negative, or so her mother told me. However, in a background such as Claudia's this kind of report is not necessarily reliable.

Both parents had wanted a second child badly; thus Claudia's arrival was a cause for rejoicing. The mother's legs had been quite swollen during pregnancy, which raises some questions about the possibility of toxemia, but she had not received medication. Delivery was at term and uncomplicated. Claudia was a big demanding baby

Reprinted with permission from The Orton Dyslexia Society, from *Annals of Dyslexia* 32:305–320. 1982.

from the start. She constantly clamored for food and needed a bottle in the middle of the night for several years. She had always been a somewhat hyperactive child. She walked without support at thirteen months and toilet training was completed without undue strain shortly before her third birthday. Speech was very slow to emerge. The child babbled to some extent, but questioning elicited that quantity was quite limited and sounds were at first poorly modulated. For the longest time she sounded as if she used some kind of "shadow" language. At two years four months Claudia named a few objects but she progressed little from then on.

It should be added that she was taken to Portugal for three weeks when she was fifteen months old. She returned there to stay nearly two months at the time of her grandfather's death when she was just over two years of age. Thus, at a time critical for language acquisition, this little girl was exposed to two different linguistic codes during an experience emotionally upsetting to her mother, and thus probably to her also.

I did my best to obtain some impression from the mother about the child's ability to process linguistic input without the assistance of visual, intonational and, above all, situational cues.

Comprehension is basic to language production; it appears early along the developmental continuum and is a prerequisite for language output. It was my impression from the mother's comments that the child presented significant gaps in comprehension. (A hearing loss had been ruled out. The audiograms showed some slight fluctuations; all, however, were within the normal range.)

Claudia, her mother says, was completely uninterested in having the simplest story read to her. Often the child was not receptive to verbal communication, but there were also times when the mother felt she did listen, but looked puzzled when one used longer and more complex linguistic constructions. The referential function of language was relatively intact; she used the names of a number of objects, but her output in general was severely impoverished; it consisted of stock phrases and some fragmented sentences. Her constructions were primitive and ungrammatical. I had the feeling that content above all was idiosyncratic and inappropriate.

Because the pediatrician continued to reassure this rather anxious mother, the child was not evaluated except for hearing, until she was nearly four years old. The neuropsychiatrist whom the parents then consulted made a diagnosis of developmental dysphasia, both receptive and expressive. He had no doubt as to the child's basically adequate intelligence; there was, apart from her speech, her entirely normal developmental history and she functioned adequately in many areas. In addition, she had scored in the average range on the performance section of the WPPSI, although there was of course considerable scatter. The neuropsychiatrist ascribed her often severe temper tantrums and her rigidity to her inferior verbal tools and felt they were also responsible for her occasional unavailability. Rather to my amazement, the child was not referred for either psychiatric or language therapy, although she was getting close to the end of the critical phase for language acquisition when early intervention, because of the greater plasticity of the brain, has a far better chance for success than later.

The parents made strenuous efforts at home to "teach" Claudia how to speak, efforts that may well have been counterproductive. At best, there were many tensions between mother and child and withholding speech provided a convenient mechanism for Claudia to express hostility. (Withholding, incidentally, was not the primary cause of the child's speech delay. Contrary to popular opinion, it rarely is.)

The mother described Claudia as rather a competent child. She dressed herself in the morning and made her own bed. There were several aspects of the history that gave me pause, although the mother did not seem to understand their significance. There was the report of frequent and, apparently completely unprovoked, explosive outbursts that seemed to reflect some inner disorganization. She had no appreciation of danger. The mother said that Claudia liked people, but it turned out that her relationships were entirely undiscriminating. She was apt to attach herself to any adult who took her fancy, even to complete strangers. I found it fascinating that up to a short while ago she had three different security blankets which she used interchangeably. (A security blanket is a substitute for mother and represents her warmth and protection—one would therefore expect that only one blanket would meet this need.) At times, the mother said, she produced some "strange" verbalizations but she glided over this comment quickly.

The regular nursery school found Claudia to be a very strange little girl. She easily separated from her mother, but she did not become attached to any teacher, she did not participate in the activities of the group, she did not form any relationship with other children. She made little or no efforts at communication. It was the teacher who insisted that Claudia be seen by the psychiatrist, who in turn sent her to us.

I spent considerable time setting up a language stimulation program for the parents to carry out at home, one that eliminated all pressure to speak and was heavily affectively loaded in that it was built around strongly emotionally-invested situations. Comprehension of language, rather than output, was stressed. Articulation was in no way emphasized. Short verbalizations were integrated into a variety of pleasurable situations, and the child's verbal output was to be taken up, expanded, and organized for her. Because her mother had told me that until Claudia was over three years old she had been unable to indicate which part of her body hurt when she was involved in some minor accident, I suggested a number of activities that served to make Claudia more familiar with her body and its parts.

It took about two months before Claudia could be seen at the office and, according to her mother, she had made progress since the language stimulation had been begun.

At the office, Claudia, by then a tall, pretty five-year-old with a rather undifferentiated face, had again no trouble with separation from her mother, but she seemed generally anxious, frantic is probably a better word. In the playroom she was moderately hyperactive. She was not withdrawn, and she showed some interest in things around her. I strongly disagreed with the mother's statement that the child related well. To begin with, she seemed totally disoriented, paying as much attention to the people on the periphery as to those working with her. When my husband entered the waiting room (there was a closed door between him and Claudia) she confused him with the person in the story that Dr. Jansky was trying to tell her.

Her doll play was very little elaborated for a child nearly five years old, her handling of toys quite unimaginative, and there was little or no sign of fantasy play. She did pretend; that is, she filled the car with sand and once she poured juice for her doll, but she never developed a theme. Her symbolic use of play material was very limited. She tuned out occasionally. Her drawing of the human body was not cohesive, but although it was quite primitive, it was not bizarre.

There was no doubt that there were severe gaps in Claudia's comprehension of speech. Her score on the Northwestern Syntax Screening Test (Lee 1969) would have been very low even for a three-year-old. She did not comprehend the story we usually tell our four-year-olds. Asked who sent the little red bike (it was the child's birthday and the bicycle was a present from her grandmother) she said "the man," meaning the postman who delivered it. As to expressive language, her articulation was not bad, speech melody was excellent, there was nothing in her utterances of the mechanical quality one so often hears in autistic children's speech. Her ability to name pictures shown to her was on the level of a not-yet four-year-old. Claudia's syntax fluctuated markedly. She sometimes reversed the order of words and phrases but one very soon heard a few rather well con-structed short sentences. She had trouble with tenses though. Despite her confusion about where people belonged and who they were, she hardly ever confused pronouns.

The content of Claudia's speech showed some echoing with a slightly questioning intonation as if she were trying to figure some-thing out. Claudia did have an ear for the idiom and would say, "Hey, cut it out," a stock phrase, but used appropriately. However, there were also utterances which made no sense at all. When asked what

Curious George was looking at, Claudia replied, "Years and garage." She smiled a little as she said it, but she was not really kidding and she continued, "Looks like a week." Asked again, this was sometime later, she said, quite surprisingly, "Unbelievable means incredible", highly abstract words. As she was playing with Mr. Potato Head, she sang a song about him over and over again, "Mr. Potato Head I love you;" she had heard it on TV. Other associations followed and one felt she was not overly eager to modify her speech in order to communicate the content to someone else. There was no doubt that this child lived in a disorganized chaotic world. One was tempted at times to look at her strange verbalizations as a defense designed to contain, yet keep at a distance, the overwhelming multiplicity of confusing stimuli with which she was unable to cope. Clinically, I got the impression of an angry child, but she clearly was at her worst in unfamiliar situations and we assumed that she functioned better in the home environment.

I saw the parents for one more interview to discuss the findings. The father wanted a label which I was, unfortunately, unable to provide. I communicated to the parents our impression that Claudia's lack of boundaries, her fluidity, seemed to make it difficult for her to retain the internal representation of different experiences, linguistic and affective. We agreed that she was basically a strong person and I agreed when the analyst suggested trying medication. She was put on Ritalin in the hope that it would help her organize herself and her world. However, medication was dropped because it was ineffective.

It was of interest that the father said Claudia did not relate much to him either, a statement which one had to accept with some reservation. Claudia may well have been angry because he adored her older sister. However that may be, the child's relationships were at best tenuous.

We felt that her present situation was too unstructured and that the child was in no way ready for kindergarten. A therapeutic nursery school appeared to be desirable and we felt she needed fairly intensive intervention.

In the fall of 1976 Claudia was placed in a therapeutic environment and she began to work twice weekly with Mrs. Howell, one of the therapists in our office. The first interoffice memo written by her after about eight weeks of tutoring read, "Hyperactivity persists, bizarre verbal responses are still in evidence." Mrs. Howell wondered whether they constituted a defense against communication. I felt that some of it sounded like an attempt to mask her massive gaps in understanding. Her receptive difficulties were glaring. At first she vehemently resisted listening to the simplest story even if the therapist acted it out for her prior to reading it. At one point she tore up the book. After this outburst, things started to improve and Claudia began pretending to read a story to the therapist. By and by she became willing to listen a little and to look at the pictures. However, not only words appeared to confuse her, but the pictures in books as well. She managed, when she acted out the story while Mrs. Howell read it to her. At best she was capable of understanding a story appropriate for a three-year-old if one paraphrased it. Cinderella was way beyond her.

However, speech production improved rapidly and her linguistic constructions became a little longer and more complex. She began to use speech as a vehicle for combatting confusion. She was apt to mix up the story she had just listened to with the next one that was being read to her and would tell herself loudly, "This is a *different* story." Soon after the book-tearing incident a remarkable conversation took place. Claudia sat primly, her legs crossed, and asked politely if the therapist had any dogs and if they were healthy. This lead to the topic of death and Mrs. Howell remarked that Claudia's Portuguese grand-father had died when the child was little. She replied, "Yes, far away, how much do sick people cry when they are dying?" It occurred to me that what she meant to say was "How much do people cry when a relative dies?" But she lacked the cognitive and syntactical competence to express the distinction.

Claudia gradually enjoyed coming to the office. The school was pleased and reported that she showed a growing capacity to retain some inner image of people and situations. It was remarkable, on the other hand, that she showed so little affection for the therapist, and, as far as I could judge, hardly any for her mother.

The following example of Claudia's speech in January was given to me by Mrs. Howell. She had commented on Claudia's braids and Claudia replied, "Christina (her sister) wears braids."

Mrs. Howell: "Tell me about Christina, does Christina sleep in the same room?"

A: I sleep inside my room alone, but once my Daddy came up everytime because I made too much noise and then I was turning on the night light and then I was pulling my covers over my head and then Dad came in.

Q: Was he mad?

A: No, he isn't angry, he just tucked me in and I say I'm already tucked in.

This shows that by no means all of her verbalizations were bizarre—many were on an adequate reality level. When asked, "Do you know where you will go next week?" (a trip to Disneyland was planned), Claudia answered, "Do you remember you were absent last Christmas?" Perhaps the fact of absence was foremost in her mind.

One of the goals of therapy is the establishing of a temporal-spatial framework. Claudia had some vague idea as to the past but none of the future. Temporal concepts were precarious.

There were times when Claudia's behavior was unacceptable. She would mess up the doll house, kick the big blocks around, and as she became more comfortable in the office she showed more of her anger, which may have meant that she was in better contact with herself and others. She became very provocative, dumping the contents of the wastepaper basket all over the floor. I felt she was jealous of the child whose session followed hers. Some fantasizing became apparent for the first time. When Mrs. Howell patted her lightly on the back, because she had completed a difficult puzzle, Claudia said angrily, "Don't touch me, you are not supposed to touch me, to touch breasts. I know *w* is for wedding."

Mrs. Howell: Will you get married?

A: Yes, to Simon in my school.

Despite her progress and the considerable improvement in both the content and the formal aspects of her expressive speech, her associations remained confused. The name of the boy whose session followed hers was Mark. Claudia would say, "Mark is a birthday, March is a month, M is for mother, you know puppets, puppets are moppets, M is for Wedding" (she turned the M around to make a W). After doing something that was naughty during the session, Claudia was heard to say, "Oh, you drive me up the wall," echoing something her mother had said, as though she were speaking her mother's lines.

Before the summer holidays, Mrs. Howell made a great effort to get the concept of separation across to her, but I don't think that Claudia took it in. She was given a little pocketbook and she was told that she could come and visit anytime. She felt, nevertheless, that separation had to do with punishment. She said to the therapist, "What does your mother do when you are bad? Slap you on the hand or spank you? Does she say, 'I'm disappointed'?"

Lessons were discontinued in the fall because the logistics were too difficult for the mother. She wrote me a note to the effect that Claudia continued to improve. But we have not heard since. The father was sent to California and took his family with him.

Let us now look at this child's protocol to see if and how it fits into some of the prevailing theories. In a paper, published fifteen years ago (de Hirsch 1967), I attempted to establish criteria for a differential diagnosis of what I called then "aphasic" and "schizophrenic" language. Modifications in terminology reflect the changes that have occurred in our thinking since. Most researchers—and I agree— consider autism a form of psychosis, distinct from schizophrenia. In schizophrenia a structure that was established, however precarious, dissolves. In autism the structure was never formed to begin with.

In order to highlight what I assumed to be distinct categories of communicative failure, I had looked, in my previous paper, at "pure"

cases—those with severe deficits in decoding and encoding of language, relatively uncomplicated by psychic pathology on the one
hand, and those in which the deficit appeared to reflect a lack of
communicative intent related to a pathological orientation to the self,
the love object and the environment on the other. I continue to believe
that we occasionally do see "pure" cases. Both are organic etiologically
but I'm quite certain now that, among children, we find all kinds of
mixtures and that the pure cases are the exception rather than the rule.

Autism

Many American researchers stress the vicissitudes of language
and cognitive development in the diagnosis and prognosis of autism.
The English psychologist, Rutter, (1965) emphasizes the frequency of
low IQ in autistic children. He maintains that the linguistic disorder is
the primary feature in autism, and that what he calls "behavioral
symptoms" are secondary to the severe linguistic deficit. He admits
later however, (Rutter 1968) that autism differs from the condition
found in uncomplicated disorders of receptive language in that autistic
youngsters, for reasons that are still obscure, do not *use* language for
social give and take. Just the same, while a massive language difficulty
is the most striking aspect of the disorder and undoubtedly affects the
total personality, it does not necessarily follow, as Rutter claims, that
the linguistic deficit causes, for instance, the insufficient separation
between self and nonself in these children. Rutter (1978) modified his
opinion, and said that the presence or absence of nonverbal communicative difficulties differentiates the autistic from the purely language
disabled. But in the last instance, he looks at autism as a cognitive and
perceptual defect and does not take any affective features into account.
However, the fact that these affective deficiencies have an organically
determined origin makes them no less relevant.

Autistic children, (I speak of course of those whose IQ falls in the
average range) unlike dysphasic ones, do not often present fluctuating
audiograms; they are rarely tone-deaf. Their auditory memory span
seems to be much longer than that of dysphasics; autistic children are
liable to repeat extensive and complex utterances heard on TV which
may or may not be meaningful. In other words, autistics manage most
of the subskills underlying language performance.

Autistic children give one the impression, on the other hand, that
they are not *available* for communication. Some turn their heads away
when spoken to; they are unwilling partners in any dialogue. They
seem, moreover, to lack a feel for the social nuances of language; how
to begin a conversation, for instance, and how to differentiate between
the way one talks to an adult or to a three-year-old.

Dysphasia

With respect to dysphasia, I assume that most of you know the American literature. I refer only to Eisenson (1968), but it might be worthwhile to discuss some of the work done outside the English speaking world, in particular that of de Ajuriaguerra (1963) in Geneva. A brilliant clinician, de Ajuriaguerra, in a longitudinal study, followed seventeen children diagnosed by him as aphasic at the age of four and a half. They presented severe deficits in all aspects of language, phonological, morphological, syntactic, and semantic. Their outstanding difficulty was with language comprehension. None of these children had experienced either separation or prolonged illness. He retested them subsequently at the age of seven and again at twelve years seven months and he was primarily interested in the following categories:

1) the children's verbal communication
2) their intellectual and academic progress
3) their social and affect development (unlike many other researchers, he does not use the term "social competence," a far more limited superficial way of looking at a very complex phenomenon).

Dysphasic children have massive difficulties with verbal comprehension and production. They manifest disregard for morphological and syntactical rules. They present severe difficulties with word-finding, gross deficits in articulation, substitutions and omissions of sounds and parts of words, telescoping, and poorly patterned linguistic detail (Masland and Case 1965). In other words, fully half of de Ajuriaguerra's group showed relatively defective speech at older ages. In 50 percent of his sample, formulation of extended discourse remained poor. Comprehension of spoken language was limited. They were "hazy" when it came to interpretation of complex messages both spoken and printed. Spelling was bizarre. Compositions were invariably barren and impoverished.

While the percentage of apparently intellectually subnormal children was high in de Ajuriaguerra's group, those who did not present marked affect disturbances were better organized intellectually than were the disturbed youngsters. Furthermore, the brighter children did rather well on the Similarity subtest of the WISC (Wechsler 1971) which requires only short verbal responses, proving that they were able to generalize. Seventy percent of these children learned to reason fairly adequately at older ages. However, since high-order linguistic concepts are a requisite for the highest forms of thought (formal operations in Piaget's sense [Piaget 1952]) it is not surprising that none of the children was capable of functioning at this level. If verbal concepts are limited, it follows that the organization of the dysphasic child's cognitive system must differ from that of his normal peers. In cases where the mathematical code as well as the verbal code is affected, academic problems are vastly more complicated. Among his twelve subjects only two remained in regular school, having repeated at least once. Some learned to read fluently but nearly all had trouble with comprehension.

As far as psychic organization is concerned, de Ajuriaguerra identified three groups of children: those whose personality structure was within normal limits (though I personally would assume that one would find mild to moderate lags in ego development); those who showed intense free-floating anxiety with defects along the entire range of ego functions; and finally a small group that presented frankly psychotic features such as abnormal psychic organization, disabling defenses, and a rigidly closed personality structure. He says that half of the last group showed marked autistic features.

No single factor accounted for improvement. Improvement depended not only on the severity of the initial condition but also on the child's inherent endowment, his vulnerability to stress, physiological and psychological, on the potential for affect development, on the timing of treatment, and on the degree of nurture from the environment, all of which in combination determined the outcome.

Discussion

The two conditions, dysphasia and autism, clearly have important features in common. Echolalia is one of them; lack of comprehension is another. I raise however the question of whether these apparently similar conditions have the same underlying dynamics. Let's examine echolalia first. Dysphasic youngsters often repeat phrases and sentences to assist them in the processing of incoming linguistic data. One can see from the expression of their faces and detect from the tone of their voices that they are groping for the meaning of what has been said, while the often mechanical and manneristic echolalia of autistic children appears to reflect a lack of communicative intent. Paralinguistic features such as the well known "flat" emotional tone of voice and the lack of appropriate stress heard in autistics suggest the same. In looking at inferior language comprehension, an outstanding symptom in both groups, we see again that dynamics may differ. Dysphasics may understand single words, but they fail mostly when it comes to processing long and complex utterances. This is not true for autistic youngsters. They miss the meaning, be it in single words or longer units because they often do not tune in.

To come back finally to Claudia. A look at her protocol shows that her pathology and that of certain other children does not fit neatly into a precise classification, either phenomenologically or theoretically.

Few people continue to believe as they did in the 40's and 50's that autism, as defined by Kanner (1943), Bettelheim (1967), and others is purely pyschogenic and related to rigid and cold parental attitudes. There is a good deal that may be said about family dynamics in Claudia's case. But her sister flourished in the same environment. Claudia must have been vulnerable from the start. Early onset of the disorder is described as a necessary criterion for both the dysphasic and autistic group. Thus, in her case, early onset is not a differentiating sign.

Claudia produced quite a few phonologically and syntactically acceptable utterances after a short period of treatment. Her relatively good articulation speaks against a severe auditory perceptual problem. Her bizarre utterances do not seem to be a matter of concreteness either—this in contrast to Kanner's example of the boy who every time something was forbidden said, "Don't throw the dog off the balcony," because he could not extract the concept of prohibition from the context in which it had originally been embedded.

I was impressed with Bartak's paper (Bartak, Rutter, and Cox 1975) which showed that there is a genetic link between dysphasia and autism. In the family background of his dysphasic group there were members who were autistic. Quite apart from stressing the genetic aspect, I want to repeat here that both conditions, dysphasia and autism, have a neurophysiological basis.

What then is the usefulness of the autistic-dysphasic dichotomy? No doubt it is useful to identify those children whose language deficit seems to be related to lack of communicative intent. Psychic disturbances appear to be preeminent; the fantasy life of these youngsters seems to take up all their available life space. They live in a world of their own and are not really part of any dialogue. Their formal speech is not too deviating, apart from paralinguistic features which carry the emotional load of communication.

Leaving aside the group of children usually called autistic, what of those who have severe and specific language deficits but who nevertheless seem engaged in the world around them and interested, up to a point, in communication? They do show deviations—those intimately tied to their difficulties with language (and I don't here talk of those whose lack of competence in every day tasks bespeaks genuine intellectual retardation). The children I mean have relatively little difficulty with nonverbal conceptualization, they are competent dealing with objects, they are sometimes very good at mechanical problems. Above all they show a capacity for relationships. A strong language program is indicated; it goes without saying that it has to be affectively loaded because the children are different enough to suffer.

But there are children, like Claudia, whose communicative difficulties are symptomatic of a more fundamental problem in grasping the universe. What one sees in Claudia is *more than* a cognitive-symbolic deficit with its accompanying behavioral manifestations. There is an instability about her inner representation of the world, a failure to integrate perceptual and, later on, affective streams already on the earliest level. Things in Claudia's universe lack boundaries and clear differentiation; this must have been a feature from way back. Her very earliest perception of her mother, and by perception I mean, of course, the elaboration of the sensory input in the brain (her mother's smell and voice) must have remained unstable and uncertain. This must have delayed or impaired object constancy, when the mother was experienced as different and distinct from the environment. For Claudia this applies to all objects—one remembers her confusion about pictures—and certainly has resulted in insecure attachment—Bowlby (1969) calls it bonding—when the mother's inner representation becomes heavily emotionally invested.

All this makes for a shaky world. It would explain Claudia's difficulty separating the person in the story read to her with the person in the waiting room. It would make above all, for her, tenuous relationships. The three security blankets belong here as well, all stemming from a host of difficulties on the earliest preverbal level.

The instability of inner representation affected Claudia on two levels. On the deepest level it affected her relationship to the world and the important people in it. Secondarily, it affected of course language and all kinds of symbols. It led to gaps in comprehension and to her often idiosyncratic speech (so marked a feature in her case), because any language loss affects the epigenesis of the ego, that is, the development of integrating, synthesizing, and organizing functions.

Certainly in a case like Claudia's it would be a mistake to label her as if she were either an autistic child or a straight-forward language casualty. Claudia was, up to a point, interested in communication. She showed some curiosity about the world. She responded to some gestures. She never acted strangely; she neither ate the playdough nor did she drink the soap bubble solution. Yet, her bizarre verbalizations were different from a specific language deficit. Not only the words, but things and people were shifting and blurred. For this child nothing was fixed, the world was like a kaleidoscope that is shaken too fast.

Probably children such as Claudia belong, neurophysiologically, in the same category as do asphasic and autistic youngsters. Nevertheless, they are different; perhaps it is a subgroup, I don't know, and I offer my explanation only tentatively. But it is important to recognize the instability of their basic experiences and feelings and the lack of boundaries which must be remedied, to some degree, by treatment.

A few words about treatment: For children such as Claudia I think that an analytical kind of therapy is not indicated. What is needed, on the other hand, is not a linguistic therapy but one that clarifies and stabilizes not only the world and her feelings about it, but also the physical self. One would work toward strengthening the lines of separation between herself and the outer world. Early efforts might be directed toward movement, with the aim of acquainting her with her own body. Not for the purpose of improving coordination by the way, but to demonstrate the relationship between self and the outside, an understanding that is basic to develop a sense of power and a co-hesiveness of the ego. Only later would one teach the personal pronoun.

It is a long road and it would have been better started years ago in Claudia's case, though I think maturation will do a lot. The very presence of a caring and inventive therapist serves as a point of reference. By way of modeling both feelings and speech, she assists the youngster in making certain fundamental experiences and clothing them in the linguistic code, thereby stabilizing both the experience and the word. The child thus learns to organize what was previously a shaky and unstructured universe.

It is essential that the same person work with the youngster over a long span of time. A psychotherapist who is experienced in the successive stages of language development, or a language clinician who is very aware of the child's needs, are possible choices.

Only with appropriate early therapy will children such as Claudia come out of their unstable universe and learn to feel and use language consensually.

Interactions between
Educational Therapist and Child

During the thirty-five years I have worked in the field of remedial education, I have read a great many reports from educational diagnosticians and therapists, reports that run more or less like this: John is repeating the third grade but he is failing in reading comprehension, spelling, and composition. His number concepts are adequate. He rates a full scale IQ of 123 on the WISC, scoring high, 16, on Similarities and very well, 15, on Block Designs but quite low on Digit Span and Coding. His visual discrimination is excellent, at least where nonverbal patterns are concerned. His Bender is acceptable for his age. However, his auditory memory span is short, his auditory discrimination and sequencing are weak. He has trouble formulating and is unable to summarize the plot of a movie he has seen the previous day. He is an agreeable youngster, very anxious to do well, but his attention fluctuates. He and his therapist have worked hard on phonics and John has mastered all of the rules. He has learned to blend. Nevertheless, his progress is remarkably slow in spite of the fact that he sees his therapist religiously for three sessions each week.

This is a sound enough report, but unfortunately it does not tell me a great deal about John, less about the therapist, and nothing about the interaction between the two.

While to outsiders the task of tutoring looks deceptively easy, you and I know that baffling situations arise, that discouragement sets in, that once in a while one has to admit that the job is beyond one.

In this presentation, I have not shied away from truisms but will attempt to conceptualize which are the forces we have to face within ourselves and the child. In looking through the literature I do not find a satisfactory definition of the remedial teacher's task; what, beyond the necessary formal qualifications and training, makes for success in remediation; which types of youngsters present the most severe challenge; and which are the pitfalls inherent in the job.

Reprinted with permission from The Orton Dyslexia Society, from *Bulletin of The Orton Society* 27:87–101. 1977.

The remedial therapist, is, of course, something of an oddity. She is not a psychotherapist, but she is not, in the usual sense, a teacher. Unlike the teacher, she works with individual children rather than with groups, and unlike the teacher, she does not deal with children who, by and large, have reached a level of development, cognitive, perceptual, linguistic, and emotional, that enables them to benefit from the teaching methods offered them in the schoolroom. The educational therapist is concerned with pathology of learning. Children are referred to her because they have failed or have been predicted to fail at school. They constitute a highly selected group.

The remedial teacher's goals are educational and while in the process of learning the child's inner situation may be modified; she is concerned with that part of the child's psychic organization that deals with reality, that is to say, with the ego. Her task is to teach the youngster not only specific skills but to delay immediate gratification, to check unruly drives, to enjoy mastery for its own sake rather than for extrinsic rewards, all of it in the framework of the specific learning situation.

In contrast, the psychotherapist works with disturbed youngsters who may not be available to learning and who, as a result of conflict, are either fixated on or have regressed to a level of development that does not permit them to give of themselves to educational demands. The psychotherapist directs himself to the child's inner situation, to his unconscious fears, his fantasies, his secret terrors, to those forces that interfere with his investment of psychic energy in tasks unrelated to his drives.

The educational therapist who sees himself as a psychotherapist is bound to fail in both roles. Goals and methods differ. It is unwise to blur the boundaries between the two approaches. Nevertheless, there are areas that overlap. As does psychotherapy, remedial work rests on a treatment alliance between the child and the adult, on a pact, spoken or unspoken, that the two will work together towards a common goal, that in spite of inevitable frustrations, occasional anger and, worse, boredom, they will stick together in the service of learning. Such an alliance cannot be taken for granted. The children who suffer from specific deficits have to work harder than their more fortunate peers. Few of them are anxious to give up play time or favorite TV programs in order to exert themselves beyond the demands required by the school.

It is true that among them are some who are very ready to form a treatment alliance. Their earliest experiences have taught them that it is safe to trust the adult. They have already acquired a measure of control; they are willing to delay gratification; they have incorporated something one might call work ethos. Above all they have a degree of autonomy that stands them in excellent stead in the remedial process.

Their early failure has not basically damaged their sense of self; they have remained, at least in the lower grades, curious and involved; and a candid and clear explanation as to what has gone wrong at school usually does wonders.

Let us assume that a severe dysnomia is a crucial factor in such a youngster's reading disorder. It makes sense to him if he finds out that his trouble evoking not only words but also the names of the letters of the alphabet and their sound equivalents is based on some difficulty with retrieval. Such a youngster might say: "*Now* I know why I can never remember the name of a movie even if I know exactly what happened, and why I had such a terrible time at first recalling the names of the boys in my class and why, when I sound out, I forget the first sound when I try to figure out the last one."

When the therapist then suggests that maybe his well-developed feel for the flow of a sentence might be a way to work around his difficulty, he is all set to try and he will, in addition, make suggestions for mnemonic devices. He knows he is in need of help and he is relieved when it is forthcoming. His unconscious works *for* him rather than draining his ability to give of himself. He senses the therapist's respect for him and enjoys his cozy relationship with her; but basically such a youngster does not work to please the adult; he works because he enjoys mastery and finds pleasure in problem solving.

On the other hand, there are many children who come to us so bruised by an endless succession of failures, so defeated, that they are convinced that nothing will succeed. The therapist is fortunate if she can show them that they have failed not because they are abysmally stupid and incompetent but because a specific teaching approach did not meet their particular needs. One boy, for instance, whose visual recall of whole words is unstable, will be pleased to find that with a solid background in phonics he no longer feels lost when he meets with an unknown word. A different youngster, for whom the fragmented kind of phonics that involves the smallest units does not work, will be delighted to find that an approach that uses larger segments, such as syllables or even sentences, will make the reading task easier. A different approach adapted to the child's very specific needs and the therapist's heavy support will often carry the day, at least if the youngster's feeling of self is intact.

Unfortunately, there are those who feel damaged and impotent, the object of forces over which they have little or no control. These feelings may go back to their earliest days and failure at school has merely confirmed their previous severe doubts about themselves. Hearty verbal reassurance on the part of the parents and the therapist is usually of little avail. Up to a point one has to protect these children from failure in the learning situation, but excessive praise and an unrealistic lowering of demands may have the opposite effect. An honest appraisal of the youngster's level of performance and a recognition of his potential strength are more helpful, at least if the relationship with the therapist is based on trust and honesty. In the last instance, it is the therapist's faith in the child and respect for him that reaches him at a deeper level and helps him to experience himself as a stronger and more capable person than he did in the past.

There are children who simply and flatly refuse to work, and one must keep in mind that overt behavior does not always give one a clue as to what is behind such a refusal. There are youngsters who do not try because they cannot afford to fail. I am now thinking of children whose fantasies of omnipotence are severely threatened by any performance that does not come up to their fantasies. Failure is intolerable because it constitutes a severe narcissistic blow. Telling this kind of child that there is really no need to excel helps little because his resistance to trying is on an irrational basis invested with large amounts of psychic energy. It is the force of the resistance that points to its irrational source, and if it is severe the therapist cannot always get through.

One observes a similar resistance, though based on different dynamics, in phobic youngsters. In spite of an often excellent relationship with the therapist and although they may be genuinely anxious for help such children do not "deliver." One sees it vividly in the many pupils who have a "thing" about writing compositions. They frequently have legitimate difficulties with the technical aspects of writing: with the handling of the pencil, with spacing, paragraphing, capitalization and punctuation or, and this is far more important, with the formulating of ideas in written form. None of it, however, accounts for their desperate fear of putting pen to paper. Realizing that their resistance derives from unconscious sources, we used to handle these situations overly permissively. On the basis of a trusting relationship, but only on this basis, we now insist that the child write at least a paragraph or two right from the start. We might allow him to use a tape recorder at first and have him take down what he dictated. We make sure that the material he writes about is invested heavily with affect, and it goes without saying that we refrain from correcting the technical aspects of his work. But we do insist that he push through, at least up to a point; that is to say, we support the healthy aspect of his personality. The relief if the child does push through is a revelation to him and the therapist. The overly permissive schools err in this respect. If the child fails to bring in his composition, he is told to deliver it in a week's or maybe in two weeks' time with the result that the youngster worries himself to death and, in some instances, has trouble falling asleep. Anna Freud (1966) says: "in the theory of education the importance of the infantile ego's determination to avoid pain, has not been sufficiently appreciated. If children lack guidance, their choice is determined not by their particular gifts but by the hope of freeing themselves as quickly as possible from anxiety and pain." To insist on delivery does not, of course, always work; much depends on the strength of the phobia and what it represents to the unconscious.

In remediation we always deal with two main variables; the severity of the specific deficit and the availability of compensatory resources. The latter is largely determined by psychological factors. In children who are fantasy-ridden and so preoccupied with daydreams that they have little or no psychic energy available for academic pursuits, psychological aspects may be more important than specific deficit. Daydreaming is, of course, much less evident in a one-to-one situation when the therapist engages the child actively in some task, but it constitutes an interference when the child is on his own, during tests, when he does his homework, or when he is part of a large group in the classroom. For a first-grader who has trouble listening, that is, processing material presented orally, the pull of fantasies becomes compelling. Involvement in daydreams is a very seductive occupation and makes him less available for listening; thus, we may be confronted with a vicious cycle even when the child's specific deficits are not particularly severe.

There is still another group that presents massive difficulties for remediation but for different reasons: compulsive youngsters. They are conscientious, there is little wrong with the treatment alliance, but they invariably get bogged down. When they are doing their home-work, they spend hours sharpening their pencils, sorting out their papers; nothing, unfortunately, happens. They get lost in innumer-able details. In the earlier grades at school they are sometimes referred to us because, in spite of their excellent background in phonics, they don't read, or read so slowly that they fall down on comprehension. The heavy emphasis on phonics fits all too well into their own doubt-ridden and cautious way of functioning. Such children don't take a chance. They refuse to guess from context and the surrounding syn-tactical configurations what their options are. They stick to details and tend to miss the point. They do not see the forest for the trees. We know, as a general principle in learning, that separate items are quickly forgotten and that only when one has a framework to fit them into will one recall the particular. Thus, the overly compulsive youngster may be at a severe disadvantage when it comes to grasping the essential of any subject.

There are, of course, conflicted, phobic and obsessive-compulsive youngsters who do manage; obviously it is also a matter of degree, but in cases in which intensive resistance and counterproductive mecha-nisms interfere drastically with the remedial process, a psychiatric referral might be indicated. It should not be done lightly and it goes without saying that it needs the parents' full cooperation which is not always easy to obtain because many of them look for educational help precisely because they feel uncomfortable about psychiatry. Parents will have to understand that the presence of specific perceptual and linguistic difficulties does not exempt children from emotional problems. On the contrary, so called organic youngsters or those who present significant developmental lags are far more vulnerable, emotionally, than are others. In addition, in nearly all cases, a succession of failures has contributed heavily to their problems. It should be added, on the other hand, that hardly ever does psychiatric intervention obviate the need for educational therapy.

So-called minimally brain-injured youngsters are being so extensively described these days that I shall not discuss them in this particular framework. A number of the children we see do, in fact, suffer from mild to severe central nervous system dysfunctions. But a far larger group, and the two may overlap, presents very specific language deficits as part of a neurophysiological lag, often, as Orton (1930) pointed out, on a familial basis. At younger ages such youngsters are poorly patterned and hyperactive. They have trouble attending and may have severe problems with impulse control, problems which in many cases are carried over into adolescence. Their perceptuomotor performance resembles that of a chronologically younger group. Spatial and temporal sequencing present difficulties. They are indifferent listeners and poor processors of input, and they have trouble conceptualizing. At kindergarten age and often later one is impressed by their emotional infantilism which may be viewed as one other aspect of their pervasive organismic immaturity. They continue to live in a somewhat egocentric universe. Aggression is crude and often nonverbal, at least at younger ages. Wish-fulfilling and magic solutions are ready at hand. An impressive number are preoccupied with food, that is, with early instinctual gratification. They have not moved from the pleasure principle to the reality principle, and they retain the infantile expectation that life should provide rewards without corresponding effort (de Hirsch 1975). Such children are not particularly good candidates for psychotherapy, mainly because they are not really conflicted. For the educational therapist they present long-term commitments. Such children may at first simply deny that something is wrong. In working with them one may find them basically friendly but explosive. They have not learned to tolerate frustration and delay gratification. They don't persist, they don't push through. For long periods of time, the therapist must "lend" them her own ego, as it were, help them incorporate her own attitudes: involvement in and devotion to a task, pride in achievement, and the courage to persist even when the going is rough. The therapist must fully exploit the child's usually heavy dependence on her because such youngsters will at first work only to please the adult. Slowly, and as the work gets more rewarding, it becomes in itself a source of pleasure and interest. Eckstein (1969) says that from having learned to love, children must proceed to love of learning.

If I were asked what kinds of children I find hardest to work with, I would say passive youngsters. Learning is in the last instance an aggressive act. Passive children are usually polite and, at least on the surface, willing to cooperate. Unfortunately, nothing much happens. Passivity may have stood such youngsters in good stead in the past; it may have kept them out of trouble. They don't appear to be angry; they yawn instead. Any therapist who has worked with passive adolescents knows that she is defeated if she fails to make the youngster carry the ball (de Hirsch 1963). Take a severe spelling disability, a subject most resistant to remediation. A clear explanation of the neurological basis of the disorder is a good thing to start out with. From then on, it is the pupil who must himself choose what avenue to pursue: reauditorization, revisualization, spelling rules, work on the roots of words and on prefixes and suffixes, using some of the ingenious suggestions presented by Carol Chomsky (1972). It must be the pupil who has to find out which approach or which combination of approaches works best for him.

It is difficult to mobilize passive children because, often enough, they are not really involved in any area, not in hobbies or sports, not in the social scene, not in the age-appropriate problems they share with their peers. They lack the capacity for excitement about a specific period in history or about some lab experiment, the kind of excitement about discovery that stays with one for the rest of one's life and that most often goes back to an intense relationship to some admired adult who has started one along the way. Because such a child's relationship to the therapist is usually shallow and does not allow for identification, the therapist cannot fire him with enthusiasm and cannot help him when the road gets rough. Here again we have a parallel with psychotherapy. Both procedures are bound to fail if the youngster is unable to form a relationship strong enough to help him tolerate the many frustrations inherent in the educational and psychotherapeutic process (de Hirsch 1963).

Identification is the mechanism that carries the child over the vicissitudes of remedial work. It implies the internalizing not only of single elements but of the basic attitudes of the model. It implies that this attitude does not remain a foreign body, as it were, but becomes integrated in the learner's way of meeting the world and becomes part and parcel of his own internalized value system.

But identification is not an end in itself. It should point the way to autonomy. I have not found a definition of autonomy, but I use the term here as it is used in some of the psychiatric literature, as an ego function, the ability to invest in work for its own sake, independent of gratification, of being loved or rewarded, and unhindered by conflict.

What does this mean for the relationship between the child and the remedial therapist? I do not in this framework want to elaborate on the task of the educational diagnostician who has to unravel or at least to describe the interactions among the many forces that determine a child's scholastic effectiveness: his inherent endowment, his vulnerability to stress, the level of his neurophysiological maturation, his developmental status: perceptual, cognitive, linguistic, and interpersonal, the emotional climate of the home that has nurtured him, the social environment that has in part shaped him, and finally the educational measures that have so far failed. In order to be effective the educational diagnostician needs extensive training in the field of developmental disorders in the broadest sense or at least a life-long experience with educationally-disabled children.

I would rather discuss the traits desirable in the person who does the actual work with the pupil. Needless to say she should be familiar with a variety of techniques and ready to adapt them to the children's specific needs. She should not be an evangelist, a person so heavily wedded to one specific approach that this would make it hard for her to modify her technique. She should be familiar with the vicissitudes of each successive developmental phase. When she is working with the preschool child, she should expect the normal negativistic behavior of the three-year-old, the bathroom talk of the four-year-old, the swaggering of the five-year-old. Without such knowledge she will hardly be in a position to judge whether or not her pupil deviates from the norm.

Needless to say, she must be familiar with the life style of the children she works with, the social group they belong to, and the social and ethnic background they spring from. I remember the indignation of a young therapist because her young Chinese charge was totally unable to express any negative feelings. The poor child would have been in trouble at home had he tried a more aggressive stance.

Identical attitudes and words may have an entirely different meaning even in the same social group. The use of the word *fuck* might reflect enormous progress in a middle class youngster who had previously resorted to hitting when he got angry; it might be entirely inappropriate in the next youngster.

Flexibility is of the essence. There are times when the famous lesson plan has to be dropped. Whatever the child brings in must be dealt with right away: a fight with his teacher, a math problem, help with the organization of a report, as long as the youngster knows that the educational task he and the therapist have decided on takes priority. Flexibility refers to content as well as to method. Most of our youngsters have to learn how to learn and the task is easier when it is relevant. Dr. Jansky taught one of our bright adolescents, who had no idea what work meant, entirely around his main and only interest in life: animals. He taught her more about zoology than she would have learned in a college course. In the process, she demonstrated to him that he could use the very same traits—ability to organize and classify material, tolerate frustration (he wrote several manuals on how to handle a cobra)—in the service of other learning tasks. In the end he accepted all the tiresome routines and drills he needed to get into an acceptable college.

We take for granted that the educational therapist possesses a degree of empathy and intuitiveness and, indeed, I know some who simply can't go wrong. But I also remember watching a therapist working with a six-year-old boy who had terrible difficulties with drive control. The two were looking at the picture of a large giraffe in a cage. The boy eyed the animal with considerable misgiving and said half jokingly: "My, that giraffe would be dangerous if she would get out." "Yes," replied the therapist, "if she clobbered one on the head with her hoofs there would be little left." The boy made no comment but when the time came for his next session, he flatly refused to go. He did not really believe, at age six, that an animal in a picture book can get out of its cage. I believe that his malaise referred to his own unruly drives and his fear lest no one protect him from "getting loose" and destroying himself or others. There was no need for the therapist to be familiar with the theoretical framework behind this kind of reasoning. Nevertheless, she should have sensed that her remark would arouse anxiety on several levels.

Unfortunately, intuition, like tact, cannot be taught. It might help the student, though, to watch someone else who instinctively chooses the right approach, not necessarily the same for each child. Learning on this level is a little like catching a disease. A sense of humor in a therapist is an enormous help. I remember a tiny creature, actually she was six years old but she looked like three, stamping her foot because she was made to wait for her turn. The student who taught her was indignant and she had a point, of course. But she entirely failed to see how comical it was when this tiny bundle of energy insisted on her rights, the same insistence that stood her in very good stead when it came to remediation.

Teaching styles differ and in general people do best if their personal style is not interfered with. I remember a fifteen-year-old who got a lot of fun out of tormenting his therapist. She never protested. She became kinder and sweeter, only her voice sounded higher and more tense. The boy got nastier by the minute. When it was over I said to the therapist: "That boy must have made you terribly mad." She was rather shocked and said: "Oh, *I* never get angry with my children." I then transferred the boy to another therapist who was entirely uncorrupted by psychiatric principles but who was pretty unflappable and who had a blessed sense of humor. When the boy started on her, she watched him for a while and then said (rather good humoredly), "Listen, buddy, I won't take it, I have no intention of being trampled on; you would think me an idiot if I let you." He sensed that she wasn't a bit afraid of his aggression and the session proceeded. By a combination of circumstances I watched the very same youngster with a third highly sophisticated therapist. Clearly, he was going to test her out, too. She took it up right away and said: "You are mad, aren't you?" And in a relatively short time the two together found out that he experienced the very fact of coming for remediation as humiliating, hence the nastiness.

What I want to say is this: there are various approaches that may be effective but it is essential for the therapist to be close to her own feelings, negative as well as positive. Some therapists need to be loved. Anna Freud (1952), herself a teacher, said: "The teacher's role is not that of a mother substitute. If she plays the mother role she will get from the child the appropriate reaction—demand for exclusive attention and affection and the wish to get rid of all the other children in the classroom." The situation involving the remedial teacher and the child is, of course, different. One of its advantages for the youngster is *not* having to share the therapist's attention with his siblings. Nevertheless, there are pitfalls in this situation. I have seen remedial tutors who were quite seductive; this might be very threatening to the child. And there is the mistake most of us make when we start in this field, the tendency subtly to side with the youngster against the parent. This is unwise for several reasons; it intensifies the child's own conflicts and it may make him feel guilty; both interfere with work rather than further it. This overlooks the fact, furthermore, that in many situations both parents and the child may be in the right.

Absence of rescue fantasies on the part of the therapist is highly desirable. One's own need to salvage a youngster constitutes a subtle kind of exploitation and might result in considerable anger if the pupil refuses to be rescued. It is just as well to realize that, for better or worse, one cannot really "shape" a child, except that occasionally one can provide, and this is true above all in the case of deprived children, a model of an adult who respects him and whom he can learn to trust in a world that is quite literally beset by dangers.

There is in all teaching a need for clarity and for structure. Absence of limits may make for severe anxiety and a few well-chosen rules are indispensable. Children cannot take toys home from the office; they must arrive and leave on time; missing sessions except for valid reasons is unacceptable. Nevertheless, there are occasions when structure must go by the board. A gift that has not been asked for might serve a useful purpose. Prolonging the session if the child has something important to communicate may be a necessity. There are therapists who structure their sessions to such a degree that they never get an inkling as to what the child is like and, above all, how he feels. A few years ago we worked with a four-year-old referred because of severe articulatory difficulties. He made remarkably little progress although he was on good terms with his rather rigid therapist. It wasn't that he was unwilling to cooperate; he was full of good will. But he was miles away during his sessions. We finally put him in front of the doll house where he became instantly and heavily involved in a play situation he himself had set up and which dealt with a vampire who sucked the boy doll's blood. It needed no probing whatsoever to learn that a vampire sucked *his* blood every night and that it was by no means safe either to fall asleep or to tell anyone about it. No wonder that these fears interfered with his freedom to learn.

While sensitivity to a youngster's anxieties is essential, it is *not* our business to interpret his fears for him (although in this particular case it was fairly evident that the child's sister, three years older, played an important part in the boy's psychic household). We have no right to get involved in psychodynamics. To begin with, we are not in a position to judge whether it is safe to weaken defenses in a youngster who may present severe psychopathology. In the second place, we cannot risk releasing affect that may result in unbearable anxiety or guilt on the part of the child; we should not open up situations we are unable to handle, and, finally and most importantly, playing around with psychodynamics might compromise our educational goals. Rawson (1974) points out that if we have our role and our responsibility clearly in mind, we do not have to become amateur psychiatrists. On the other hand, we cannot afford to slam down the lid. It is essential to find out whether something is very wrong and we must listen to what the child has to say even on a nonverbal level.

It is very much our business, though, to deal with the child's feelings as they are reflected in the actual learning situation. A child comes in looking like thunder, for instance. He does not say anything but it is evident that he is boiling. Maybe he had a fight with a teacher, maybe he felt humiliated by a classmate, maybe his therapist, unbeknownst to herself, had hurt his feelings during the last session. In such a situation one *must* ask: "Hey, what's the matter?" If the youngster is not encouraged to vent his rage, the session will be unproductive because his mind will be somewhere else. It is entirely justifiable to tell a child who is dreaming: "You are quite somewhere else, aren't you? Is that the way it sometimes feels in class when you say you can't follow the teacher?" Assisting the youngster to recall and recognize what it *felt* like at certain moments might help him on the occasion when the situation recurs.

If the child is late for a couple of sessions it behooves us to find out why. There might be a valid practical explanation; on the other hand, his school report may have been abysmally poor and he might deny even to himself that something is wrong and assure himself and the therapist that "everything is O.K." It is essential for the therapist to find out whether this particular youngster meets unpleasant feelings and situations by denying them. And she might file away this tentative hypothesis for an occasion when something similar occurs during the remedial session.

There is finally the separation problem. It is, of course, a mistake to discontinue remedial work before gains are consolidated. But it is unwise to hang on. Separation may be as painful for the therapist as it is for the child (above all for the therapist who needs to be loved or adored). Fortunately, most children know surprisingly clearly when it is time to be weaned and they cheerfully discard the therapist when the job is done.

Kubie (1967) said that it is often difficult to know whether one has succeeded or failed with a particular child. Gains may show up later, rather than right away; on the other hand, an improved report card might mask lack of essential progress. The fact is, no one has yet found a way to measure with any degree of precision the many variables that go into educational progress. Just the same, one should at least try to find out why one has failed with a youngster one has done one's best to help. Is the pupil afraid to succeed? Why did a particular technique work with one child and not with the next one, although their deficits were quite similar? Why did the first youngster compensate for his weaknesses and the next one, equally intelligent, fail to do so? Maybe we have succeeded with the first pupil because we managed to infuse either the subject matter or the relationship with enthusiasm. But why didn't we manage to do just that for the second child?

One thing is certain: In the process of learning, affective and cognitive streams flow together. In this particular child the affect that carried language was negative but it was strong enough to provide the energy needed to produce verbalizations in an emotionally heavy loaded situation.

To go back to the interactions between the child and the therapist, a strongly positive relationship will allow her to make realistic demands; such demands, as long as they are in the child's range, reflect the therapist's respect for the youngster. Respect is probably the most important single feature in the remedial relationship. I agree with Jansky (1972) when she says: "the teacher's confidence in the child's ability to learn will be experienced by him as a confirmation of his basic intactness and each small successful step will prove it."

To sum up, the learning ability of the children we work with either has not developed or has been damaged. The goal in remediation is not to liberate the drives but to contribute to the growth of that aspect of psychic organization that deals with reality. It is silly to deny that the road is often rough.

Identification is the mechanism that helps the educationally handicapped child to submit to sometimes irksome demands. It should go a long way towards a wish for mastery.

What, in the last instance, are the goals of education? Surely not the amassing of information. It is sobering to remind oneself of the innumerable facts one has forgotten. I believe that there are fundamentally two goals and I have not found that extrinsic rewards are effective in reaching them.

1) Learning how to learn. This includes the mastering of tools. But it means, above all, to learn how to grasp the underlying structure of the information presented. This does not depend only on cognitive and linguistic factors, although a level of maturation is a prerequisite; it depends also on teaching. Many children can get hold of it in a one-to-one situation. They learn from the therapist how to go after essentials, after the principles, after the pattern.

2) Getting excitement out of learning is the second goal. It means among other things that the pupil be actively involved in the process, that he be willing to work on the techniques that will enable him to tear out the heart of a learning experience, and that with luck these tools become interesting and challenging in and by themselves. To achieve it, the pupil must internalize the teacher's attitudes and values by a process that goes forward on a conscious and an unconscious level.

Maybe Emerson (1940) put it best when he said: "If he can communicate himself, he can teach, but not by words. He teaches who gives and he learns who receives. There is no teaching until the pupil is brought into the same state in which you are: a transfusion takes place. He is you and you are he. There is a teaching and by no unfriendly chance or bad company can he lose the benefit."

References

Allen, I. 1952. The history of congenital auditory imperception. *The New Zealand Medical Journal* 51:239–274.

Apert, E. 1924. *Bulletin Médicine* 241.

Arnold, G.E. 1957. Tachephyemia: The neglected language disability. *Talk Magazine* 38(2):10.

———. 1960. Studies in tachyphemia. *Logos* 3(1,2).

———. 1965. Cluttering: Tachyphemia *in* Luchsinger, R. and Arnold, G. (eds). *Voice, Speech, and Language* Belmont CA: Wadsworth.

Atkins, S. 1969. Psychoanalytic considerations of language and thought. *Psychoanalytic Quarterly* 38:549–582.

Austin, M. and Morrison, C. 1963. *The First R: The Harvard Report on Reading in Elementary Schools.* New York: Macmillan.

Bachman, F. 1927. Über Kongenitale Wortblindheit. *Abhandlungen aus dem Neurologie, Psychiatrie, Psychologie* 40:1.

Badal, 1888. Contribution à l'étude des cécités, psychiques; alexie, agraphie, nemianopsie inferieure, trouble du sens de l'espace. *Archives of Ophthamology.* 8:97.

Balkanyi, C. 1964. On verbalization. *International Journal of Psycho-Analysis* 45:64–74.

Baratz, J.C. 1969. Language and cognitive developments of Negro children. *American Speech and Hearing Association* 11:87.

Barrett, T. 1965. *Reading Teacher* 18:276.

Bartak, L., Rutter, M., and Cox, A. 1975. A comparative study of infantile autism and specific receptive language disorder. I: The children. *British Journal of Psychiatry.* 26:127–145.

Bateman, B.D. 1973. Educational implications of minimal brain dysfunctions. *Annals of the New York Academy of Science* 205:245–250.

Beebe, H.H. 1944. Auditory memory span for meaningless syllables. *Journal of Speech and Hearing Disorders* 9:273–276.

Bench, J. 1968. Sound transmission to the human foetus through the maternal abdominal wall. *Journal of Genetic Psychology* 113:85.

Bender, L. 1938. A visual motor Gestalt test and its clinical application. *Research Monograph No. 3* American Orthopsychiatry Association.

———. 1949. Psychological problems of children with organic brain disease. *American Journal of Orthopsychiatry* 19:404–415.

———. 1951. *Quarterly Journal of Child Behavior* 3:449.

———. 1953. Childhood schizophrenia. *Psychiatric Quarterly* 27.

———. 1955. *Psychopathology of Children with Organic Brain Disorders.* Springfield Ill.: Charles C. Thomas.

———. 1958. Problems in Conceptualization and Communication with Developmental Alexia. *Psychopathology of Communication.* New York: Grune and Stratton.

_____. 1960. Genetic data in evaluation and management of disordered behaviour in children. *Diseases of the Nervous System* 21(2).

_____. 1966a. Plasticity in developmental neurology *in* Hoch, P. and Zubin, J. (eds.). *Schizophrenia*. New York: Grune and Stratton.

_____. 1966b. The concept of plasticity in childhood Schizophrenia *in* Hoch, P.H. and Zubin, J. (eds.). *Psychopathology of Schizophrenia*. New York: Grune and Stratton.

Bender, L. and Yarnell, H. 1941. An observation nursery. *American Journal of Psychiatry* 97:1158.

Benton, A. 1940. Mental development of prematurely born children: a critical review of the literature. *American Journal of Orthopsychiatry* 10:719–746.

_____. 1959. *Left-Right Discrimination and Finger Localization: Development and Pathology*. New York: Hoeber.

Bentzen, F. 1963. Sex ratios in learning and behaviour. *American Journal of Orthopsychiatry* 33:92–98.

Berko, J. 1958. The child's learning of English morphology. *Word* 14:150.

_____. 1960. The acquisition of grammatical categories in children. *Word* 16–287.

Bernstein, B. 1961. Social class and linguistic development: a theory of social learning *in* Halsey, A.J.H., Fland, S., Anderson, C.A. (eds.). *Education, Economy and Society*. New York: The Free Press.

Berry, M. 1969. *Language Disorders of Children*. New York: Appleton-Century-Croft.

Bettleheim, B. 1967. *The Empty Fortress: Infantile Autism and the Birth of the Self*. New York: Free Press.

Birch, H.G. 1964. The problem of "brain damage" in children *in* Birch, H.G. (ed.) *Brain Damage in Children, the Biological and Social Aspects*. Baltimore: Williams and Wilkins.

Birch, H. and Belmont, L. 1965. Lateral dominance, lateral awareness, and reading disability. *Child Development* 36:57.

Birch, H. and Gussow, J. 1972. *Disadvantaged Children, Health, Nutrition and School Failure*. New York: Harcourt Brace.

Blanchard, P. 1946. Psychoanalytic contributions to the problem of reading disabilities *in* Esiler, R. et. al (eds.). *The Psychoanalytic Study of the Child Volume II*. New York: International Universities Press.

Blau, A., Slaff, B., Easton, K., Welkowitz, J., Springarn, J., Cohen, J. 1963. The psychogenic etiology of premature births. *Psychosomatic Medicine* 25:201–211.

Blegen, S. 1952. The premature child. *Acta Paediatrica* Supplement 88.

Bloom, L. 1970a. *Form and Function in Emerging Grammars* Cambridge: M.I.T. Press.

_____. 1970b. *Readings in Language Development*. New York: Simon and Schuster.

Bluemel, C.S. 1930. *Mental Aspects of Stuttering*. Baltimore: Williams and Wilkins Co.

Bluemel, C.S. (n.d.) *Stammering and Allied Disorders*. New York: Macmillan Company.

Blumenthal, A.L. 1907. Language and Psychology. New York: John Wiley.

Borel-Maisonny, S. 1951a. Les troubles du langage dans les dyslexies et les dystortographiese. *Enfance* 5:400.

_____. 1951b. Les dyslexies: definition, examen, classement, rééducation. *Folia Phoniatrica* 3:86.

_____. 1954. Quelques observations sur les rhythmes pathologiques. *International Association of Logopedics and Phoniatrics* International Speech and Voice Therapy Conference.

Bowlby, J. 1969. *Attachment and Loss. Vol. I. Attachment*. New York: Basic Books.

Bradley, C. 1955. Organic factors in the psychopathology of childhood *in* Hoch, P. and Zubin, J. (eds.) *Psychopathology of Childhood*. New York: Grune and Stratton.

Braine, M.D.S. 1963. The ontogeny of English phrase structure: first phase. *Language* 39:1.

Brodbeck, A.J. and Irwin, O.C. 1946. The speech behavior of infants without families. *Child Development* 17:145.

Brown, R. 1958. *Words and Things* New York: The Free Press.

_____. 1964. The acquisition of language *in* Riach, D.Mck., and Weinstein, F.A. (eds.). *Disorders of Communication. Research Publications Association of Nervous and Mental Disease* 42:56.

Brown, R. and Bellugi, U. 1964. Three processes in the child's acquisition of syntax. *Harvard Education Review* 34:133.

Buhler, C. and Hetzewr, H. 1935. *Testing Children's Development from Birth to School Age.* New York: Farrar and Rinehart.

Burdin, G. 1940. Surgical treatment of stammering. *Journal of Speech Disorders* 5:43.

Burks, H. 1957. The effect of learning of brain pathology. *Exceptional Children* 24:169–172, 174.

_____. 1960. The hyperkenetic child *Exceptional Children* 27:18–26.

Caplan, H. 1952. Body image concept in child development. *Quarterly Journal of Child Behavior* 4.

Caplan, H., Bibace, R., and Rabinovitch, M.S. 1963. Paranatal stress, cognitive organization and ego function. *Journal of the American Academy of Child Psychiatry* 2:434–450.

Carrell, J. and Bangs, J. 1957. Disorders of speech comprehension associated with idiopathic language retardation. *The Nervous Child* 9:64–76.

Carroll, J.B. 1961. Language development in children. *in* Saporta, S. (ed.) *Psycholinguistics: A Book of Readings.* New York: Holt.

Cazden, C. 1966a. Subcultural differences in child language: An interdisciplinary review. *Merrill-Palmer Quarterly* 12:185–219.

_____. 1966b. Some implications of research on language development for preschool education. Paper presented at National Council of Teachers Learning Programs for the Disadvantaged.

_____. 1968a. The acquisition of noun and verb inflections. *Child Development* 39:433.

_____. 1968b. Three sociolinguistic views of the language and speech of lower-class children-with special attention to the work of Basil Bernstein *Developmental Medicine and Child Neurology* 10:600.

_____. 1972. *Child Language and Education.* New York: Holt, Rinehart, and Winston.

Chall, J., Roswell, F., Alshan, L., and Bloomfield, M. 1965. Paper read at Annual Meeting of American Education Research Association. Chicago.

Chess, S. 1944. Developmental language disability as a factor in personality distortion in childhood. *American Journal of Orthopsychiatry* 14:483.

Chomsky, C. 1972. Stages in language development and reading exposure *Harvard Educational Review* 42(1):1–33.

Chomsky, N. 1959. Review of "Verbal Behavior" by B.F. Skinner. *Language* 35:26.

_____. 1965. *Aspects of the Theory of Syntax.* Cambridge: MIT Press

Clark, R.M. 1959. Maturation and speech development. *Logos* 2.

Cleland, D. 1953. Seeing and reading. *Optometry* 30:467–481.

Clements, S.D. 1973. Minimal brain dysfunction *in* Sapit, S. and Nitzburg, A.C. (eds.). *Children with Learning Problems.* New York: Brunner/Mazel.

Cohen, T.B. 1963. *American Journal of Orthopsychiatry* 33:330.

Coleman, R. and Deutch, C. 1964. *Perceptual Motor Skills* 19:43.

Connelly, K. 1972. Learning and the concept of critical periods in infancy. *Developmental Medicine and Child Neurology* 14:705–714.

Conrad, K. 1948. Beitrage zum Probleme der Parietalen Aleixie. Archiv Psychiatrie und Nervenkrankenheit 181:19.

Coriat, I. 1942–43. Psychoanalytic conception of stuttering. *Nervous Child* 2.

Coriat, J.H. 1927. The oral erotic components of stammering. *Journal of Psychoanalysis* 8.

Cruttendon, A. 1970. A phonetic study of babbling. *British Journal of Disorders of Communication* 5:110.

Daniels, J.C. and Diack, H. 1959. The phonic word method. *Reading Teacher* 13:14–21.

Davis, D.M. 1939. Relation of repetitions in speech of young children to certain measures of language maturity and situational factors. *Journal of Speech Disorders* 4:303.

de Ajuriaguerra, J. 1963. Le troubles du langage. *Confin. neurol.* 23:91–107.

———. 1966. Speech disorders in children *in* E.C. Carterette (ed.). *Brain Function.* Berkeley: University of California Press.

de Ajuriaguerra, J., Guignard, R., Jaeggi, A., Kocher, R., Maquard, M., Paumier, A., Quinnodoz, D., and Liotis, E. 1963. Organization pyschologique et trouble du development du langage: Etude d'un groupe d'enfants dysphasique *in Probleme de Psycholinguistique.* Paris: University of France Press.

de Hirsch, K. 1952. Specific dyslexia or strephosymbolia. *Folia Phoniatrica* 4:231–248.

———. 1953. Developmental word deafness and speech therapy. *Bulletin of the Orton Society* 3:11–20.

———. 1954. Gestalt psychology as applied to language disturbances. *Journal of Nervous and Mental Diseases* 120(3,4):257–261.

———. 1957. Tests designed to discover potential reading difficulties at the 6-year-old level. *American Journal of Orthopsychiatry* 27:566–567.

———. 1961a. Diagnosis of developmental language disorders. *Logos* 4(13):9.

———. 1961b. Concepts related to normal reading processes and their application to reading pathology. *Journal of Genetic Psychology* 102:227–285.

———. 1961c. Studies in tachyphemia: Diagnosis of developmental language disorders. *Logos* 4:3–9.

———. 1963. Two categories of learning difficulties in adolescents. *American Journal of Orthopsychiatry* 33(1):87–91.

———. 1961d. Diagnosis of developmental language disorders. *Logos* 4(1).

———. 1965. The concept of plasticity and language disabilities. *Speech Pathology and Therapy* 8:12–17.

———. 1967. Differential diagnosis between aphasic and schizophrenic language in children. *Journal of Speech and Hearing Disorders* 32:3–9.

———. 1970. Language deficits in children with developmental lags. *The Psychoanalytic Study of the Child* 30:95–126.

de Hirsch, K. and Jansky, J. 1957. Word deafness. *Journal of the South African Logopedics Society* 4:13–15.

de Hirsch, K., Jansky, J., and Langford, W.S. 1966a. Comparisons between prematurely and maturely born children at three age levels. *American Journal of Orthopsychiatry* 36:616–626.

de Hirsch, K., Jansky, J. and Langford, W.S. 1966b. *Predicting Reading Failure.* New York: Harper and Row.

de Hirsch, K. and Langford, W.S. 1950. Clinical note on stuttering and cluttering in young children. *Pediatrics* 5:934–939.

Denckla, M.B. 1978. Minimal brain dysfunction *in* Chall, J. and Mirsky, A. (eds.) *Education and the Brain.* Chicago: National Society for the Study of Education and University of Chicago Press.

Despert, L. 1946. Discussion of irrelevant and metaphorical language in early infantile autism. *American Journal of Psychiatry* 103:242.

Deutsch, M. 1960. Minority-group and class status, as related to social and personality factors in scholastic achievement. *Society for Applied Anthropology Monograph 2*

Di Carlo, S. 1964. *in* Rappaport, S. (ed.). *Childhood Aphasia. Pathway School Symposium, Part 2.* Philadelphia: Livingston Publications.

Diak, H. 1960. *Reading and the Psychology of Perception.* Nottingham: Peter Skinner.

Doll, E.A. 1940. *The Oseretsky Tests of Motor Proficiency.* Minneapolis: Educational Publishers.

Douglas, J. 1956. Mental ability and school achievement of premature children at 8 years of age. *British Medical Journal* 1, 4977:1210–1214.

Douglas, J. 1960. Premature children at primary schools. *British Medical Journal* 51:1008–1013.

Drew, A. 1956. Neurological appraisal of familial congential word-blindness *Brain* 79(3):440–450.

Drillien, C. 1964. *The Growth and Development of the Prematurely Born.* Baltimore: Williams and Wilkins.

Dwornicka, B., Jasienska, J., Smolary, W., and Wawryk, R. 1964. Attempt of determining the foetal reaction to acoustic stimulation. *Acta Otolaryngology* 57:571.

Eckstein, R. and Motto, R.L. (n.d.). *From Learning for Love to Love of Learning.* New York: Brunner/Mazel.

Edelheit, H. 1968a. Panel Report: Language and ego development. *Journal of the American Psychoanalytic Association* 16:113–122.

———. 1968b. Language and ego development. *Journal of the American Psychoanalytic Association* 16:13.

———. 1969. Speech and psychic structure. *Journal of the American Psychoanalytic Association* 17:381–412.

Eisenberg, R.B. 1970. The development of hearing in man. *American Speech and Hearing Association* 12:119.

Eisenson, J. 1968. Developmental aphasia (dyslogia). A postulation of a unitary concept of the disorder. *Cortex* 4:184–200.

Ekstein, R. 1965. Historical notes concerning psychoanalysis and early language development. *Journal of the American Psychoanalytic Association* 13:707–730.

Elmas, P.D., Siqueland, E.R., Jusczk, P., and Vigorito, J. (n.d.). Speech perception in infants. *Science* (n. vol.):303–306.

Emerson, R.W. 1940. Spiritual laws *in Complete Essays and Other Writings.* New York: Random House.

Ervin-Tripp, S., and Slobin, D.I. 1966. Psycholinguistics *Ann. Rev. Psychol.* 17:435.

Eveloff, H. 1971. Some cognitive and affective aspects of early language development. *Child Development* 43:1895.

Ewing, A. 1940. *Differential Diagnosis of Aphasia in Children.* London: Oxford University Press.

Fabian, J.A. 1951. Clinical and experimental studies of school children who are retarded in reading. *Quarterly Journal of Child Behavior* 3:15.

Fairbanks, G. 1940. *Voice and Articulation.* New York: Harper and Brothers.

Farnham-Diggory, S. 1966. Self, future, and time: a developmental study of the concepts of psychotic, brain-damaged, and normal children. *Soc. Res. Child Dev.* 31 Monograph Serial 103.

Fay, W.H. and Butler, B.V.F. 1968. Echolalia, IQ, and the developmental dichotomy of speech and language systems. *Journal of Speech and Hearing* 11:365.

Fischer, M.S. 1932. Language patterns of pre-school children. *Journal of Experimental Education* 1:70.

Fisher, J.H. 1905. *Ophthalmological Review* 20:61.

Fisichelli, R.M. 1950. A study of prelinguistic speech development of institutionalized infants. Doctoral dissertation. Fordham University.

Florensky, J.A. 1933. Zur Frage der functionellen Sprachstörungen Paraphrasie und Tachylalie. *Zeitschrift Neurologie* 148:59.

Frank, A. 1969. The unrememberable and the unforgettable. *This Annual* 24:48–77.

Freedman, A., Braine, M., Heimer, C., Kowlessar, M., O'Connor, W., Wortis, H., and

Goodman, B. 1960. The influence of hyperbilirubinemia on the early development of the premature. *Psychiatric Research Report. American Psychiatric Association* 13:108–127.

Freeman, F. 1958. *Guiding Growth in Handwriting, Evaluation Scale.* Columbus OH: Parker Zaner-Bloser.

French, E.L. 1953. Psychological factors in cases of reading difficulties. Paper presented at the 27th Annual Conference of the Secondary Education Board, New York.

Freud, A. 1946. *The Ego and the Mechanism of Defense.* New York: International University Press.

_____. 1952. The role of teacher. *Harvard Education Review* 22:229:234.

_____. 1965. *Normality and Pathology in Childhood.* New York: International Universities Press.

_____. 1974. A psychoanalytic view of developmental psychopathology. *Journal of the Philadelphia Association of Psychoanalysis* 1:7–17.

Freud, S. 1911. *Formulations on the Two Principles of Mental Functioning.* S.E. 12:215–226.

_____. 1957. *The Unconscious. Standard Edition XIV.* London: Hogarth.

Freund, H. 1934. Uber die Beziehungen zwischen Stottern und Poltern. *Monatsschrift fur Ohrenheilk* 12:68.

_____. 1952. Studies in the interrelationship between stuttering and cluttering. *Folia Phoniatrica* 4(3).

Friedlander, B.Z. 1970. Receptive language development in infancy. *Merrill-Palmer Quarterly* 16:7–52.

_____. 1972. Time sampling analysis of infants natural learning environment in the home. *Child Development.*

_____. 1973. Receptive language anomaly and language/reading dysfunction in "normal" primary school children. *Psychology in the Schools* 10:12–18.

Friedman, D.C. 1968. *Personality Development in Infancy.* New York: Holt, Rinehart and Winston.

Frisk, M., Takkunen, R.L, and Holmstrom, G. 1964. Small prematures at 6–7 years of age. *Annales Paediatric Fenniae* 10:79–83.

Froeschels, E. 1942–43. Pathology and therapy of stuttering. *Nervous Child* 2:148.

_____. 1946. Cluttering. *Journal of Speech Disorders* 2:31.

_____. 1948. *Twentieth Century Speech and Voice Correction.* New York: Philosophical Library, Inc.

_____. 1949. Pure word deafness in a child. *Quarterly Journal of Child Behavior* 1:228–240.

Fry, D.B. 1966. The development of the phonological system in the normal and deaf child. *in* Smith, F. and Miller, G.A. (eds.) *The Genesis of Language.* Cambridge: M.I.T. Press.

Furth, H.G. 1974. The concept of the "school for thinking," *in The Learning Disability Child. Proceedings of a Symposium on Current Operation, Remediation and Evaluation.* Dallas: University of Texas Health Science Center.

Galifert-Granjou, N. 1951. Le probleme de l'organisation spatiale dans les dyslexies d'evolution. *Enfance* 5:445–479.

Gann, E. 1945. *Reading Difficulty and Personality Organization.* New York: King's Crown Press.

Gates, A. 1936. *Teachers College Record* 37:679.

Gerstman, J. 1958. Psychological and phenomenolical disorders of body image. *Journal of Nervous and Mental Disease* 126:49.

Gesell, A. 1945. *The Embryology of Behavior-The Beginning of the Human Mind.* New York: Harper and Brothers.

Gesell, A., Halverson, H., Thompson, H., Ilg, F., Castner, B., Ames, L. Amatruda, C. 1940. *The First Five Years of Life.* New York: Harper and Brothers.

Gibson, E.J. 1963. Perceptual development *in* H.W. Stevenson (ed.) *Child Psychology.* National Society for the Study of Education Yearbook. Part 1. Chicago: University of Chicago Press.

———. 1969. *Principles of Perceptual Learning and Development.* New York: Appleton-Century-Crofts.

Gillingham, A. 1946. Remedial Training of Children with Specific Disability in Reading, Spelling, and Penmanship. Distributed by the author.

———. 1949. Auditory Failure in Reading and Spelling. *Independent School Bulletin.*

Gletiman, L. 1973. *Metalinguistic Capacity.* Position paper presented at the meeting of the Language Panel on Head Start. Sponsored by the Rand Corporation. Washington, D.C.

Goldenberg, S. 1950. An exploratory study of some aspects of idiopathic language retardation. *The Journal of Speech and Hearing Disorders* 15:221–233.

Goldfarb, W. 1961. *Childhood Schizophrenia.* Cambridge: Harvard University Press.

Goldstein, K. 1939. *The Organism.* New York: The American Book Company.

———. 1948. *Language and Language Disturbances.* New York: Grune and Stratton.

———. 1953. Personal communication.

Goldstein, K. and Scheerer, M. 1941. Abstract and concrete behavior: An experimental study with special tests. *Psychological Monographs* 53.

Goodenough, F. 1926. *Measurement of Intelligence by Drawing.* New York: World Book Company.

Goodman, K. 1972. Reading: The key is in the children's language. *Reading Teacher* 25:505–508.

Greenacre, P. 1953. *Trauma, Growth and Personality.* London: Hogarth.

Grewel, F. 1959. How do children acquire the use of language? *Folia Phoniatrica* 3:193.

———. 1970. Cluttering and its problems. *Folia Phoniatrica* 22:301–310.

Grossman, W. and Bennet, S. 1969. Anthropomorphism. *The Psychoanalytic Study of the Child* 24:78 New York: International Universities Press.

Gutzman, H. 1898. Das Stottern. *Eine Monographie fur Aertze, Padagogen und Behorden* Frankfort: M.J. Rosenheim.

———. 1910. Ueber Stottern als Herdsymptom. *Med.-Pedagog. Monatschr.* 20:248.

Hallgren, B. 1950. Specific dyslexia. *Acta Psychiatrica et Neurologica* Supplement 65:1.

Halpern, E. 1970. Reading success by children with visual-perceptual immaturity: explorations within Piaget's theory. Paper read at 47th Annual Meeting of the American Orthopsychiatric Association, San Francisco.

Hardy, W.G. 1965. On language disorders in young children: a reorganization of thinking. *Journal of Speech and Hearing Disorders* 30:3–16.

Harper, P. 1964. Personal communication.

Harper, P., Fisher, L., and Rider, R. 1959. Neurological and intellectual status of prematures at three to five years of age. *Journal of Pediatrics* 55:679–690.

Harris, A.J. 1957. Lateral dominance, directional confusion, and reading disability. *Journal of Psychology* 44:283

———. 1958. *Harris Test of Lateral Dominance. Manual for Administration and Interpretation.* New York: Psychological Corporation.

Head, H. 1926. *Aphasia and Kindred Disorders of Speech.* London: Cambridge University Press.

Henig, M. 1949. *Elementary School Journal* 50:41.

Hermann, K. 1961. *Reading Disability.* Springfield, Ill: Charles C. Thomas.

Hertzig, M., Bortner, M., and Birch, H. 1969. Neurologic findings in children educationally designated as "brain damaged." *American Journal of Orthopsychiatry* 39:437–446.

Hertzig, M.E., Birch, H.G., Thomas, A., and Murdez, O.A. 1968. Class and ethnic differences in the responsiveness of preschool children to cognitive demands. *Society for Research in Child Development* Serial No. 117, No. 33(1) Chicago: University of Chicago Press.

Hess, J., Mohr, G., and Bartelme, P. 1934. *The Physical and Mental Growth of Prematurely Born Children.* Chicago: University of Chicago Press.

Hess, R. and Shipman, V. 1965. Early experiences and the socialization of cognitive modes in children. *Child Development* 36:869–86.

_____. 1966. Influences upon early learning *in* Hess, R.D. and Bear, R.M. (eds.). *Early Education: Current Theory, Research and Action.* Chicago: Aldine Publishing Co.

Hinshelwood, J. 1895a. *Lancet* 1:83.

_____. 1895b. Word blindness and visual memory. *Lancet* 2:1564.

_____. 1896a. "Word blindness and visual memory." (Letter to the editor). *Lancet* 1:196.

_____. 1896b. A case of dyslexia: a peculiar form of word blindness. *Lancet* 2:1451.

_____. 1898. A case of "word" without "letter" blindness. *Lancet* 1:422.

_____. 1900. Congenital word blindness. *Lancet* 1:1506.

_____. 1904. A case of congenital word blindness. *British Medical Journal* 2:1303.

_____. 1907. *British Medical Journal* :1229.

_____. 1917. *Congenital Word Blindness.* London: Lewis.

Hoberman, S. and Goldgarb, W. 1963. Speech reception thresholds in schizophrenia. *Journal of Speech and Hearing Research* 6:101–106.

Houston, S. 1970. A reexamination of some assumptions about the language of the disadvantaged child. Child Development. 41:947–963.

Howard, P. and Worrell, C. 1952. Premature infants in later life. *Pediatrics* 9:577–584.

Ilg, F.L. and Ames, L.B. 1965. *School Readiness.* New York: Harper and Row.

Irwin, O.C. 1946. Development of speech during infancy. *Journal of Experimental Psychology* 36:43.

Izmuzi, H. 1963. Studies of premature children. *Japanese Journal of Educational Psychology.*

Jackson, J.H. 1958. *Selected Writings of Hughlings Jackson.* Taylor, I. (ed.). New York: Basic Books.

Jakobson, R. 1962. *Selected Writings. I.* The Hague: Mouton and Co.

Jakobson, R. and Halle, M. 1956. *Fundamentals of Language.* The Hague: Moulton and Co.

Jansky, J. 1955. Word deafness viewed as one aspect of an inclusive syndrome. Paper written for City College, New York.

_____. 1960. Congenitally word deaf children. Master's thesis. College of City of New York.

_____. 1971. The contribution of certain kindergarten abilities to second grade reading and spelling achievement. Doctoral thesis. Teachers College. Columbia University.

_____. 1972. Untitled paper presented at Symposium, Neuropsychiatric Institute Princeton NJ.

Jansky, J. and De Hirsch, K. 1972. *Preventing Reading Failure.* New York: Harper and Row.

Jeruchimowicz, R., Costello, J., and Bagur, J. 1971. Knowledge of action and object words: A comparison of lower and middle class Negro preschoolers. *Child Development* 42:455–464.

Johansson, B., Wedenberg, E., and Westin, B. 1964. Measurement of tone response by the human foetus. *Acta Otolarynyg.* 57:188.

Johnson, W. 1938. Role of evaluation in stuttering behavior. *Journal of Speech Disorders* 3:85.

_____. 1942. Study of onset and development of stuttering. *Journal of Speech Disorders* 7:21.

Kagan, J. 1969. Continuity in cognitive development during the first year. *Merrill-Palmer Quarterly* 15:101.

Kagan, J., Moss, H.A., and Sigel, I.E. 1960. Conceptual style and the use of affect labels. *Merrill-Palmer Quarterly.*

Kainz, F. 1956. *Psychologie der Sprache (Vierter Band, Spezielle Sprachpsychologie).* Stuttgart: Ferdinand Enke Verlag.

Kanner, L. 1943. Autistic disturbances of affective contact. *Nervous Child* 2:217–250.

Kapelman M., Kaplan, E., and Gauber, R.L. 1970. A study of learning disorders among disadvantaged children. *in* Chess, S. and Thomas, H. (eds.). *Annual Progress in Child Psychiatry and Child Development* New York: Brunner Mazel.

Kaplan, B. 1959. The study of language in psychiatry *in* Arieti, S. (ed.). *American Handbook of Psychiatry, Vol. III.* New York: Basic Books.

Kaplan, D.M. and Mason, E.A. 1960. Maternal reactions to premature birth viewed as an acute emotional disorder. *American Journal of Orthopsychiatry* 30:539–552.

Karelitz, S. and Frischelli, V.R. 1969. Infants' vocalizations and their significance. *Clinical Proceedings* Children's Hospital, Washington, D.C. 25:11.

Kasanin, J.S. 1944. *Language and Thought in Schizophrenia.* San Francisco: University of Caifornia Press.

Kastein, S., and Fowler, E. 1959. Language development among survivors of premature birth. *Archives of Otolaryngology* 69:131–135.

Katan, A. 1961. Some thoughts about the role of verbalization in early childhood. *Psychoanalytic Study of the Child* 16:184–188.

Katz, D. 1951. *Gestalt Psychology.* London: Metheun and Co.

Kawi, A. and Pasamanick, B. 1958. Association of factors of pregnancy with reading disorders in childhood. *Journal of the American Medical Association* 166:1420–1423.

Kerr, J. 1897. School Hygiene, Mental, Moral, and Physical Aspects. Howard Medal Prize Essay June 1896. *Journal of the Royal Statistical Society* 60:613.

———. 1900. Minutes of Meeting of Bradford Medico-Chirurgical Society April 24, 1900. 1:1446.

Kimball, M. and Dale, P. 1971. The relationship between color naming and color recognition ability of preschoolers. *Child Development*

Klingman, O. 1956. Discussion *in* Neurology and psychiatry in childhood. *Research in Nervous and Mental Disease* 34:390.

Knobloch, H. and Pasamanick, B. 1960. Environmental factors affecting human development before and after birth. *Pediatrics* 26:210–218.

———. 1962. Mental subnormality. *New England Journal of Medicine* 266:1045–1051, 1092–1097, 1155–1161.

Koch, H. 1964. A study of twins born at different levels of maturity. *Child Development* 35:1265–1282.

Koehler, W. 1933. *Psychologische Probleme.* Berlin: Springer.

Koffka, K. 1953. *Principles of Gestalt Psychology.* New York: Harcourt, Brace and Co.

Kolansky, H. 1967. Some psychoanalytic considerations of speech in normal development and psychopathology. *This Annual* 22:274–295.

Kopp, H. 1943. *Nervous Child* 2:107.

Koppitz, E. 1964. *The Bender Gestalt Test for Young Children.* New York: Grune and Stratton.

Korte, W. 1923. Uber die Gestaltauffassung im indirekten Sehen. *Zeitschriffte Psychologie* 93:17–82.

Kubie, L. 1967. The utilization of preconscious functions in education *in* Bower, E. and Hollister, W. (eds.). *Behavioural Science Frontiers in Education.* New York: John Wiley and Sons.

Kugelman, M. 1946. Psychomatic study of 50 stuttering children. *American Journal of Orthopsychiatry* 16:127.

Kurlander, L.F. and Colodny, D. 1965. "Pseudoneurosis" in the neurologically handicapped child. *American Journal of Orthopsychiatry* 35:733–738.

Kussmaul, A. 1877. *Ziemssen Cyclopedia of the Practice of Medicine on Disturbances of Speech.* 14:771.

———. 1910. *Die Störungen der Sprache.* Leipzig: F.C.W. Vogel.

Laffal, J. 1965. *Pathological and Normal Language*. New York: Atherton.

Langford, W.S. 1955. Developmental dyspraxia. *Bulletin of the Orton Society* 5.

Langman, M.P. 1960. The reading process: A descriptive, interdisciplinary approach. *Genetic Psychology Monographs* 62:3–40.

Lashley, K. 1954. *in* Jeffries, L.A. (ed.). *Cerebral Mechanisms of Behavior*. New York: John Wiley and Sons.

Lawrence, M. 1960. Minimal brain injury in child psychiatry. *Comprehensive Psychiatry* 1:360–369.

Lee, L.L. 1969. *Northwestern Syntax Screening Test*. Evanston: Northwestern University Press.

Leischner, A. 1951. Über den Verfall der menschlichen Sprache. *Archiv Psychiatrie und Nervenkrankenheit* 187:250–267.

Lennenberg, E. 1964a. Speech as a motor skill with special reference to nonaphasic disorders *in* Bellugi, U. and Brown, R. (eds.). *The Acquisition of Language Society for Research in Child Development Monographs* 29:115

––––––. 1964b. A biological perspective of language *in* Lennenberg, E.E. (ed.). *New Directions in the Study of Language*. Cambridge: M.I.T. Press

––––––. 1966. The natural history of language *in* Smith, F., and Miller, G.A. (eds.). *The Genesis of Language*. Cambridge: MIT Press.

––––––. 1967. *The Biological Foundations of Language*. New York: John Wiley and Sons.

––––––. 1968. The effects of age on central nervous system disease in children. Paper read at Eastern Regional Society for Research in Child Development Meeting, Clark University, Worcester, MA.

Leopold, W.F. 1953. Patterning in children's language learning. *Language Learning* 54.1.

Leshan, L. 1952. Time orientation and social class. Journal of Abnormal Social Psychology 47:589–592.

Lesser, S.R. and Easser, R.B. 1972. Personality differences in the perceptually handicapped. *Journal of the American Academy of Child Psychiatry* 11:458–466.

Lewis, M.M. 1951. *Infant Speech*. New York: Humanities Press.

––––––. 1963. *Language, Thought and Personality in Infancy and Childhood*. London: Harrop.

Lieberman, A. 1900. *Poltern*. Berlin: Coblenz.

Lieberman, A.M., Cooper, F.S., Shankweiler, D.P., and Studderet-Kennedy M. 1967. Perception of the speech code. *Psychological Review* 74:431–461.

Lieberman, P. 1967. Intonation, Perception and Language. Cambridge MA: MIT Press.

Liss, E. 1950. The dynamics of learning. *Quarterly Journal of Child Behavior* 2:140.

Los Angeles County Medical Association. 1940. *Report of the Ophthamological Section of the Los Angeles County Medical Association*.

Lowe, A. and Campbell, R. 1965. Temporal discrimination in aphasoid and normal children. *Journal of Speech and Hearing Research* 8:313–314.

Lubchenco, L., Horner, F., Reed, L., Hix, I., Metcalf, D., Cohig, R., Elliot, H., and Bourg, M. 1963. Sequelae of premature birth. *American Journal of Diseases of Children* 106:101–115.

Luchsinger, R. 1959. Die Verebung von Sprache und Stimmstörungen. *Folia Phoniatrica* 11:7–64.

Luria, A.R. 1961. *in* Tizard, J. (ed.). *The Role of Speech in the Regulation of Normal and Abnormal Behaviour*. New York: Pergamon Press.

Mahler, M.S. 1963. Thoughts about development and individuation. *The Psychoanalytic Study of the Child*. 18. New York: International Universities Press.

––––––. 1971. A study of the separation-individuation process. *This Annual* 26:403–424.

Malmquist, E. 1963. Figurel, J.A. (ed.) *Reading as an Intellectual Activity. International Reading Association Conference Proceedings* 8:204.

Masland, M.W. 1960. Personal communication.

––––––. 1967–68. Listening skills and reading performance. Conference on Progress in

Reading. *Proceedings of Fifth Annual Study Congress of United Kingdom Reading Association.* Edinburgh.

Masland, M.W. and Case, I. 1965. Limitation of auditory memory as a factor in delayed language development. Paper read at meeting of International Association of Logopedics and Phoniatrics. Vienna 13th Congress.

Masland, R. 1965. The neurological substrata of communicative disorders. Paper read at Convention of American Speech and Hearing Association. Chicago.

Mason, A.W. 1967–68. Follow up of educational attainments in a group of children with retarded speech development and in a control group *in* Clark, M. and Maxwell, S. (eds.). *Reading: Conference on Progress in Reading. Proceedings of Fifth Annual Study Congress of the United Kingdoms Reading Association.* Edinburgh.

McCarthy, D. 1954. Language development in children *in* Carmichael, L. (ed.) *Manual of Child Psychology* (2nd edition). New York: John Wiley and Sons.

———. 1958. Language development. Opening address at the Summer Symposium of the Cleveland Hearing and Speech Center.

McDonald, E.T., and Baker, H.K. 1951. Cleft palate speech. *Journal of Speech and Hearing Disorders* 16:9–20.

McFie, J. 1952. Cerebral dominance in cases of reading disability *Journal of Neurology, Neurosurgery, and Psychiatry* 15:194–199.

McGraw, M. 1951. *The Neuromuscular Maturation of the Human Infant.* New York: Columbia University Press.

McNeill, D. 1966. Developmental psycholinguistics *in* Smith, F. and Miller, G.A. (eds.). *The Genesis of Language.* Cambridge: MIT Press.

Menyuk, P. 1958. The role of distinctive features in children's acquisition of phonology. *Journal of Speech Research* 11:138.

———. 1967a. "Innovative" linguistic descriptions of the language acquisition of children who acquire language normally and those whose language acquisition is deviant. Paper presented in Pittsburgh.

———. 1967b. Children's learning and recall of grammatical and non-grammatical phonological sequences. Paper presented at the New York meeting of the Society for Research in Child Development.

———. 1968. Speech pathology: some principles underlying therapeutic practises. Paper presented at American Speech and Hearing Association Meeting.

———. 1971. The developmental implications of deviant language acquisition. Paper presented at the Annual Meeting of the Association for Research in Nervous and Mental Disease, New York.

Merrimann, A.C. 1966. Loundes County, Alabama. TICEP Health Survey Statement prepared for the U.S. Senate Subcommittee on Employment, Manpower and Poverty. Washington DC: Government Printing Office.

Moffitt, A.R. 1971. Consonant cue perception by twenty- to twenty-four-week-old infants. *Child Development* 42:717.

Monroe, M. 1928. *Genetics Psychology Monograph* 4:335.

———. 1932. *Children who Cannot Read.* Chicago: University of Chicago Press.

———. 1935. *Education* 56:7

Morgan, W.P. 1896. A case of congenital word blindness. *British Medical Journal* 1378.

Mottier, G. 1951. Über Untersuchung der Sprache lesegestörter Kinder. *Folia Phoniatrica* 3(3):170.

Myklebust, H.R. 1954. *Auditory Disorders in Children.* New York: Grune and Stratton.

Myklebust, H.R. and Boshes, B. 1960. Psychoneurological learning disorders in children. *Archives of Pediatrics* 77:247–256.

Nakzima, S., Okamoto, N., Mural, J., Tanaka, M., Okuno, S., Maeda, T. and Shimizu, M. 1962. The phoneme systematization and the verbalization process of voices in childhood. *Shinrigan-Hyoron* 6:1.

Nance. L. 1946. Differential diagnosis of aphasia in children. *The Journal of Speech Disorders* 2:219–223.

Nettleship, E. 1905. *Ophthalmological Review* 20:61.

Ombredane, A. 1951. *L'Aphasie et l'Elaboration de la Pensee Explicite*. Paris: Presse Universitaire de France.

Oppé, T. 1960. Emotional aspects of prematurity. *Cerebral Palsy Bulletin* 2:233–237.

Orton, S.T. 1925. "Word Blindness" in school children. *Archives of Neurology and Psychiatry* 14:581.

———. 1928a. A physiological theory of reading disability and stuttering in children. *New England Journal of Medicine* 199:1046.

———. 1928b. Specific reading disability—strephosymbolia. *Journal of the American Medical Association* 90:1095.

———. 1929. The "sight reading" method of teaching reading as a source of reading disability. *Journal of Educational Psychology* 20:13.

———. 1930. Familial occurrence of disorders in acquisition of language. *Eugenics* 3:140.

———. 1931. Special disability in spelling. *Bulletin of the Neurological Institute of New York* 1:159.

———. 1932. Some studies in the language function. *Proceedings of the Association for Research in Nervous and Mental Disease* 13:614.

———. 1937. *Reading, Writing and Speech Problems in Children*. New York: W.W. Norton and Co.

———. 1943. Visual functions in strephosymbolia. *Archives of Ophthalmology* 30:707.

Orton, S.T. and Gillingham, A. 1933. Special disability in writing. *Bulletin of the Neurological Institute of New York* 3(1,2).

Osgood, C.E. 1957. Motivational dynamics of language behavior *in* Jones, M.R. (ed.). *Nebraska Symposium of Motivation*. Lincoln: University of Nebraska Press.

Oseretsky, N. 1931. *Angewandle Psychologie* Supplement.

Owen, F., Adams, P., Forrest, T., Stolz, L., and Fisher, S. 1971. Learning disorders in children: sibling studies. *Society for Research in Child Development* Serial 144 36:4. Chicago: University of Chicago Press.

Paine, R.S. 1965. Organic neurological factors related to learning disorders *in* Hellmuth, J. (ed.). *Learning Disorders*. Spec. Child Public. of Seattle Sequin School. 1:1–29.

Palmer, F.H. 1970. Socioeconomic status and intellectual performance among Negro preschool boys. *Developmental Psychology* 3:1.

Palmer, M.F. 1940. The speech development of normal children. *Journal of Speech Disorders* 5:185.

———. 1949. Speech disorders in cerebral palsy. *Nervous Child* 8:193–202.

Pasamanick, B. and Knobloch, H. 1960. Brain damage and reproductive casuality *American Journal of Orthopsychiatry* 30:298–305.

Peacher, W.G. 1950. The etiology and differential diagnosis of dsyarthria. *Journal of Speech and Hearing Disorders* 15:252–265.

Pearson, G.H.J. 1952. A survey of learning difficulties in children. *Psychoanalytic Study of the Child* 7:322–386.

———. 1954. *Psychoanalysis and the Education of the Child*. New York: Norton and Co.

Peller, L.E. 1965. Language and development *in* P.B. Neubauer (ed.). *Early Childhood Education*. Springfield Ill: Charles C. Thomas.

———. 1966. Freud's contribution to language development. *Psychoanalytic Study of the Child* 21:448–467.

Penfield, W. and Roberts, l. 1959. *Speech and Brain Mechanisms*. Princeton: Princeton University Press.

Piaget, J. 1932. *The Moral Judgment of the Child*. New York: Free Press.

———. 1952. *The Origins of Intelligence in Children*. New York: International University Press.

———. 1971. *The Science of Education and the Psychology of the Child*. New York: Viking Press.

Pick, A. 1913. Aphasie. *Handbuch der Normalen und Pathologischen Physiologie* 15(2):Hälfte: 1416–1524.

———. 1931, Reissued in 1973. *Aphasia*. Springfield Ill: Charles C. Thomas.

Pinchon, E. 1948. Psychophysiologie du langage. *Folia Phoniatrica* 1:140.

Povich, E., Baratz, J. 1967. An investigation of syntax development of Head Start children: a developmental sentence types analysis. *American Speech and Hearing Association*.

Provence, S. and Lipton, R. 1926. *Infants in Institutions*. New York: International Universities Press.

Quay, L.C. 1971. Language dialect, reinforcement and the intelligence test performance of Negro children. *Child Development* 42:5.

Rabinovitch, R. 1959 *in* Arieti, S. (ed.). *American Handbook on Psychiatry I*. New York: Basic Books.

Rabinovitch, R. 1960. Pre-Conference Institute, International Reading Association.

Rappaport, S.R. 1961. Behaviour disorder and ego development in a brain injured child. *Psychoanalytic study of the Child* 16:423–448.

———. 1964. Childhood aphasia. *Pathway School Symposium* Cambridge MA: MIT Research Laboratory of Electronics.

Rawson, M.B. 1974. The self concept and the cycle of growth. *Bulletin of the Orton Society* 24.

Reed, H. 1963. Some relationships between neurological dysfunction and behavioral deficits in children *in Conference on Children with Minimal Brain Impairment*. Easter Seal Research Foundation. Chicago: National Society of Crippled Children and Adults.

Rider, R., Taback, M. and Knobloch, H. 1955. Association between premature birth and socio-economic status. *American Journal of Public Health* 45:1022–1028.

Riley, C.M. 1952. Familial autonomic dysfunction. *Journal of the American Medical Association* 49:1532–1535.

Riley, C.M., Day, R., and Langford, W. 1949. Central autonomic dysfunction with defective lacrimation. Report of five cases. *Pediatrics* 4:479–481.

Riley, C.M., Freedman, A.M., and Langford, W.S. 1954. Further observations on familial dysautonomia. *Pediatrics* 14:475–480.

Robbins, S.D. 1935. Relation between the short auditory memory span disability and disorders of speech. *Laryngoscope* 45:545.

———. 1940. Dysarthria and its treatment. *Journal of Speech Disorders* 5:113–120.

Robinson, H.M. 1956. The findings of research on visual difficulties and reading *in Reading for Efficient Living. International Reading Association Conference Proceedings* 3:107–111.

Robinson, N. and Robinson, H. 1965. A follow-up study of children of low birth weight and control children at school age. *Pediatrics* 35:25–433.

Roman-Goldzieher, I. 1962. Handwriting and speech. *Logos* 2:29–39.

Rosen, V.H. 1966. Disturbance of representation and reference in ego development *in* Loewenstein, R.M., Newman, L.M., Shur, M., and Solnit, A.J. (eds.). *Psychoanalysis—A General Psychology*. New York: International Universities Press.

———. 1967. Disorders of communication in psychoanalysis. *Journal of The American Psychoanalytic Association* 15:467–490.

Rousey, C.L. 1969. A theory of speech. Presented at the Annual Meeting of the American Association of Psychiatric Clinics for Children, and at the Winter Meeting of the American Psychoanalytic Association, 1970.

Rubenstein, B.O., Farlik, M.L., Levitt, M., and Eckstein, R. 1959. Learning impotence: a suggested diagnostic category. *American Journal of Orthopsychiatry* 29(2):315–323.

Rutherford, B.R. 1944. A comparative study of loudness, pitch, rate, rhythm, and quality in speech of children handicapped by cerebral palsy. *Journal of Speech Disorders* 9:263–271.

Rutter, M. 1965. Influence of organic and emotional factors on origins, nature and outcome of child psychosis. *Developmental Medicine and Child Neurology* 7(5):518–528.

———. 1968. Concepts of autism: A review of research. *Journal of Child Psychology and Psychiatry* 9:1–25.

———. 1978. Language disorders and infantile autism *in* Rutter, M. and Schopler, E. (eds.). *Autism: A Reappraisal of Concepts and Treatment.* New York: Plenum.

Scheerer, M. 1944. *Genetic Psychology Monographs* 9:232.

Schilder, P. 1942. *Mind: Perception and Thought in their Constructive Aspects.* New York: Columbia University Press.

———. 1944. Congenital alexia and its relation to optic perception. *Journal of Genetic Psychology* 65:67–68.

———. 1950. *Image and Appearance of the Human Body.* New York: International Universities Press.

———. 1964. *Contributions to Developmental Neuropsychiatry.* New York: International Universities Press.

Scholnick, F.K. and Adams, M.J. 1973. Relationships between language and cognitive skills. *Child Development* 44:741–746.

Shiller, J. and Silverman, W. 1961. Uncomplicated hyperbilirubinemia of prematurity. *American Journal of Diseases of Children* 101:587–592.

Silver, A. 1950. Diagnostic value of three drawing tests for children. *Journal of Pediatrics* 37:129.

———. 1951. *Bulletin of The Orton Society* 1:3.

———. 1952. Postural and writing responses in children. *Journal of Pediatrics* 41:493–498.

Simon, J. 1954. Contributions a la Psychologie de la Lecture. *Enfance* 5:438–447.

Skinner, B.F. 1957. *Verbal Behavior.* New York: Appleton-Century-Croft.

Snow, C. 1972. Mothers' speech to children learning language. *Child Development* 43:549.

Sperry, B., Staver, N., Reiner, B. and Ulrich, D. 1958. Renunciation and denial in learning difficulties. *American Journal of Orthopsychiatry* 28(1):98–111.

Stamback, M. 1951. Le probleme du rythme dans le development de l'enfant et dans les dyslexies d'evolution. *Enfance* 5:480.

Steward, M. and Steward, D. 1973. The observation of Anglo-Mexican and Chinese-American mothers teaching their young sons. *Child Development* 44:329–337.

Stewart, W. 1968. Continuity and change in American Negro dialects. *Florida FL Reporter* 7:1.

Stodolsky, S.S. 1965. Maternal behavior and language and concept formation in Negro preschool children: an inquiry into process. Doctoral dissertation. University of Chicago.

Stouffer, S. 1950. *Social Psychology in World War II.* Princeton: Princeton University Press.

Strauss, A. 1954. Aphasia in children. *American Journal of Physical Medicine* 32:93–99.

Strauss, A.A. and Kephart, N.C. 1955. *Psychopathology and Education of the Brain-Injured Child. Vol. 2.* New York: Grune and Stratton.

Strauss, A.A. and Lehtinen, L. 1948, 1950. *Psychopathology and Education of the Brain-Injured Child. Vol. 1.* New York: Grune and Stratton.

Subirana, A. 1961a. Relationship between handedness and language functions. Paper read at Neurological Congress in Rome.

———. 1961b. The problem of cerebral dominance. *Logos* 4:67.

Sullivan, H.S. 1959. *Clinical Studies in Psychiatry.* New York: Norton.

Symmes, J. and Rapoport, J.L. (n.d.) Unexpected reading failure. *American Journal of Orthopsychiatry* 42:82–91.

Tanner, J.M. 1961. *Education and Physical Growth.* London: University of London Press.

Taylor, O. 1971. Recent developments in sociolinguistics: some implications for ASHA. *American Speech and Hearing Association* 13:341.

Teicher, J.D. 1951. Preliminary survey of motility in children. *Quarterly Journal of Child Behavior* 3:460.

Templin, M. 1953. Norms on a screening test of articulation for ages three through eight. *Journal of Speech and Hearing Disorders* 18:323–331.

_____. 1966. The study of articulation and language development during the early school years *in* Smith, F., Miller, G.A. (eds.). *The Genesis of Language.* Cambridge: MIT Press.

Thelander, H., Phelps, J., and Kirk, E. 1958. Learning disabilities associated with lesser brain damage. *Journal of Pediatrics* 53:405–409.

Thomas, A. et al. 1963. *Behavioral Individuality in Early Childhood.* New York: New York University Press.

Thomas, C.J. 1908. The aphasia of childhood and educational hygiene. *Public Health* 21:90.

Thompson, B. 1963. *Journal of Educational Research* 56:376.

Thompson, L.J. 1947. Special disabilities in children with organic brain pathology. *North Carolina Medical Journal* 8:224.

Tinker, M.A. 1936. Eye movements in reading. *Journal of Educational Research* 30:241.

Tizard, J. (ed.) 1961. *The Role of Speech in the Regulation of Normal and Abnormal Behavior.* New York: Liveright.

Todd, G. and Palmer, B. 1968. Social reinforcement of infant babbling. *Child Development* 39:591.

Tolpin, M. 1978. Self-objects and oedipal objects: A crucial developmental distinction *in* A. J. Solnit (ed.). *The Psychoanalytic Study of the Child.* New Haven: Yale University Press.

Toriyman, M., Matsuzaki, and Hayashi, H. 1966. Some observations on auditory average response in man. *International Audiology* 5:234.

Torkewitz, G., Birch, H., and Cooper, K. 1972. Responsiveness to simple and complex auditory stimuli in the human newborn. *Developmental Psychobiology* 5:7.

Uddenberg, G. 1955. Diagnostic studies in prematures. *Acta Psychiatrica et Neurologica Scandinavica* Supplement 104.

Van Hoosan, M. 1965. *Reading Teacher* 18:507.

Vernon, M.D. 1952. *A Further Study of Visual Perception.* Cambridge: Cambridge University Press.

Vygotsky, L.S. 1962. *Thought and Language.* Cambridge MA: MIT Press.

Waelder, R. 1960. *Basic Theory of Psychoanalysis.* New York: International Universities Press.

Wattenberg, W. and Clifford C. 1964. Relational of self-concepts to beginning achievement in reading. *Child Development* 35:461.

Wechsler, D. 1971. *Wechsler Intelligence Scale for Children.* New York: International Universities Press.

Weil, A.P. 1961. Psychopathic personality and organic behavior disorders. *Comprehensive Psychiatry* 2:83–95.

_____. 1970a. The basic core. *This Annual* 25:442–460.

_____. 1970b. Children with minimal brain dysfunction. *Psychosocial Process Journal of Jewish Board of Guardians* 1:80–97.

_____. 1973. Ego strengthening prior to analysis. *This Annual* 28:287–301.

Weiner, M. and Feldman, S. 1963. *Education and Psychological Measurement* 23:807.

Weiss, D. 1935. Über die Frage des Polterns und seine Kombination mit Stottern. *Mitt. über Sprach und Stimmheilk* 1:1.

_____. 1950a. Basic considerations on cluttering. Lecture given at New York Society for Speech and Voice Therapy.

_____. 1950b. Der Zusammenhang zwischen Poltern und Stottern. *Folia Phoniatrica* 2:225.

_____. 1964. *Cluttering.* Englewood Cliffs, NJ: Prentice-Hall.

———. 1967. Cluttering. *Folia Phoniatrica* 19(4):233–283.

Wepman, J. 1939. Familial incidence in stammering. *Journal of Speech Disorders* 4:199–214.

———. 1958. *Auditory Discrimination Test.* Chicago: Language Research Associates.

Werner, H. 1940. *Comparative Psychology of Mental Development.* New York: Harper Brothers.

———. 1952. Toward a General Theory of Perception. *Psychological Review* 59:5.

———. 1957. The concept of development from a comparative and organismic point of view. *in* Harris, D.B. (ed.). *The Concept of Development.* Minneapolis: University of Minnesota Press.

———. 1966. The "latent content" of Heinz Werner's comparative-developmental approach *in* Wapner, S. and Kaplan, B. (eds.) *Papers in Memoriam.* Worcester, MA: Clark University Press.

Werner, H. and Kaplan, B. 1963. *Symbol Formation.* New York: John Wiley and Sons.

Werner, H. and Strauss, A. 1941. Pathology of figure background relations in the child. *Journal of Abstract Social Psychology* 36:236.

Wernicke, D. 1901–3. Der aphasische Symptomen Komplex. *Deutsche Klinik* 6:487–556.

Wertheimer, M. 1922. Untersuchungen zur Lehre von der Gestalt. *Psych. Torschriffte* 1:47–58.

———. 1941. Gestalt theory. *Social Research* 2:1.

West, R., Nelson, S. and Berry, M. 1939. Heredity of stuttering. *Quarterly Journal of Speech* 25:23.

West, R., Kennedy, L., and Carr, A. 1937. *The Rehabilitation of Speech.* New York: Harper and Brothers.

Wiener, G. 1962. Psychologic correlates of premature birth. *Journal of Nervous and Mental Disease* 134:129–144.

Wiener, G., Rider, R., Oppel, W., Fisher, L., and Harper, P. 1965. Correlates of lowbirth weight: psychological status at six to seven years of age. *Pediatrics* 35:434–444.

Williams, J. 1965. Auditory figure ground among dysphasic children. Paper read at Convention American Speech and Hearing Association. Chicago.

Winitz, H. 1967. Dimensions of the articulatory learning process. Paper presented at Pittsburgh.

Wood, N.E. 1959. *Language Disorders in Children.* Chicago.

Worster-Drought, C. 1943. Congenital auditory imperception (congenital word deafness) and its relation to idioglossia and allied speech defects. *The Medical Press and Circular* 210:411–417.

———. 1953. Dysarthria. *Speech* 17:48–57.

Wortis, H. and Freedman, A. 1965. The contribution of social environment to the development of premature children. *American Journal of Orthopsychiatry* 35:57–68.

Wyatt, G. 1957. Speech and interpersonal relations. Mimeographed report—limited circulation.

———. 1958a. Mother-child relationship and stuttering in children. Doctoral dissertation. Boston University.

———. 1958b. A developmental crisis theory of stuttering *in Language and Speech* Vol. 1. London.

———. 1965. Special language disorders in preschool children. *Pediatrics* 36(4):637–647.

Wyatt, G. and Herzan, H. 1962. Therapy with stuttering children and their mothers. *American Journal of Orthopsychiatry* 32(43):645–659.

Yeni-Komshain, G., Chase, R.A., Mobley, R.L. 1968. The development of auditory feedback monitoring: II. *Journal of Speech Research* 2:307.

Zangwill, O. 1960. *Cerebral Dominance and its Relation to Psychological Functioning.* London: Oliver and Boyd.

———. 1962. Dyslexia in relation to cerebral dominance *in* Money, J. (ed.). *Reading Disability.* Baltimore: The Johns Hopkins Press.

Zazzo, R. 1951. *Enfance* 5:385.

Zentay, 1937. Motor disorders of the central nervous system and their significance for speech. Part I. Cerebral and cerebellar dysarthrias. *Journal of Speech Disorders* 2:131–138.

INDEX

Abstract functioning, 126; at six years, 40–41; testing, 42

Absurdities, understanding verbal vs. pictorial, 41

Academic failure, 53, 130

Achievement, attitudes toward, 98

Adolescence, two categories of learning difficulties in, 125–30

Age, meanings of clinical phenomena and, 141–42, 155 n.7, 244

Alexia, 20

Allen, I., 207

Anger in adolescents with learning disabilities, 129

Anoxia at birth, 43

Anxiety: absence of limits and, 135, 278; in adolescents with learning disabilities, 129; in children with central nervous system disorders, 29; inability to express fears and, 29; in mothers of prematurely born, 79; plasticity and, 135; sensitivity to, 279; separation, 245

Aphasia, 140; motor, 225–33; reading and sensory, 16

Aphasic language in children, differential diagnosis between schizophrenic language and, 235–41

Aphasic, meaning of term, 235

Aphasoid children, 235–39

Articulation: cause of errors in, 8–9; competence in, 9; testing, 64

Attention, inability to focus on task or gestalt, 43

attitude, "I don't care," 96

Audiometric testing, 196

Auditory discrimination, 64, 132–33, 134; of aphasic and schizophrenic children, 240; poor spellers and, 51

Auditory feedback, 5

Auditory memory span, 40, 63; asphasic children's short, 240; of autistic children, 262; of dyslexics and dyslalics, 105. *See also* Nonsense syllables

Auditory sequencing, 142–43; to predict scholastic performance, 51

Auditory stimuli, time lag in response to, 199, 210

Autism, 262; differentiating dysphasia and, 160; features in common with dysphasia, 264–65; genetic link with dysphasia, 265

Autistic speech, 7

Babbling, 245; deaf babies and, 5; expressive sounds and, 4; functions of, 5; stimulation of, 5; transition to language from, 6–7

Background. *See* Figure-from-ground differentiation

Behavioral disturbances: children referred for, 88; after school failure, 35

Bellevue-Wechsler Scale for Children, 36

Bender Gestalt test: anoxia at birth and, 43; dyslexics and, 107, 112, 119; in familial dysautonomia, 214; as a predictive test at kindergarten age, 50–51, 90; for visuomotor function, 38, 63, 197

Bender, L., 131, 177–78

Berko, J., 10

Black children's speech, 13

Blacks: teacher's attitude toward dialect of, 99; transformations of the language code for adult, 13

Blanchard, P., 113

Block designs, copying, 41